Electrotherapy Explained

Principles and practice

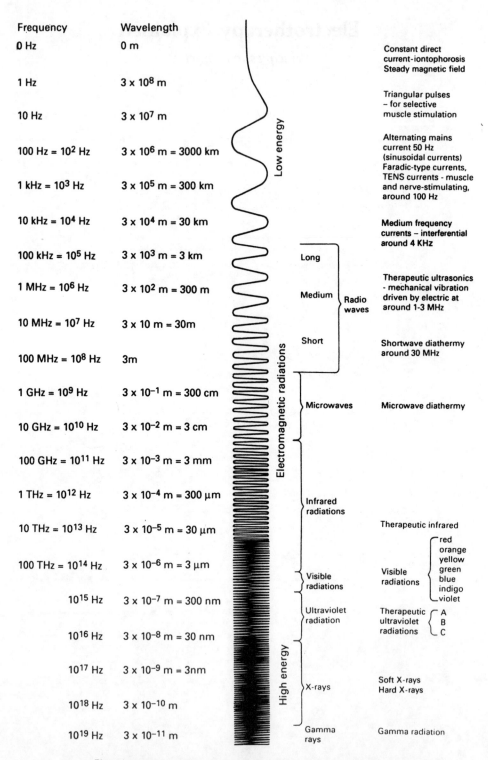

Frequency	Wavelength			
0 Hz	0 m			Constant direct current-iontophorosis Steady magnetic field
1 Hz	3×10^8 m			Triangular pulses – for selective muscle stimulation
10 Hz	3×10^7 m			
100 Hz = 10^2 Hz	3×10^6 m = 3000 km		Low energy	Alternating mains current 50 Hz (sinusoidal currents) Faradic-type currents, TENS currents - muscle and nerve-stimulating, around 100 Hz
1 kHz = 10^3 Hz	3×10^5 m = 300 km			
10 kHz = 10^4 Hz	3×10^4 m = 30 km			Medium frequency currents – interferential around 4 KHz
100 kHz = 10^5 Hz	3×10^3 m = 3 km	Long		
1 MHz = 10^6 Hz	3×10^2 m = 300 m	Medium	Radio waves	Therapeutic ultrasonics - mechanical vibration driven by electric at around 1-3 MHz
10 MHz = 10^7 Hz	3×10 m = 30m	Short		
100 MHz = 10^8 Hz	3m			Shortwave diathermy around 30 MHz
1 GHz = 10^9 Hz	3×10^{-1} m = 300 cm	Microwaves		Microwave diathermy
10 GHz = 10^{10} Hz	3×10^{-2} m = 3 cm			
100 GHz = 10^{11} Hz	3×10^{-3} m = 3 mm			
1 THz = 10^{12} Hz	3×10^{-4} m = 300 µm	Infrared radiations		
10 THz = 10^{13} Hz	3×10^{-5} m = 30 µm			Therapeutic infrared
100 THz = 10^{14} Hz	3×10^{-6} m = 3 µm	Visible radiations	Visible radiations	red orange yellow green blue indigo violet
10^{15} Hz	3×10^{-7} m = 300 nm	Ultraviolet radiation	Therapeutic ultraviolet radiations	A B C
10^{16} Hz	3×10^{-8} m = 30 nm			
10^{17} Hz	3×10^{-9} m = 3nm			
10^{18} Hz	3×10^{-10} m	X-rays		Soft X-rays Hard X-rays
10^{19} Hz	3×10^{-11} m	Gamma rays		Gamma radiation

Electromagnetic radiations (label along wave)

High energy

Electric and magnetic fields – electromagnetic radiations

Electrotherapy Explained

Principles and practice

John Low BA(Hons), MCSP, DipTP, SRP
Acting Principal, School of Physiotherapy, Guy's Hospital, London

Ann Reed BA, MCSP, DipTP, SRP
Senior Lecturer, Institute of Health and Rehabilitation, Polytechnic of East London

Foreword by

Mary Dyson PhD, MIBiol, CBiol
Reader in Biology of Tissue Repair, Guy's Hospital, London

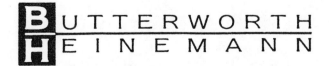

Butterworth-Heinemann Ltd
Linacre House, Jordan Hill, Oxford OX2 8DP

 PART OF REED INTERNATIONAL BOOKS

LONDON   OXFORD   BOSTON
MUNICH   NEW DELHI   SINGAPORE   SYDNEY
TOKYO   TORONTO   WELLINGTON

First published 1990
Reprinted 1991, 1992 (twice)

British Library Cataolouging in Publication Data
Low, John
Electrotherapy.
1. Medicine. Electrotherapy
I. Title   II. Reed, Ann
615.845

ISBN 0 7506 0049 7

Typeset by Latimer Trend & Co Ltd, Plymouth
and printed in England by Clays Ltd, St Ives plc

Contents

Foreword

Electrotherapy Explained — Principles and Practice was written by John Low and Ann Reed primarily as a textbook for BSc and Diploma students of Physiotherapy. The authors have tried, and in my opinion succeeded, in bridging the gap between theory and practice, and have done so in a manner which is both enlightening and entertaining. The main strength of the book is that it *explains*, as far as possible given the current state of knowledge, both how electrotherapy works, and its value in diagnosis. Principles are stated lucidly and succinctly, the subject matter being arranged in logical groupings to aid understanding and simplify access to the vast body of information that the text contains. The debt owed to the past has not been forgotten, and the development of the various electrotherapeutic agents has been described, putting present day usage into historical perspective.

The authors have deliberately avoided using a didactic approach, and wherever possible provide all the information required for the practitioner to arrive at an appropriate course of treatment in a logical fashion. The evidence, for the physical and physiological mechanisms proposed, is set out in a comprehensive and constructively critical manner. Where mechanisms are uncertain, this is clearly indicated. I hope that this will focus attention on the urgent need for more research, and will encourage physiotherapists and their colleagues in related disciplines to initiate and take part in it. The book is illustrated with line diagrams which are easy to understand and recall; I anticipate that they will be much used both by students and their tutors. Published work used by the authors in preparing the text is listed at the end of each chapter, making the book a valuable source of references.

John Low and Ann Reed each have over two decades of practical experience as teachers and users of electrotherapy. Their book is a much needed response to the absence of a comprehensive explanatory textbook written at a level suitable for degree-level physiotherapy students. It will also make a welcome and much-consulted addition to any practising physiotherapists's working library, and will be of particular value to those wishing to bring their knowledge of electrotherapy up to date.

In my opinion, *Electrotherapy Explained* lives up to the promise of its title, and I am delighted that the authors have found the time and dedication needed to write this masterly book which will enable them to share their experience as teachers with a wider audience than those privileged to be their pupils.

Mary Dyson, PhD, MIBiol, CBiol, FCSP (Hon.)
August 1990, London.

Preface

Electrotherapy has tended to be a subject confused by traditional naming systems, jargon and didactic statements which have perhaps not always been justified by reason or research. In this book we have attempted to demystify electrotherapy for the physiotherapy student.

We have tried to give a fairly complete coverage of the field describing the most common modalities known to us to be employed by physiotherapists. Our intention is to explain how these modalities work and their effects upon the patient. We have used a different approach to some electrotherapy texts. In the initial chapter of each section we have tried to lay the foundations of the principles of modern electrotherapy, because we feel that a thorough understanding of these principles will ultimately lead to safer and more effective clinical practice. Therefore, the book builds up from the basics without, we hope, sacrificing accuracy to give a description of the types of energy available to the therapist. We have classified treatments of the same kind together so that the book is divided into sections devoted to electrical, mechanical, thermal and radiation energy.

The nature, production, effects and uses on the body tissues of each modality are explained and illustrated with what we hope is a reasonably comprehensive range of references to support the points made. With the very welcome involvement of physiotherapists in research, we hope to give undergraduates access to the vast amount of literature upon which they are encouraged to base their final clinical intervention. For postgraduates and practitioners our aim is to stimulate a vigorous search for answers.

We are well aware of the inherent dangers in explaining 'how things work' and in an attempt to communicate our ideas easily we may have been deliberately less precise than we could have been in some instances. We have tried to use the words that would convey the most meaning in the hope that a thorough understanding of even the more difficult concepts might be reached. Perhaps some of the ideas we offer will ultimately be shown to be too simple or just plain wrong, but we console ourselves that even these explanations can lead to debate and serve as a stepping stone to greater accuracy. Many treatments that have faded from use over the years are now returning in an appropriately modern guise, with new rational explanations. One such example is the use of low-frequency electrical stimulation following the development of the pain gate theory.

Rather than producing a step-by-step guide to technique, we have aimed for a description of the principles, the modalities and practical applications of their use. We believe that if the modality is well understood there can be a wide variation in acceptable technique and treatment within the confines of safe and effective practice.

After many years of teaching electrotherapy we both felt the need to attempt such a book. For our omissions and failings we apologize. However, our sincere hope is that we will have made electrotherapy more comprehensible for some which, in turn, will raise the standards of safe and effective treatment for our patients — the aim of us all.

John Low and Ann Reed, 1990

1.

Electrical charges within the body

At its simplest level electrotherapy can be defined as the treatment of patients by electrical means. By implication this means that electrical forces are applied to the body bringing about physiological changes for therapeutic purposes. However, in addition to these external forces electrical charges are generated within the body by normal physiological processes. Between these two sets of electrical forces there will be interaction. Before embarking on the study of external electrical forces on the body it is useful to consider the charges that are generated physiologically within the body.

CHARGES GENERATED BY THE BODY

The body tissues are organized systems of cells which are bathed in fluid. About two-thirds of the body weight is due to water and rather more than half of this is found inside the cells. The electrical properties of the body tissues depend on the fact that numerous ions are dissolved in this water, and on the fact that water molecules are electric dipoles which may adhere to some of the ionic compounds and surfaces to modify their behaviour.

The division between intra- and extracellular fluid is maintained by the cell membrane; this consists of a double layer of lipids in which globular proteins are scattered. The lipid bilayer is arranged so that the hydrophobic (water-hating, hence water-repellent) ends of both layers of lipid molecules face inwards and are thus not in contact with the intra- and extracellular fluid. Some of the globular proteins extend through the thickness of both layers. These arrangements allow water molecules and some solutes to pass passively through the membrane—either by diffusion or by carrier-mediated transport. Other solutes may be moved across the membrane by active transport; that is, energy is used to move the substance against its concentration gradient. Alterations of the globular proteins are considered to be the main way in which the permeability of the membrane to different substances can be controlled.

It is the balance of ions that determines the charges found on the surface of

1

cells. All cells tend to maintain high concentrations of potassium ions (K^+) and low concentrations of sodium ions (Na^+) in their intracellular fluid. The extracellular fluid contains plenty of both ions, but more Na^+ than K^+. The cell membrane allows the passage of both these ions to some extent, but has an active transport mechanism that brings K^+ into the cell and expels Na^+. This sodium–potassium (Na^+–K^+) 'pump' uses energy to move these ions against their passive gradients. The passive gradient will depend on the relative concentration of each ion on each side of the membrane—they will tend to diffuse from high to low concentration—as well as on the electrical forces across the membrane: negative charges attract positive ones and similar charges repel one another.

These two driving forces are linked by the Nernst equation which gives the maximum electromotive force that is generated by any given ratio of concentration of a particular ion. This can be used to predict the electromotive forces due to any particular concentration of each type of ion separated by a cell membrane.

The difference of potential across a normal cell membrane at rest, known as the resting membrane potential, has the inside of the cell negative relative to the outside. The potential varies in the cells of different tissues, being anything between -60 and -90 mV. In nerves and smooth muscle fibres it is usually about -70 mV, for skeletal muscle cells -80 mV and for glial cells -90 mV (Bray *et al.*, 1986). This electrical potential—electrical pressure—across the cell membrane is due to the fact that such membranes are much more permeable to K^+ than to Na^+. Thus K^+ can get out of the cell much more easily than Na^+ can get in. The Na^+–K^+ pump ejects three ions of sodium for every two of potassium that it takes in. The result of both mechanisms is a deficiency of positive charges inside the cell compared to the outside, hence the membrane potential.

As well as the Na^+–K^+ pump other ions, such as CA^{2+} and H^+, are also moved by an active transport process. In all cases adenosine triphosphate (ATP) is utilized by means of an enzyme (adenosine triphosphatase; ATPase) which is activated by the appropriate ions to supply the energy needed.

The resting membrane potential of nerves

Neurons consist of a cell body and several extensions which convey the nerve impulses to and from the cell body. A resting membrane potential is present across the membrane of the cell body and across the whole length of the processes—nerve fibres—the longest of which is usually called the axon.

The resting membrane potential is ultimately due to the Na^+–K^+ pump, but it must be understood that the quite large potential can be built up by the pump because of the different permeability of the nerve membrane to Na^+ and K^+. The pump ejects Na^+ from inside the fibre membrane, which cannot easily return from the extracellular fluid because the membrane is not easily penetrated by Na^+. Thus there is a high concentration of Na^+ outside the fibre which provides a (chemical) diffusion force to try to drive the Na^+ back into the fibre. K^+ move much more easily across the fibre membrane so that, although pumped in, they can readily leak out again down their chemical concentration gradient. Both sodium and potassium are positively charged ions so that the excess of Na^+ outside as well as the K^+ that leak out give a net positive charge which tends to repel other positive charges, i.e. further outflow of K^+. Thus the exit of K^+ is limited by, or balanced by, the electrical force. The result is a relatively high concentration of K^+ inside the fibre and Na^+ outside, with the total number of positive charges being much greater outside, leading to a potential across the membrane of -70 mV. Notice that the Na^+ tend to be driven into the nerve fibre both by their own chemical concentration gradient and by the electrical force across the membrane (Miles, 1969). These ideas are illustrated in Figure 1.1.

The membrane is not completely impermeable to Na^+, but the small inward flow can be controlled by the Na^+–K^+ pump. The situation is like that of a ship at sea in which the lower parts are below the water level but contain air able to pass freely in and out, like K^+. The seawater, like Na^+, is kept out by the hull and the small amount that does leak in is easily removed by the bilge pumps, an active transport mechanism. Thus different compounds—air and seawater—are separated by the ship's hull; due to the greater density of water a pressure difference is developed across the hull. If the hull is holed, water will rush in with great force because of the pressure difference, but if the hole is then quickly blocked the small quantity of additional water is ultimately removed by the bilge pumps to restore the situation.

In many tissues the individual cells are connected by gap junctions which allow some electrical conduction between cells. This does not occur in skeletal muscle or nerve tissue (Finean *et al.*, 1978). There are, of course, many other ions in the intra- and extracellular fluid, particularly negatively charged chloride ions (Cl^-) and large negatively charged organic (proteinate) ions. Many other positive ions, notably calcium, are also present.

The nerve impulse

The nerve impulse is a wave of electrochemical activity which passes along the nerve fibre using energy already stored as part of the membrane potential. It is a reversal of the membrane potential from -70 to $+30$ mV which occurs very briefly—taking about 1 ms—and spreads along the fibre without decrement. It is called the action potential.

The impulse is initiated by depolarization of the fibre membrane due to chemical disturbance at a synapse or receptor or to some other disturbance such as an electrical pulse. Depolarization means that the potential difference across the membrane is reduced from the -70 mV of the resting membrane. However, the impulse is only triggered when depolarized by about 10–15 mV (i.e. to about -55 mV). Once this threshold is reached the impulse, or action potential, is generated automatically and spreads along the nerve fibre at a rate that is characteristic of that particular fibre. If the impulse is initiated normally it will pass only in one (orthodromic) direction, but if the middle of a nerve

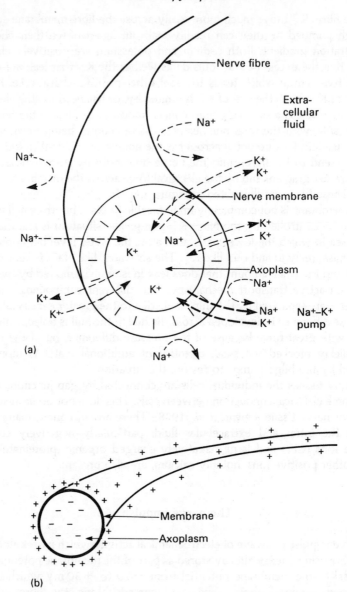

Fig. 1.1(a) Sodium ions maintained on the outside; (b) the membrane potential.

fibre is artificially stimulated two impulses will travel away from the point of stimulation, one in each direction, orthodromic and antidromic.

The effect of depolarization beyond the threshold level is to cause the membrane to become much more permeable to Na^+ by opening special channels or gates. (This probably occurs by an alteration of the configuration of certain proteins embedded in the bilayer membrane.) These voltage-dependent sodium gates open widely to allow Na^+ to rush into the fibre, causing an abrupt local reversal of membrane polarity. Since these sodium gates are opened by the voltage change—the depolarization—they allow rapid acceleration of the depolarizing process: a positive feedback effect. The result is a very rapid depolarization of the membrane. However, K^+ channels are also caused to open by the depolarization, but only after a delay. The Na^+ gates close automatically but again, after a similar delay. Consequently, the rush of Na^+ into the fibre is soon stemmed and there is a loss of K^+ from the fibre; thus the membrane repolarizes again. Once the process is started, rapid depolarization followed by a relatively slow repolarization occurs automatically and takes several milliseconds. It must be understood that a very small proportion of the available Na^+ enters the fibre before repolarization occurs, and those ions that do are ultimately removed by the Na^+–K^+ pump. Even without the activity of the pump the impulse can occur many hundreds of times before the membrane potential is significantly altered. The ship analogy used above is appropriate; many small rushes of water could be allowed into the hull before the ship is in danger of sinking even if the bilge pumps are not working.

The impulse will travel along the length of the fibre because the depolarization—altered charge on the membrane—spreads in all directions. Since the voltage-dependent sodium gates are opened once the threshold is reached the electrical charge spreading along the surface of the membrane causes the next area of the fibre to depolarize and so on. Once the impulse has passed, that particular part of the fibre membrane is refractory, i.e. it cannot be stimulated until it has repolarized (Fig. 1.2).

The first part of the action potential (Na^+ ions rushing in) is analogous to a line of dominoes set up so that when the end domino is pushed over it falls against the next which falls against the next and so on. A wave of falling dominoes thus travels along the prearranged line. Such a system has the characteristics of the initial part of the nerve impulse in that energy is stored in the upright position of the domino, like the store of energy in the membrane potential. Also the domino has to be disturbed sufficiently to bring its centre of gravity outside its base—beyond the threshold—from which point it accelerates downwards, tipping over the next domino as it goes. The falling domino has the same positive feedback properties—rapid acceleration to the limit of the system—as the reversal of membrane polarity due to the inrush of sodium ions. Of course, the nerve membrane potential is automatically reset but the domino line needs the attention of a dextrous human hand to reconstruct it.

The speed of propagation of the nerve impulse along the nerve fibre varies in different nerves. Generally, the larger the nerve fibre diameter the lower its electrical resistance, hence larger currents and faster conduction. Further, many nerve fibres are surrounded by an electrically insulating sheath, the myelin sheath, interrupted at intervals by the nodes of Ranvier which are areas with much less insulation. The electrical potential of the nerve impulse travels along the membrane but only triggers the depolarization at the nodes of Ranvier because the intervening membrane has too much resistance (Fig. 1.3). Thus the nerve impulse can be described as skipping from node to node (saltatory conduction) using less energy and travelling much faster. This is like replacing

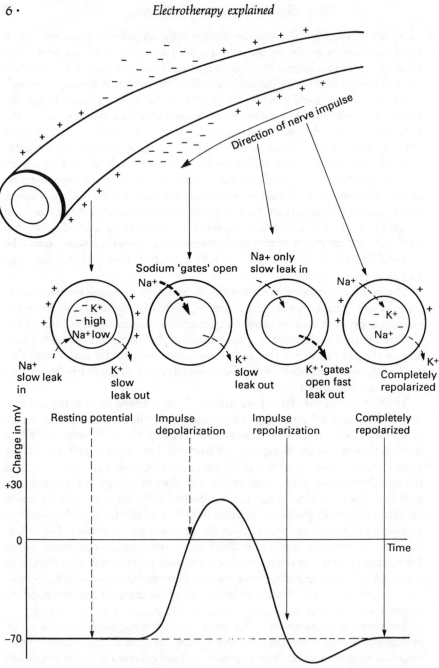

Fig. 1.2(a) The passage of a nerve impulse;

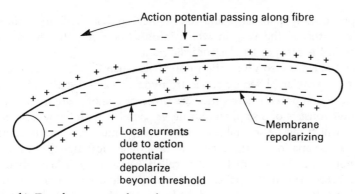

Action potential passing along fibre

Local currents due to action potential depolarize beyond threshold

Membrane repolarizing

Fig. 1.2(b) Depolarization and repolarization.

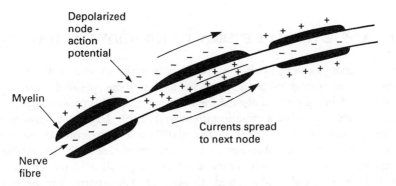

Depolarized node - action potential

Myelin

Nerve fibre

Currents spread to next node

Fig. 1.3 Section through a myelinated nerve fibre.

the usual size of dominoes with very tall ones that fall over a greater distance and thus pass the 'falling wave' more rapidly. The action potential will actually be spread over many nodes of Ranvier at any one time, for instance an impulse travelling at 100 m/s may occupy some 5 cm of axon length (Bray *et al.*, 1986).

The nerve impulse is thus an 'all-or-none' event. If it is triggered by a disturbance of the nerve membrane beyond threshold then an identical impulse travels along the nerve fibre whatever the size of the disturbance. Further, the velocity of the impulses is always the same in any given nerve. Therefore the transfer of information in the nervous system or variations in muscle contraction are all 'coded' by the number and frequency of these nerve impulses.

Nerve impulses can be recorded at the surface to investigate their average conduction rates in peripheral nerve conduction studies.

Electric charges generated by muscle cells

Like nerves, muscle fibres also produce an electrical disturbance which occurs when they contract. When many muscle fibres contract in unison the electrical signal produced is quite large and can be measured at the body surface. An example of this is the way in which information about the heart can be provided in the form of an electrocardiogram.

Skeletal muscles also give action potentials when they contract and these can be picked up, amplified by an electromyograph and displayed in a similar way. The action potentials recorded are those of one or more motor units. A motor unit consists of a single motor nerve together with the muscle fibres it supplies, which can be several hundred in a large muscle. There is, therefore, considerable variation in the recording of an electrical signal from a single motor unit—a spike potential, as it is called. On average it lasts about 4 ms (Walsh, 1988). When the patient performs a voluntary muscle contraction both the number of motor units and the frequency of firing increase, leading to a more complex recording (see Chapter 4).

THE APPLICATION OF ENERGY TO THE BODY FOR THERAPY

Physical energy can be applied to the body in various forms (Table 1.1). The most obvious is mechanical energy, in the form of some appreciable mass, such as the hand, being pressed against the body surface. If this pressure varies at a suitable rate it is called a vibration (therapy 1, Table 1.1). If the frequency of vibration occurs between about 30 and 20 000 cycles per second, i.e. hertz, it is detected as sound when it strikes the tympanic membrane of the ear. At higher frequencies the sensory nerves cannot detect the vibration so we are unaware of it; it is then called ultrasound (therapy 2). This energy can be passed through the body tissues generating heat and causing other effects where it is absorbed.

If the atoms and molecules of the object placed against the skin are given more motion—that is, the object is made hotter—this heat energy can be transferred to the skin and tissues. The tissues are thus heated by conduction (therapy 3). If the molecules of the object in contact have less motion than those of the tissues then heat is conducted from the tissues to the object, thus cooling the tissues (therapy 4).

Where particles on or near the skin are given an electric charge this can cause ions in the tissues to move. The movement of charges is an electric current in the tissues (therapy 5). If these currents are varied, either in intensity or direction at a suitable frequency, e.g. 50 Hz, it can disturb the ionic balance across nerve or muscle membranes, causing a nerve impulse or muscle contraction to occur (therapy 6). Increasing the frequency of current change to, say, 4000 Hz will allow the ions to pass easily through the tissues without stimulating nerve or muscle. However, if two such currents are passed through the tissues slightly out of phase they interfere to produce an amplitude-modulated current of low frequency which will stimulate nerve and muscle (therapy 7). Still higher frequencies, in the megahertz range, will allow large currents to pass through the tissues, producing significant heating spread throughout the tissues (therapy 8).

When the movement of electrons is made to occur at very high frequencies

Table 1.1   Forms of energy applied to the body

	Mechanical	*Electrical*	*Radiation*
Continuous Low- frequency Medium- frequency High- frequency Still higher frequencies	Pressure Vibration Sound Ultrasound Heat	Constant current Low-frequency currents Medium-frequency currents High-frequency currents Electron oscillation	 Radiowaves Microwave Infrared Visible Ultraviolet X-rays γ-rays

Therapies	1. Pressure and
	   vibration
	2. Ultrasound
	3. Conduction
	   heating
	4. Cold therapy
		5. Direct current
		6. Muscle-stimulating
		   currents and trans-
		   cutaneous nerve
		   stimulation
		7. Interferential
		   therapy
		8. Shortwave
		   diathermy
			9. Microwave
			10. Infrared
			11. Laser
			12. Ultraviolet

energy is given off in the form of electromagnetic radiations. These radiations can enter the tissues and cause effects when they are absorbed. Thus where the electron movement is at frequencies of thousands of millions of cycles per second (GHz) it produces radiations called microwaves (radar) which lead to heat when absorbed in the tissues (therapy 9). At higher frequencies they are called infrared and are absorbed at the skin surface but still cause heating (therapy 10). Higher still give radiations which stimulate the retina of the eye, i.e. they are visible. Beyond the visible—ultraviolet (therapy 12)—cause marked biological changes when absorbed at the skin surface, i.e. sunburn.

Applied electric charges

The effects on the body of applied electric charges depend on the intensity and nature of the resulting current in the tissues. They can be rather simply summarized as having three basic effects, each of which may have various complex physiological and therapeutic consequences.

1 Chemical changes occur in the tissues as a result of the application of unidirectional or direct current. Such effects are described in Chapter 2 and Appendix B. If the current is sufficiently great tissue destruction will occur.
2 Excitable tissues, nerves and muscles, can be stimulated by currents that

vary at a suitable rate. The change in current has to be quick enough to unbalance the ions around cell membranes, but not so quick that they do not allow time for the cell to respond. This may lead to many effects such as muscle contraction and altered pain perception.

3 Significant heating can be generated in the body tissues if high-frequency evenly alternating currents are applied because the rate of change is too high to allow time for excitable cells to respond and the polar or chemical effects are insignificant due to the even alternation, so that relatively high current intensities can be applied. High currents cause significant heating in the tissues because they dissipate much more energy than low current intensities. The heating will actually depend on the square of the current intensity (Joule's law: $H \propto I^2Rt$, where $H =$ heat, $I =$ current, $R =$ resistance and $t =$ time).

These three effects, which may overlap, can be described in terms of recognized therapeutic modalities as:

1 Direct current.
2 Nerve- and muscle-stimulating currents.
3 Diathermy.

In addition to these three main effects, there is now evidence that various forms of electrotherapy are capable of restoring normal cell membrane potential, and affecting tissue growth and repair.

In conditions of inflammation the cell membrane potential is reduced, which allows K^+ ions to escape into the extracellular fluid. This has the effect of attracting water by osmosis, which results in oedema which in turn can lead to pain. It is theorized that a pulsating magnetic field restores the negative charge to these cells, which re-establishes the K^+ and Na^+ balance and hence normal cell permeability (Hayne, 1984). Dyson (1985) states that ultrasonically induced membrane pertubation may increase calcium transport into mast cells, which activates them to release agents which initiate repair.

Acoustic streaming caused by ultrasound is known to change diffusion rates and membrane permeability which may alter rates of protein synthesis and hence repair (Dyson and Suckling, 1978). Laser therapy, which has been used successfully to accelerate wound healing (Dyson and Young, 1986), may work in the same way.

Kidd *et al.* (1988) has demonstrated the plastic adaptation of motor neurons using eutrophic electrotherapy – see Chapter 3.

REFERENCES

Bray J. J., Cragg P. A., MacKnight A. D. C. *et al.* (1986). *Lecture Notes on Human Physiology*. London: Blackwell Scientific Publications.
Dyson M. (1985). Therapeutic applications of ultrasound. In *Biological Effects of Ultrasound Clinics in Diagnostic Ultrasound* (Nyborg W. L., Ziskin M. C., eds) Edinburgh: Churchill Livingstone, pp. 121–33.

Dyson M., Suckling J. (1978). Stimulation of tissue repair by ultrasound: a survey of the mechanisms involved. *Physiotherapy*, **64**, 105–8.

Dyson M., Young S. (1986). Effect of laser therapy on wound contraction and cellularity in mice. *Lasers Sci.*, **1**, 125–30.

Finean J. B., Coleman R., Michell R. H. (1978). *Membranes and their Cellular Functions* 2nd edn. London: Blackwell Scientific Publications.

Hayne C. R. (1984). Pulsed high frequency energy—its place in physiotherapy. *Physiotherapy*, **70**, 459–66.

Kidd G. L., Oldham J. A., Stanley J. K. (1988). Eutrophic electrotherapy and atrophied muscle: a pilot clinical trial. *Clinic. Rehab.*, **2**, 219–30.

Miles F. A. (1969). *Excitable Cells*. London: Heinemann Medical Books.

Walsh J. C. (1988). Electrophysiology. In *Electrophysical Agents in Physiotherapy: Therapeutic and Diagnostic Use* (Wadsworth H., Chanmugan A. P. P., eds). Marrickville, NSW Australia: Science Press.

2.

Therapeutic direct current

HISTORY

The discovery of electricity came piecemeal, from the production of static charges on glass bulbs in the early 18th century, through the various means of producing a steady current—such as the voltaic pile—to more and more sophisticated means of varying and reversing the current. At each stage medical use was recommended, tried and much benefit was usually claimed. In 1786 Luigi Galvani stimulated the nerves and muscle of frogs with electric charges. When his work was published in 1791 it gave an enormous impetus to scientific experimentation in this realm. As a consequence Humboldt called the steady current 'galvanism' to distinguish it from frictionally generated static charges. Galvanic currents—continuous direct currents—came to be widely used therapeutically and even more extensively to introduce medication into the body tissues. As early as 1833 Fabre-Palaprat exploited this idea—nowadays called iontophoresis—and many subsequent claims were made for its effective use, often under strange-sounding names such as 'cataphoric medication' or 'endosmosis'. Stephane Le Duc in France popular-

12

ized iontophoresis in the early years of the 20th century and is sometimes described as its originator; for a detailed description of the history of iontophoresis see Licht (1983).

NATURE (see Appendix A)

Direct current refers to a current passing continuously in the same direction. For the purposes of definition direct current (DC) is considered to pass for more than 1 s (Alon, 1987), and is sometimes called constant current or galvanism.

TRANSMISSION

Current is passed to the body tissues by means of wet pads, sponges or a bath of suitable solution. Thus the conduction current generated in the apparatus is changed to a convection current in the wet pads and tissues. At the junction of the metal electrode (a conductor) with the electrolyte of the pad chemical changes will occur—the changes of electrolysis. The nature of these changes depends on the constituents of the electrolyte and the metal of the electrodes (see Appendix B). The general result is the formation of acids at the positive electrode (anode) and bases at the negative electrode (cathode). Although these reactions occur at the junction of the electrode with the electrolyte, i.e. where the metal electrode touches the conducting gel or wetted pad in treatment situations, their effects can spread to the skin causing chemical damage. Such a chemical burn is far more likely to occur close to the negative terminal (cathode) as a result of the alkalis formed there. The magnitude of these changes depends on the current density, that is the current intensity per unit area (mA/cm^2); also, because of the spread of chemicals through the wetted pad, the changes will depend directly on the total time that the current is flowing.

The current in any circuit depends on the voltage and inversely on the resistance, Ohm's law (see Appendix A). The major resistance in a DC system applied to the body is the epidermis; thus the area of contact with the epidermis will determine the total resistance: the larger the cross-sectional area, the smaller the resistance. The value of this resistance will determine the current for any given voltage. Therefore what matters from a therapeutic point of view is the current per unit area, that is the current density.

IONTOPHORESIS

Iontophoresis involves the movement of ions across biological membranes by means of an electric current for therapeutic purposes. It is also called ion transfer.

Electrotherapy explained

Mechanism of iontophoresis

If a voltage is applied to an electrolyte a convection current will flow. This consists of positively charged ions moving towards the negative pole and negatively charged ions moving to the positive pole.

If a drug is in an ionic form, i.e. it has a charge, it can be made to travel in either direction depending on the polarity applied. Atoms and molecules in an electrolyte are constantly gaining or losing electrons to become ions and then reverting to their non-ionized form. There is also considerable random movement of particles. When an electric charge is applied it results in a steady drift of appropriately charged ions in each direction. If the electrolyte is divided by membranes—as in the therapeutic situation—then many more ions are driven through the membranes than would pass through due to random particle (brownian) motion.

This is the situation that occurs when applying iontophoresis. The tissues are effectively a continuous electrolyte with the solution of the wet pad or sponge which contains the ionized drug (Fig. 2.1). Thus positively charged ions can be made to drift away from the positively charged pole towards the negative pole (from left to right in Fig. 2.1) and will pass through the skin and into the tissues, and vice versa for negatively charged ions. Some will lose their charge in the tissues and become chemically active. Hence some of the drug has been locally introduced into the tissues.

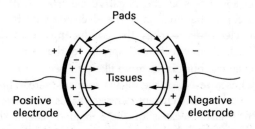

Fig. 2.1 Movement of ions during iontophoresis.

The effects of any drug introduced by iontophoresis are likely to be either local in the skin under the active electrode or systemic because when the drug enters the tissue fluid it is disseminated throughout the body tissues. This has been demonstrated by the iontophoresis of radioactive material (O'Malley and Oester, 1955).

The number of ions entering the tissues from any given area of active electrolyte is proportional to both the current density and the time of application. In fact the number of ions transferred has been shown to be proportional to the cube root of the product of current density and time of application (Trubatch and Van Harreveld, 1972; Fig. 2.2). For practical purposes the current density is limited by the skin tolerance, which usually allows between 0.1 and 0.3 mA/cm^2; dosage can thus be reasonably expressed for a given treatment area in terms of total current in mA multiplied by the time in minutes.

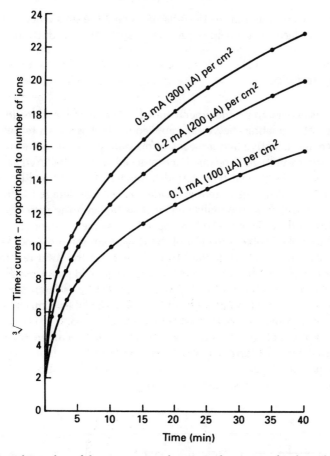

Fig. 2.2 The relationship of dosage to time (duration) of treatment for three different current densities. The number of ions introduced into the tissues is proportional to the cube root of the product of time and current density, e.g. for 100 μA the current passing for 5 min = 500; cube root for 500 = 7.94. Other points are found in a similar way.

The concentration of ions in the solution used will obviously have an effect on the number of ions available; it has been shown, however, that concentrations of about 1 or 2% are as satisfactory as higher concentrations.

It must be understood that tissue penetration by ions used therapeutically is not a simple matter. Specific conductivity and pH of the solutions used, as well as the presence of non-drug ions which will compete with the drug, are all factors which have an influence. Furthermore some ions, such as zinc or silver, form precipitates which are insoluble and may limit penetration.

In spite of the generalization made above that iontophoresis would only lead to skin or systemic effects, there have been many suggestions that drugs act on deeply placed structures beneath the site of application (Kahn, 1975; Wadsworth and Chanmugan, 1980). There is also some evidence from animal experiments (Glass *et al.*, 1980) in which higher concentrations of radiolabelled substance were found in the deep tissues below the sites where iontophoresis had taken place than would occur due to systemic introduction.

PRODUCTION

All that is needed to provide therapeutic DC is a steady unidirectional voltage, a means of regulating the voltage applied to the tissues via terminals marked positive and negative and a means of measuring the current flow.

The mains voltage is rectified and reduced; a potential divider is placed in parallel with the patient (Fig. 2.3); this divider can be altered by moving the control knob. With the potential divider at zero no voltage is applied so that no current will flow; the milliammeter in series with the patient will indicate zero current flow. Suppose 50 V is applied across the resistance and the knob is turned to make contact one-fifth of the way along the resistance, as shown in Figure 2.3: then 10 V is applied to the tissues. If the total resistance of the patient and the meter were 5000 Ω then 2 mA would pass through the tissues and be shown on the meter (10/5000 = 0.002: Ohm's law). Similarly, if the connection is moved to halfway and 25 V is applied then 5 mA will flow. Thus the current to the patient can be regulated from zero.

Many pieces of apparatus have a switch to connect a different circuit, giving a different range of current, e.g. 0–10 mA or 0–100 mA. Note that the current in the patient depends not only on the voltage but also on the patient's resistance, so if skin resistance falls current will rise.

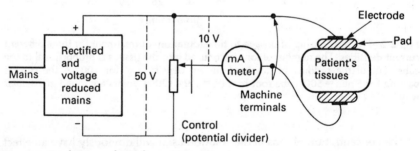

Fig. 2.3 Production of DC for patients.

PHYSIOLOGICAL EFFECTS AND THERAPEUTIC USES

Low-density currents have been used for the effects they cause in the skin and for iontophoresis, usually for periods of 10–30 min. The current density is kept to a level that does not cause tissue damage or patient discomfort. Traditionally this is said to be below about 0.33 mA/cm^2 (2 mA/in^2) but Cummings (1987) uses between 0.1 and 0.5 mA/cm^2.

Direct current

Sensory stimulation

During the passage of such currents the patient is aware of a mild tingling or prickling sensation, which may merge into a mild irritation or itching. If sufficient current has passed for long enough an erythema of the skin will be evident under both electrodes, and is more marked under the negative (cathode). In the past this irritating effect was used for relief of pain. This erythema is confined to the area of the applied electrode.

Hyperaemia

Since this erythema is confined it indicates a capillary hyperaemia, unlike that due to heat in which arteriolar dilatation occurs. The initial erythema lasts for about 20 min or so but may be made to recur over a period of several hours, even a day later, by another stimulus such as heat or washing in hot water (Kovacs, 1949). The mechanism of this erythema has not been fully elucidated; it differs from the erythemas produced by chemical stimuli such as an inflammatory or ultraviolet radiation-provoked erythema. The evident erythema has in the past led to the idea that vasomotor stimulation and increased circulation may promote improved nutrition of the area and speed up the resolution of inflammatory products (Kovacs, 1949); there seems to be no significant evidence to support this.

Relief of pain

The relief of pain has long been claimed as a result of such DC treatments. Sensory stimulation of cutaneous nerve endings (due to the electrochemical changes) inhibiting pain by means of the 'pain gate' theory could reasonably account for this phenomenon (see Chapter 3). Older theories concerned the decreased nerve excitability in the region of the positive pole—anelectrotonus as it was called. The positive charge on the outside of the nerve fibre relative to the inside was said to be augmented by the positively charged anode. The repulsion of H^+ and K^+ ions in the area has also been suggested to account for this pain relief (Wadsworth and Chanmugan, 1980).

Acceleration of healing

Direct currents of low intensity applied in 2-h spells three times a day have been used in the treatment of skin ulcers of various kinds. This treatment, using one electrode (negative for the first 3 days) over the ulcer and the other electrode about 25 cm from the lesion, appears to be successful in accelerating the healing rate (Gault and Gatens, 1976). Battery-powered sources were used which could be set to deliver a fixed current, and safety devices were incorporated to ensure that this was not exceeded; the total current used could be varied between 0.2 and 1 mA so that the current density for most ulcers would be very low.

Other studies have given similar encouraging results (Wolcott *et al.*, 1969). The mechanism of this effect has not been elucidated but it has been suggested (Binder, 1981) that an antibacterial effect of DC, shown to occur in vitro, increased circulation, or otherwise that the triggering of growth and repair may account for it.

High-voltage pulsed currents have also been successfully used to accelerate healing (see Chapter 3). Chronic skin ulcers healed at a rate of 44.8% per week in a controlled trial of this treatment (Kloth and Feeder, 1988).

While the mechanism for such effects has not been fully explained there is evidence that proliferation and/or migration of epithelial and connective tissue cells involved in wound repair can be increased by an electric field. This has been demonstrated on pigs (Alvarez *et al.*, 1983). It has also been suggested that the skin 'battery potential'—the outside of the epidermis being negative to the dermis in normal skin—could be involved in wound healing (Foulds and Barker, 1983). It may be that these small potentials are augmented by the various forms of DC which therefore accelerate repair.

Many studies have shown increased rates of bone formation where a small DC has been applied to the bone with electrodes implanted in the tissues (Becker *et al.*, 1977). Here, again, the mechanism is not clear. The effects of polarity are unresolved. A recent study (Brown *et al.*, 1988) found that positive pole high-voltage pulsed currents applied to experimentally induced wounds delayed healing during the first 4 days but increased healing during days 5–7. For a recent review see Weiss *et al.*, 1990.

Tissue destruction

At higher current densities DC will cause tissue damage. Coagulation of protein occurs under the positive pole and liquefaction under the negative. These effects will occur if the current density is high, such as would happen if a bare wire or needle electrode were placed on or in the skin (Kovacs, 1949). This effect has been used in the deliberate destruction of unwanted tissue such as warts. It is best known for its use in the removal of unwanted hair; with a large positive dispersive electrode applied in a convenient place, the fine-needle negative electrode is introduced into the hair follicle and a current applied to liquefy and destroy the hair-bearing epithelium.

Electrophoresis

Anodal galvanism used to be used as a treatment for local oedema as it was considered to have a drying effect on the underlying tissue.

Iontophoresis

The physiological and therapeutic effects of iontophoresis depend on the nature of the drugs introduced into the tissues. A very large number of substances have been used for a vast range of therapeutic purposes over the years, most of them with little success. This has, perhaps, tended to diminish recognition of the fewer, effective applications.

Local anaesthesia

Local cutaneous anaesthesia can be achieved by the iontophoresis of a suitable agent such as lignocaine or procaine. The time of anaesthesia can be increased considerably by the addition of adrenaline. A study which compared iontophoresis with subcutaneous infiltration and topical application (Russo *et al.*, 1980; quoted by Boone, 1981) found that infiltration produced the longest-lasting anaesthesia—an average of 22.2 min—while iontophoresis caused anaesthesia of the same depth but lasting 14.5 min on average; topical application caused only a short 2.1-min effect. This has been used therapeutically in the treatment of herpes zoster and trigeminal neuralgia, but how successfully is not clear. Although little used in physiotherapy departments, this technique could be valuable for patients who have a strong aversion to hypodermic needles for inducing local anaestheisa. It is used sometimes for minor ear or eye surgery in which hypodermic injection is especially painful. The application of this form of treatment needs particular care in technique because skin anaesthesia is induced during the passage of the current (see below).

Relief of idiopathic hyperhidrosis

Perhaps the most successful use of iontophoresis is in the treatment of idiopathic hyperhidrosis. This distressing condition usually affects the palms and soles and sometimes the axillae. It can be sufficiently severe to interfere with the patient's work. Topical application of various antiperspirants may be ineffective so that surgical treatment—sympathectomy for hands and feet or skin removal for axillary hyperhidrosis—remains the only other option.

Glycopyrronium bromide iontophoresis has been shown to be a simple, safe and effective treatment (Abell and Morgan, 1974), particularly for the hands and feet. Exocrine sweat glands in the palms and soles are innervated by the sympathetic system but stimulated by acetylcholine so that the introduction of an anticholinergic agent (glycopyrronium bromide) into the skin will suppress sweating immediately. This effect lasts a variable length of time; Abell and Morgan (1974) found a mean of 33.7 days for the palm in 16 patients and 47.2 days for the soles in 4 patients. Later it was suggested that few patients need treatment repeated more often than every 4 to 6 weeks (Morgan, 1980).

The length of post-treatment anhidrosis varies not only between patients but in successive treatments of the same patient. One of us (JL) treating two patients with a standard technique found mean periods of dryness to be 30 and 38 days, with a range of 17 to 62 days.

Treatment of the axillae has been less successful in the sense that dryness persisted for only a short period, 7.3 days (Abell and Morgan, 1974). This, and the fact that women and children seem on average to have shorter periods of anhidrosis, suggests that the drug may be held in the epidermis and released slowly, so that more is held by the thicker epidermis (Abell and Morgan, 1974).

Other drugs have been used with the same effect, e.g. poldine methylsulphate (Grice *et al.*, 1972). Using tap water iontophoresis—that is, simply DC—has been described as successfully producing anhidrosis (Grice *et al.*, 1972, Midtgaard, 1986). The anode is used as the active electrode. Older texts refer to a drying effect of the anode but this is based on the observed effect when the metal electrode is implanted in the tissues. The sweat-reducing effect is likely to be due to obstruction of the sweat duct by the deposition of keratin (Abell and Morgan, 1974). Unfortunately, anhidrosis due to tap water iontophoresis seems to last only a few days so that repeated treatments are needed (Grice *et al.*, 1972; Abell and Morgan, 1974; Morgan, 1980). However Midtgaard (1986) and Akins *et al.* (1987) claimed periods of 4 weeks' freedom from sweating. Akins *et al.* (1987) in testing the Drionic unit found that it took on average 14 days of treatment before sweating was inhibited and there were significant side-effects.

Application of antibiotics

The application of antibiotics to avascular areas by iontophoresis has been studied. Ear chondritis following burn injury has been succesfully treated by iontophoresis of gentamicin sulphate (LaForrest and Cofrancesco, 1978). Another method of dealing with chronic infection is metallic silver iontophoresis (Becker and Spadaro, 1978). Chronic non-healing ulcers have been treated with xanthinol nicotinate, a capillary dilator, and histamine diphosphate, which presumably acted similarly; both are quoted by Boone (1981).

Application of anti-inflammatory drugs

Anti-inflammatory drugs used to treat tendinitis and bursitis when delivered by iontophoresis were described as successful by several workers (quoted in Cummings, 1987). The advantages of this method of delivery over conventional injection are the painlessness and sterility of the treatment: absolute sterility is clearly very important for the introduction of anti-inflammatory agents. The disadvantages are that there is even less certainty of their efficacy and it is a time-consuming, hence expensive, method. The major doubt is whether these drugs reach the inflamed tissues, particularly if they are relatively deeply placed structures such as ligaments. However, a study of rhesus monkeys has shown that therapeutic dosages can be delivered to deeply placed joint structures (Glass *et al.*, 1980).

Neurogenic pain

Iontophoresis of vinca alkaloids (vincristine) has been used and recommended for the treatment of chronic pain syndromes. This drug has been found to block transport processes in peripheral nerve axons, i.e. the movement of substances in the nerve fibre cytoplasm, without affecting nerve conduction. The treatment is applied over the painful or hyperaesthesic area. A small controlled trial of patients with long-standing post-herpetic neuralgia (Layman *et al.*, 1986) applying treatment three times per week for 4 weeks found immediate improvement in 9 of 10 patients treated and 1 control. However, at the 6-week follow-up only 6 of the 10 treated patients were considered still to be improved and these 6 had some pain. In spite of this improvement over the controls it was considered that the value of the treatment had not been confirmed. (This opinion was partly due to the side-effects that occurred—skin irritation and burning, especially under the indifferent electrode—but it is not clear why these problems were allowed to occur.)

Other uses

Numerous other drugs have been reported to show specific therapeutic effects when given by iontophoresis. Hyaluronidase has been used for the reduction of local oedema, but there remains considerable doubt about its stability and usefulness (Boone, 1981). Zinc iontophoersis in the treatment of ischaemic ulcers and for allergic rhinitis has been recommended and used in the past. The dramatic skin erythema and weal produced by ethylmorphine hydrochloride (Renotin) or histamine iontophoresis was at one time widely used in the treatment of a large number of conditions (Kovacs, 1949; Taylor, 1949), but there seems to be no objective evidence of its effectiveness, with the result that this treatment is rarely used at present. Iodine and chlorine have been used to increase the extensibility of scar tissue in association with passive stretching (Tannenbaum, 1980; Cummings, 1987). Copper iontophoresis has been used for the treatment of fungal skin infections (tinea pedis) and salicylate for the relief of pain in rheumatic diseases, with no apparent evidence of any advantage over other simpler forms of treatment.

The therapeutic effectiveness of iontophoretically administered drugs has been purely a matter of opinion in the last 50 years or so when the fashion for it was at a peak. This has led to many unsupported claims of therapeutic efficacy and a subsequent backlash of scepticism. There is now though good evidence for some treatments, notably for hyperhidrosis, and the advantages of iontophoresis over local injection—it is non-invasive, there is no damage to tissues and it is sterile—may be important in the future.

PRINCIPLES OF APPLICATION

The principles of applying DC are the same whether it is the effect of the current alone that is intended or the iontophoresis of specific ions. The aim is to produce a uniform current density throughout the skin area to be treated. It is necessary to provide a complete circuit: current must enter and leave the tissues at separate sites (Fig. 2.4). For most treatments, only one site is of therapeutic interest, called the active electrode, while the other, designated the dispersive or indifferent electrode, is usually made to cover a much larger

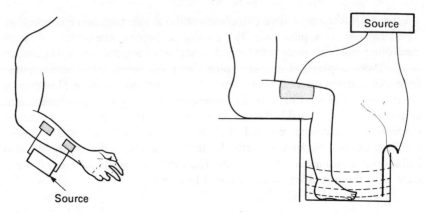

Fig. 2.4 A complete circuit for the application of DC.

area—$2\frac{1}{2}$ times the area of the active electrode (Wadsworth and Chanmugan, 1980). This is done by applying the current through a container of water (or solution) or by using pads of suitable absorbant material to hold the water or solution. This material can be lint, gauze, sponge or suitable towelling. The pad must be thick enough to contain sufficient water; it should be at least 1 cm thick when lightly compressed. Such a thickness will usually ensure that it maintains good contact with the irregular skin surface and provides enough electrolyte to dilute harmful chemicals formed at the electrolyte–electrode junction.

The current is applied to the pad by some form of malleable metal electrode, aluminium foil or other metal sheet, which is made slightly smaller—1 cm all round—than the pad. This is to reduce the likelihood of the bare electrode touching the skin. The wire should be connected to the metal electrode by some suitable clip or the bare wire simply twisted together through a hole in the metal. In either case the connection should make as little irregularity on the pad side of the electrode as possible so that the current spreads evenly over the whole area of the electrode. For the same reason the electrode should be flat and have rounded corners.

The pad and electrode are best secured in position by means of an elastic bandage, such as a crêpe bandage, to ensure an even pressure over the whole area of the pad and hence uniform current density. In order to prevent the bandage being wetted, thus transmitting current to the adjacent tissues, it is best to separate the bandage from the wet pad by a suitably sized piece of waterproof material such as polythene.

It is possible to treat the extremities by immersing the part to be treated in a container of water. The current is led in by an electrode clipped to the side of the container; the size of this electrode does not matter but it should be situated well away from the immersed body part (Fig. 2.4).

It is necessary to explain the nature of the treatment to the patient as well as the sensation (a mild prickling leading to a gentle warmth) that will be felt. It is very important to warn the patient to report any local increase in sensation or any painful sensation at once since there is a risk that a chemical burn may occur. Any increase of local current density may cause this chemical damage very rapidly; it may occur if there is an area of low skin resistance such as a cut, abrasion or papule. It can also occur if the skin resistance is uneven because some parts are covered with grease or due to uneven pressure from creases in the pad. It is therefore essential to examine the area for cuts and abrasions, establish by pinprick that the patient has normal pain sensation in the whole area of skin being treated and that he or she fully understands the need to report abnormal sensations.

As the outer horny layer of the epidermis provides the main ohmic resistance to the current flow it is helpful to reduce this resistance by wetting and warming the skin prior to treatment by means of a warm soak or wash which also serves to remove excess surface oil or grease. Much of the current probably passes through the dermis via the sweat glands.

If a water bath is used for one electrode or two baths are used, one for each electrode (monopolar baths), it is important additionally to warn the patient not to remove a limb from the bath during treatment since this will break the circuit, interrupting the current and causing a marked sensory shock and perhaps muscle twitch. While not usually dangerous this may alarm the patient. It will also be noted that the current density is higher in the skin close to the surface of the water, hence there will be more sensation in this area. This is due to the fact that current can pass both in the tissues and through the water in the bath but where the limb emerges at the surface all the current must pass through the tissues, thus the path of lowest resistance is through the skin near the surface of the water. This effect can be reduced by protecting this surface line by applying a thin coat of petroleum jelly to the skin.

When applying the current it is essential to increase the intensity slowly and never to switch on or off with the intensity control above zero, as this can cause abrupt sensory and motor stimulation—a shock. The passage of the current is reputed to reduce the skin resistance during the first few minutes of treatment (Wadsworth and Chanmugan, 1980) so that the reading on the meter may increase a little without the control being moved. If the meter should indicate a sudden increase in current it is important to turn the control down slowly and inspect the area since this indication of lowered resistance may signal the beginning of a chemical burn. Prior to treatment the bare ends of the leads can be held in water and the intensity turned up until the maximal current required for that treatment is shown on the milliammeter. This checks that the increase in current is smoothly progressive and that the milliammeter is functioning. If there is any doubt about the polarity of the terminals they may be tested at the same time (see Appendix B).

The technique for the application of iontophoresis involves ensuring that the drug to be driven into the skin is placed beneath the correct electrode. Positively charged ions must obviously be placed under the positive electrode and negative ions under the negative. All the ions mentioned above that are used therapeutically are positively charged, hence they should be placed under the positive electrode—except for acetate, chloride, iodide and salicylate, which are all negatively charged. Sometimes the solution used is quite expensive—glycopyrronium bromide, for example—so that it is economical to use small quantities of the drug. When the hands and feet are being treated for hyperhidrosis a suitably sized pad and electrode can be enclosed with the hand or foot in a small plastic bag rather than using a shallow bowl or tray of solution. The plastic bag prevents the solution being squeezed out of the pad and wasted.

DOSAGE

The introduction of ions into the tissues by iontophoresis depends on both current density and time, already noted and described (see Fig. 2.2). Many texts simply suggest total currents rather than current densities, and approximate times (Wadsworth and Chanmugan, 1980; Forster and Palastanga, 1985). As can be seen from Figure 2.2, increasing the time of treatment for any given current density makes proportionally smaller increases in ionic transfer. Thus it seems that the rather approximate dosage recommendations are quite reasonable for iontophoresis, since current densities that are detectable and yet are comfortably tolerable will be in the region of 0.1–0.2 mA/cm^2 and even if the extremes of these current densities are used the number of ions transferred less than doubles between 10 and 40 min.

Using glycopyrrolate for hyperhidrosis it has been suggested that 12 mA for 12 min is appropriate for one adult hand; that is, a current density of 0.08–0.1 mA/cm^2 (Morgan, 1980) or 15–20 mA for 15 min (Wadsworth and Chanmugan, 1980). Since the current is limited by the patient's tolerance this should always be at a comfortable level and the dosage made up by compensating with the time of treatment. Thus the dosage can be expressed in 'mA min', i.e. total current multiplied by the treatment time. Personal experience (JL) suggests that dosages of between 100 and 200 mA min are appropriate for each hand or foot and this conforms with the dosages suggested above. It must be remembered that systemic as well as local effects occur and these are unwanted and unpleasant side-effects (see below). The dosage must be kept below the level at which these effects occur, which varies from patient to patient. It is sensible to give a low dose (less than 100 mA min) for the initial treatment and assess the effects. With children the initial dose should be even less—50–70 mA min. Most adults seem able to have both hands or both feet treated at one session without serious side-effects.

Treatments that produce an immediately detectable effect—such as anhidrosis due to glycopyrrolate or anaesthesia due to lignocaine or the weal plus erythema due to Renotin—will indicate their own effective dose at the end of treatment. If the effect of treatment is inadequate then it may be continued for a longer time. Renotin treatment requires only 2–6 mA for 4 min to produce the effect (Taylor, 1949). Again the initial dose should be low: 1.125 mA for 3 min for a 30 cm^2 pad (Wadsworth and Chanmugan, 1980).

For other iontophoretic treatments the dosage is similar to that for hyperhidrosis but often longer times are suggested—5 mA for a 100 cm^2 pad, i.e. 0.05 mA/cm^2, for 20–30 min has been suggested for iodine (Tannenbaum, 1980) and acetate (Wadsworth and Chanmugan, 1980). Many writers give only the total current, not current density, but since most treatments are given over areas of 50–200 cm^2 the 5–20 mA current usually suggested represents currents of about 0.1 mA/cm^2. The times suggested vary from 10 to 30 min.

When direct current is used for pain relief and not for iontophoresis the recommended dosage varies depending on polarity. If the cathode (negative pole) is being used to achieve a pain-relieving effect then relatively high current densities of 0.5–0.8 mA/cm^2 for 10–20 min have been suggested. If the positive pole is to be used then lower current densities of 0.15–0.25 mA/cm^2 for 15–30 min have been suggested (Wadsworth and Chanmugan, 1980).

DANGERS

1 Chemical damage to the tissues, a chemical burn, can occur as a result of the current density becoming too high. This can arise in a multitude of ways. Low skin resistance due to cuts or abrasions, uneven pressure or thickness of pads have already been mentioned. There is also danger of a burn if a bare piece of the metal lead or electrode inadvertently touches the skin.

2 A shock can occur if the circuit is broken so that the current is interrupted, such as would happen if the current is switched off without being turned down slowly. This may happen in a number of ways—such as a lead breaking during treatment or the patient removing a hand from the bath—but with the relatively low currents employed there is no damage, except that the patient will suffer an alarming shock.

3 Some patients experience a skin irritation caused by hypersensitivity to the chemicals produced by the current. It can usually be prevented by washing the treated part after treatment.

4 Systemic effects can occur, especially if large areas are treated by iontophoresis. With anti-cholinergic drugs these can take the form of headaches, abdominal pains or mild dryness of the mouth. Patients should be warned to avoid vigorous exercise immediately after treatment, and if the symptoms are severe the area of treatment should be reduced. Pregnancy is a contraindication. Histamine can cause a change in blood pressure and also headaches.

REFERENCES

Abell E., Morgan K. (1974). The treatment of idiopathic hyperhidrosis by glycopyrronium bromide and tap water iontophoresis. *Br. J. Dermatol.*, **91**, 45–60.

Akins D. L., Meisenheimer J. L., Dobson R. L. (1987). Efficacy of the Drionic unit in the treatment of hyperhidrosis. *J. Am. Acad. Dermatol.*, **16**, 828–33.

Alon G. (1987). Principles of electrical stimulation. In *Clinical Electrotherapy* (Nelson R. M., Currier D. P., eds) Norwalk, Connecticut, USA: Appleton Lange, pp. 29–80.

Alvarez O. M., Mertz P. M., Smerbock R. V. *et al.* (1983). The healing of superficial skin wounds is stimulated by external electric current. *J. Invest. Dermatol.*, **81**, 144–8.

Becker R. O., Spadaro J. A., Marino A. A. (1977). Clinical experience with low intensity direct current stimulation of bone growth. *Clin. Orthop.*, **124**, 75–83.

Becker R. O., Spadaro J. A., Marino A. A. (1977). Clinical experience with low intensity direct current stimulation of bone growth. *Clin. Orthop.*, **124**, 75–83.

Becker R. O., Spadaro J. A. (1978). Treatment of orthopaedic infections with electrically generated silver ions. *J. Bone Joint Surg.*, **60A**, 871–81.

Binder S. A. (1981). Application of low- and high-voltage electrotherapeutic currents. In *Electrotherapy* (Wolfe S. L., ed.) New York: Churchill Livingstone, pp. 1–24.

Boone C. (1981). Applications of iontophoresis. In *Electrotherapy* (Wolfe S. L., ed.) New York: Churchill Livingstone, pp. 99–121.

Brown M., McDonnell, M. K., Menton D. M. (1988). Electrical stimulation effects on cutaneous wound healing in rabbits. *Phys. Ther.*, **68**, 955–9.

Cummings, J. (1987). Iontophoresis. In *Clinical Electrotherapy* (Nelson R. M., Currier D. P., eds) Norwalk, USA: Appleton & Lange, pp. 231–41.

Forster A., Palastanga N. (1985). *Clayton's Electrotherapy: Theory and Practice* 9th edn. London: Bailliere Tindall.

Foulds I., Barker A. (1983). Human skin battery potentials and their possible role in wound healing. *Br. J. Dermatol*, **109**, 515–22.

Gault W. R., Gatens P. F. (1976). Use of low intensity direct current in management of ischaemic skin ulcers. *Phys. Ther.*, **56**, 265–8.

Glass J. M., Stephen B. L., Jacobsen S. C. (1980). The quantity and distribution of radiolabelled dexamethasone delivered to tissues by iontophoresis. *Int. J. Dermatol.*, **19**, 519–25.

Grice K., Sattar H., Baker H. (1972). Treatment of idiopathic hyperhidrosis with iontophoresis of tap water and poldine methosulphate. *Br. J. Dermatol.*, **86**, 72.

Kahn J. (1975). Calcium iontophoresis in suspected myopathy. *Phys. Ther.*, **55**, 376–7.

Kloth L. C., Feeder J. A. (1988). Acceleration of wound healing with high voltage, monophasic, pulsed current. *Phys. Ther.*, **68**, 503–8.

Kovacs R. (1949). *Electrotherapy and Light Therapy* 6th edn. London: Henry Kimpton.

LaForrest N. T., Cofranesco C. (1978). Antibiotic iontophoresis in the treatment of ear chondritis. *Phys. Ther.*, **58**, 32–4.

Layman P. R., Argyras E., Glynn C. J. (1986). Iontophoresis of vincristine versus saline in post-herpetic neuralgia. A controlled trial. *Pain*, **25**, 165–70.

Licht S. (1983). History of electrotherapy. In *Therapeutic Electricity and Ultraviolet Radiations* 3rd edn (Stillwell G. K., ed.) Baltimore: Williams & Wilkins, pp. 1–64.

Midtgaard K. (1986). A new device for the treatment of hyperhidrosis by iontophoresis. *Br. J. Dermatol.*, **114**, 485–8.

Morgan K. (1980). The technique of treating hyperhidrosis by iontophoresis. *Physiotherapy*, **66**, 45.

O'Malley E. P., Oester Y. T. (1955). Influences of some physical chemical factors on iontophoresis using radio-isotopes. *Arch. Phys. Med. Rehab.*, **36**, 310.

Russo J., Lipman A. G., Comstock T. J. *et al.* (1980). Lidocaine anaesthesia: comparison of iontophoresis, injection and swabbing. *Am. J. Hosp. Pharmacol.*, **37**, 843–7.

Tannenbaum M. (1980). Iodine iontophoresis in reducing scar tissue. *Phys. Ther.*, **60**, 792.

Taylor G. A. (1949). A new drug for iontophoresis. *Physiotherapy*, **49**.

Trubatch J., Van Harreveld A. (1972). Spread of iontophoretically injected ions in a tissue. *J. Theor. Biol.*, **36**, 355–66.

Wadsworth H., Chanmugan A. P. P. (1980). *Electrophysical Agents in Physiotherapy*. Marrickville, Australia: Science Press.

Weiss D. S., Kirsner R., Eaglstein W. H. (1990). Electrical stimulation and wound healing. *Archives of Dermatology*, **126**, 222–5.

Wolcott L. E., Wheeler P. C., Hardwicke H. M. (1969). Accelerated healing of skin ulcers by electrotherapy: preliminary clinical results. *South. Med. J.*, **62**, 795–801.

3.

Nerve and muscle stimulation

PRINCIPLES

The major difficulty encountered in describing the currents used for the therapeutic and diagnostic stimulation of excitable tissue (nerves and muscles) lies in making sense of the plethora of terms that clutter this subject. There are many terms which have come to have specific meanings which are neither consistent nor informative. Many are eponymous, like galvanism, derived from inventors or popularizers, while others are trade names fabricated to sound impressive. Furthermore there is considerable overlap between terms. It is therefore essential to understand the nature and form of the pulses of current that are employed in electrotherapy.

All stimulators of nerve tissue (except implanted stimulators) are in fact transcutaneous electrical nerve stimulators (TENS), but this term is applied only to low-intensity battery-operated sensory nerve stimulators used for pain control. Such names as faradic, sinusoidal, diadynamic and accommodation currents have been used historically to specify certain pulse shapes and hence indicate certain effects. The nature of the electrical pulses and the physiological effects will be described first and the traditional names attached subsequently.

Firstly it is important to understand the effects of electric charges on the tissues in general terms. These effects depend on the *rate of change* of the electric pulse:

1 If there is no change, or only a very slow change, and the current is unidirectional there will be a steady flow of ions into and within the tissues causing chemical changes at the electrode–tissue junction, as described in Chapter 2.
2 If the rate of change is somewhat faster and the pulse has a long enough duration the ionic balance across excitable membranes is disturbed stimulating nerves and muscles (see Chapter 1). If the current is unidirectional it will also lead to chemical changes, as above, but if it is evenly alternating no such changes can occur because any change in one direction is immediately cancelled when the current reverses.
3 If the rate of change is very fast there is insufficient time for transmembrane excitation to occur so that much larger currents can be employed, which can lead to significant heating. This is the basis of diathermy (see Chapter 10).

The extent of the physiological changes will obviously depend on the current intensity; higher currents cause greater effects. The intensity will also determine whether any single electrical pulse has enough energy to provoke a nerve impulse. Thus a given rate of rise, duration and fall of pulse may be too rapid to cause nerve stimulation at a low current intensity, but may do so at a higher intensity.

It is convenient to describe the unit of stimulating current as a 'pulse' of current or current phase. This will cause one (or two) nerve impulses. The simple graphs given in Figure 3.1 illustrate the relationship of time and current intensity and hence the rate of change of current. Thus in (a) a slow rise, steady, unidirectional current, and a slow fall illustrate the direct current used in galvanic current or iontophoretic treatments (see Chapter 2). If the rise is made rapid—i.e. there is a high rate of change—then nerve stimulation occurs leading to a nerve impulse, shown in (b) (see Chapter 1). This will happen both when the current rises and when it falls. If the time for which the current flows is made shorter, say 1 ms, as in (c) then there is no time for the nerve membrane to recover and only a single nerve impulse results. The consequence of (b) and (c) would be to stimulate sensory nerves giving a series of single nerve impulses recognized consciously as a series of little shocks. Similarly motor nerves would be stimulated leading to a series of single muscle twitches. If these stimuli are repeated every 10 ms they will cause a steady tingling sensation as they stimulate sensory nerves and a tetanic muscle contraction as they stimulate the motor nerves; this is shown in (d) (see also Chapter 1). Such currents at low intensities produced by small battery-operated electronic stimulators are used for pain control in TENS stimulators. At higher intensities they are used for muscle stimulation, when they are known as faradic stimulators.

The actual strength of muscle contraction or sensory effect will depend on the numbers of nerve fibres stimulated, which depends on the intensity of current. Greater current intensity will spread further in the tissues and hence

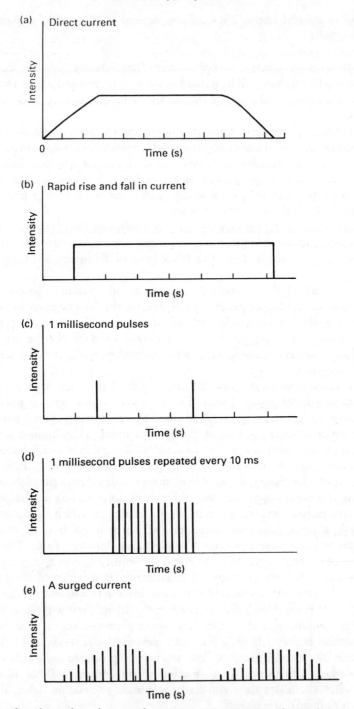

Fig. 3.1 The relationship of time and current. (a) Direct current; (b) rapid rise and fall in current; (c) 1 ms pulses; (d) 1 ms pulses repeated every 10 ms; (e) surged current.

activate more nerves. If the intensity is increased from zero over a period of a second or so and then decreased to zero again and this sequence is repeated, a series of rhythmical contractions and relaxations will occur like normal physiological muscle action (Fig. 3.1e). This is called a surged current or surging the current; American sources refer to this as 'ramping'. It is simply current modulation and can be done automatically, i.e. electronically or manually.

It will be seen that all the currents shown in Figure 3.1 are unidirectional or monophasic so that all would have chemical effects. The individual pulses, except (a), would be described as 'square wave' pulses but there are other monophasic pulses which are not in this form, e.g. triangular. These single pulses or phases can be fully described by their:

1 *duration* in seconds, milliseconds (ms) or microseconds (μs);
2 *intensity* in milliamps (mA) or voltage (V);
3 *shape*—rate of rise and fall. This is simply how the intensity changes with time.

The term peak current intensity, or peak voltage or peak phase, refers to the highest current/voltage that occurs during the pulse. The mean (average) current/voltage will be less.

The pulse (phase) charge is easily calculated. The charge is the quantity of electric charge in coulombs (C) (see Appendix A). Thus a 1 ms pulse of 1 mA average intensity would have a charge of 1 μC.

If a series of pulses are considered the pulse rate can be expressed in pulses per second (pps) or the pulse frequency in hertz (Hz). The same information is given by describing the pulse interval, or interpulse interval, expressed in ms or s. Thus a series of 10 ms pulses separated by 90 ms pulse intervals will have a frequency of 10 Hz (Fig. 3.2).

So far consideration has only been given to unidirectional pulses. Many pulses used therapeutically are biphasic. Current passes first in one then in the opposite direction (Fig. 3.3a). Such discrete pulses may be separated by various pulse intervals like monophasic phases or they can be continuous (Fig.

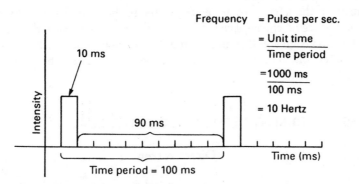

Frequency = Pulses per sec.

= $\dfrac{\text{Unit time}}{\text{Time period}}$

= $\dfrac{1000 \text{ ms}}{100 \text{ ms}}$

= 10 Hertz

Fig. 3.2 Relationship of frequency (*f*) to time period. $f =$ pps $=$ unit time/time period $= 1000/100$ ms $\doteq 10$ Hz.

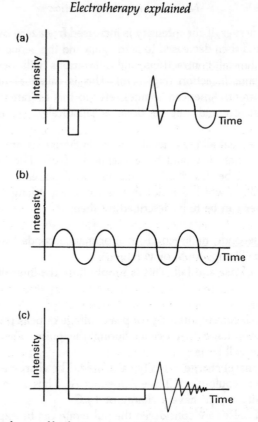

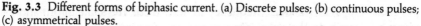

Fig. 3.3 Different forms of biphasic current. (a) Discrete pulses; (b) continuous pulses; (c) asymmetrical pulses.

3.3b). When such continuous pulses follow a sine curve the therapeutic current is called a sinusoidal current. The mains current is in this sinusoidal form. Due to the constantly changing direction, such currents are called alternating currents. These are evenly alternating but it is common to have uneven alternations, which may be of unequal intensity, unequal duration or asymmetrical shape (Fig. 3.3c).

Clearly if the alterations are equal in charge there will be no total current flow and hence no chemical changes. If the alternations are such that current in one direction is greater than in the other there will be a net current flow in the former direction. In many clinical sources the difference may be so small as to have little effect.

TYPES OF CURRENT USED THERAPEUTICALLY

Direct current

This refers to any unidirectional current but it is often used to mean *constant direct current*, that is, an unvarying current also known as *galvanism* or a *galvanic current* (see Chapter 2).

Interrupted direct current

If the continuous unidirectional current is interrupted it gives a series of pulses or phases of unidirectional current which can be of any duration or shape, repeated at any frequency. Certain durations, shapes and frequencies have acquired particular names so that although any unidirectional pulse is an interrupted direct current (IDC), the term is customarily used to describe only the longer-duration pulses.

Long duration (of 1 ms or more)

Square wave pulses.   These are pulses of any duration between 1 and 600 ms separated by pulse intervals of anything from 1 ms to several seconds (Fig. 3.2 and Fig. 3.5). Such pulses can stimulate motor and sensory nerves and can be used to stimulate denervated muscle.

Accommodation pulses.   Triangular, trapezoidal, sawtooth, serrate, slow-rising, shaped, selective and accommodation pulses are all synonymous terms. Again, these are relatively long-duration pulses, usually 600 to 1000 ms, separated by pulse intervals of one-half to several seconds (Fig. 3.5). These pulses are used to selectively stimulate muscle (as opposed to nerve) tissue and they are able to do so because of differences in muscle and nerve accommodation, hence the names (see Chapter 1).

Short duration (of 1 ms or less)

Faradic-type pulses.   Pulses of 0.1–1 ms are repeated at 30–100 Hz. With pulses repeated at 100 Hz the time period for each cycle is 10 ms, so with a 1 ms pulse the rest period is 9 ms (Fig. 3.4 and Fig. 3.5). These pulses may be unidirectional and are thus short duration IDC, or they may be biphasic. Pulses were originally generated by an induction coil and interrupter which, because it was an electromagnetic device, was called a faradic coil. The pulses produced were unevenly alternating (biphasic; Fig. 3.4c). The effective nerve stimulus is the spike of voltage, which can be about 1 ms in duration; the rest of the pulse, having much lower voltage, does not cause nerve stimulation.

Although the alternations are uneven in shape they are identical in total charge so that no chemical changes will occur. The repetition rate is dictated by the mass and elastic properties of the mechanical interrupter and is often about 60 Hz. Faradic currents are a succession of these pulses which unmodified would produce a tetanic contraction (Fig. 3.4b). Treatment by faradic current or faradic-type pulses is often called 'faradism'.

TENS.   It has already been pointed out that all nerve-stimulating pulses are TENS but the term is usually restricted to pulses of relatively low intensity used to control pain. Almost all such generators are battery-operated. A variety of pulse forms are available. A few are monophasic, i.e. short pulse IDC, but the majority are symmetrically or asymmetrically biphasic (Fig. 3.4d and Fig. 3.5). Pulse durations, often fixed for a given source, can be any length from 0.02 to 0.4 ms. The frequency is usually variable and ranged from 2 to 200 Hz, most devices giving various frequencies around 100 Hz. Voltage, and

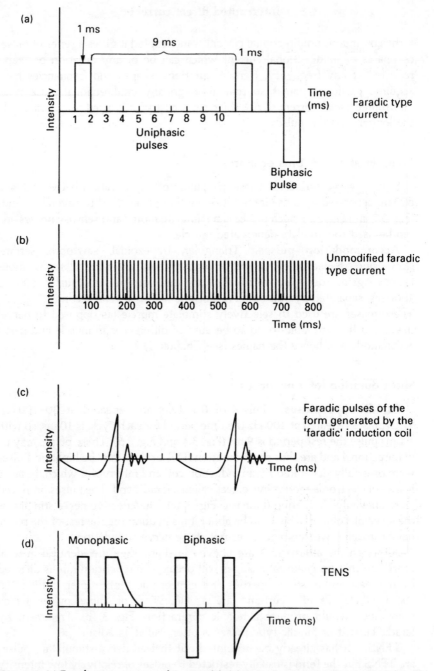

Fig. 3.4 (a) Faradic-type current; (b) unmodifed faradic-type current; (c) faradic pulses of the form generated by the faradic induction coil; (d) TENS.

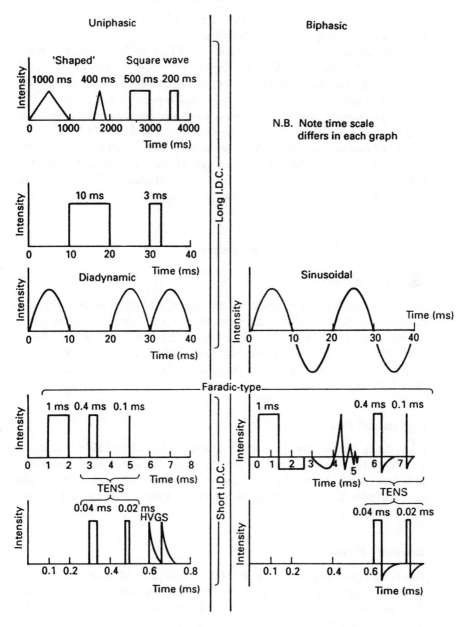

Fig. 3.5 Comparison of low-frequency currents: pulses, shapes and durations. Note that the time scale differs in each graph.

thus the applied current, can be varied but is limited to low intensities: the maximum peak current is about 100 mA.

High-voltage galvanic stimulation (HVGS) or high-voltage pulsed galavanic stimulation (HVPGS). These are pulses formed of twin peaks, each of very short duration (5–7 µs), occurring together in about 100 µs. They have very high voltages leading to high peak currents, around 2000 mA, but very low average current. Repetition rates can be varied between 2 and 100 Hz (Fig. 3.5). This current will be described and discussed later.

All unidirectional currents can cause chemical changes as described in Chapter 2 and Appendix B but the magnitude of these changes depends on both the current and the time for which it flows. In many of the short duration pulses there is so little total time that the chemical effects are negligible.

Evenly alternating

Sinusoidal currents

Sinusoidal currents refer to an evenly alternating sine wave which is the mains current form (Fig. 3.5). Since mains current in the UK is of 50 Hz the current will have 100 pulses or phases of 10 ms each, 50 in one direction and 50 in the other. This current will stimulate motor and sensory nerves but, of course, is only applied therapeutically at no more than about 80 V—not the 240 V of the UK mains.

Diadynamic currents

Diadynamic currents are sinusoidal in shape with a pulse of 10 ms duration at 100 or 50 Hz. Various other combinations of this same pulse duration are sometimes available (see Fig. 3.26). Such pulses have been popularized, mainly in continental Europe. Diadynamic current is simply rectified and modified mains alternating current.

'Russian' currents

This is an alternating sine wave of 2500 Hz applied at 50 bursts per second— i.e. 10 ms bursts of 25 cycles each—with 10 ms intervals between each burst. Since each biphasic pulse lasts only 0.4 ms it needs a high current to produce nerve stimulation (Alon, 1987). It is used for muscle re-education and strengthening.

Interferential currents

These are alternating sine wave currents of about 4000 Hz. When two such currents of slightly different frequencies are made to pass through the same area of tissue they 'interfere' producing a resultant current which varies, giving a pulse of sufficient duration and intensity to stimulate nerves. The frequency and intensity of this 'beat', as it is called, can be varied to cause different levels of stimulation (Fig. 3.27a).

High-frequency currents

High-frequency currents of millions of hertz are used therapeutically but they cannot stimulate nerve or muscle, because they change too rapidly. They can be safely applied at a high current intensity to produce tissue heating (see Chapter 10).

It can be seen why the terms *low-frequency*, *medium-frequency* and *high-frequency* currents came to be used. Faradic, TENS and sinusoidal, at frequencies around 50–100 Hz are known as low-frequency currents. Interferential, at about 4000 Hz and 'Russian', at about 2500 Hz, are called medium-frequency currents and shortwave diathermy, at about 30 MHz, is a high-frequency current. Figure 3.5 is a composite diagram illustrating the overlap between currents and their names.

PRODUCTION OF ELECTRICAL PULSES

There are several different methods of therapeutic electrical pulse generation which have been used in the past. Faradic currents from an induction coil have already been mentioned, but modern pulse generators are based on integrated circuits of transistors, resistors and capacitors.

The pulse felt at the wrist is simply a wave of fluid, i.e. blood pressure, which is generated by the action of the heart. An electrical pulse—using the word in another context but similar sense—is produced by the same basic mechanism. As the heart contracts (ventricular systole) the pressure in the arteries rises and causes the blood to flow at a higher pressure for a time while the aortic valve is open. When it closes the pressure in the arteries falls (ventricular diastole). This cycle is repeated at a rate determined by the sinoatrial node. Thus a system exerting a pressure (voltage) causes a flow (current) which is turned on and off by a valve (switch). The time for which the pressure is exerted, i.e. heart muscle contraction, is controlled by the rhythmicity of the sinoatrial node acting as a timing device. In a modern pulse generator the mains current is applied via a transformer (see Appendix C) to provide a suitably reduced voltage; it is rectified and smoothed. The switch is a transistor which can turn the current on or off very rapidly, and the timing device is a capacitance–resistance circuit.

A capacitance–resistance circuit is analogous to a sandglass eggtimer. If a capacitor is allowed to discharge through a resistance, the time it takes depends on both the size of the capacitor and the resistance. A large capacitor stores more electrons for a given voltage than a small one. The larger the resistance the smaller the current, for a given voltage (Ohm's law; see Appendix A), therefore the capacitor will take longer to discharge. Note that both current and voltage will fall exponentially (Fig. 3.6). In exactly the same way the more grains of sand the eggtimer holds, the longer they will take to pass through the narrow neck, and the smaller the neck the longer the flow of sand will take (Fig. 3.6). The importance of such circuits lies in the fact that by a suitable choice of capacitor and resistance almost any length of time for their discharge can be arranged. Thus it is possible to time pulses of voltage to last a few microseconds or for several seconds. Not only can the voltage pulse be timed but the period when it is off can be similarly controlled, so that a train of pulses can be generated with identical pulse lengths and pulse intervals. Further, the train of pulses itself can be timed to occur in bursts or surges of pulses separated by timed rest periods.

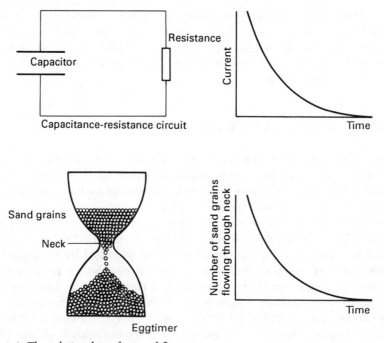

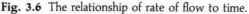

Fig. 3.6 The relationship of rate of flow to time.

The way in which the transistor acts as an electronic switch is illustrated in Figure 3.7. When no base current is flowing the transistor is off in the sense that there is a high resistance between collector and emitter. If a small current is applied through the base it will decrease the resistance of the path between collector and emitter to allow a flow of current, turning the switch on. If the base current is made large enough it will reduce the resistance in the collector–emitter pathway to zero. Quite a small base current will have a large effect on the collector–emitter current so that small changes in base current can be made to turn the transistor completely off—acting as a switch.

By applying the output from one timing circuit with a transistor to another similar circuit and feeding back the output of that to control the first circuit it is

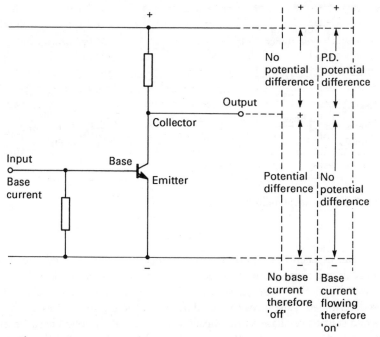

Fig. 3.7 The transistor as a switch.

possible to produce a continuously oscillating current. Such a circuit is called an astable multivibrator or, more expressively, a flipflop circuit. (It flips from one state—a pulse of current—to the other state—no current.) Figure 3.8 shows such a circuit.

To see how this circuit works, assume that transistor 1 is not conducting because no base-to-emitter current is flowing, the base being negative. There is therefore no voltage drop across the collector resistance 1 so that the collector is at the voltage of the positive line. At the same time transistor 2 is on because the base is slightly positive allowing a base emitter current to flow. Thus current flows through the collector–emitter path of transistor 2, resulting in a potential difference across collector resistance 2 and hence the collector voltage will be negative. These assumptions are made to give a starting point in the cycle.

The capacitor C_2 now charges through the resistance R_2 at a rate proportional to their sizes, as explained above. As the left-hand plate of the capacitor becomes positive, emitter-base current starts to flow in transistor 1 to turn it on. This allows collector current to flow so that the collector voltage becomes negative.

This negative voltage is transferred by capacitor C_1 to transistor 2 to turn it off. Capacitor C_1 will now charge through R_1 until transistor 2 is conducting again. Once this happens the process repeats, with transistor 2 causing a negative potential to be applied to the base of transistor 1 to turn it off again. Thus one transistor is fully conducting while the other is fully off and vice versa.

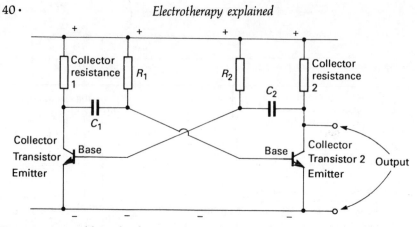

Fig. 3.8 An astable multivibrator circuit.

It can be seen that altering the resistance of R_1 and R_2 will alter the pulse intervals and pulse duration respectively. This can be easily done by means of a switch on the pulse generator which can be altered to select different predetermined resistances to give different predetermined times. Such a circuit would start to oscillate automatically once voltage is applied because the state of conduction of one or other transistor is bound to be slightly greater, thus turning the other off and starting the on–off cycle. The output from transistor 2 could have the form shown in Figure 3.9.

The 'flipover' from conducting to not-conducting and vice versa in these transistors can be very rapid. This is because quite small changes in base current will cause large changes in collector current and once the base current starts to diminish and thus reduce the collector current, making the collector more positive in one transistor, this immediately has the effect of increasing the base current of the other transistor, turning it on still further. This positive feedback ensures that the changeover from conducting to not-conducting is almost instantaneous. It is therefore justifiable to show the pulses as square wave, as in Figure 3.9.

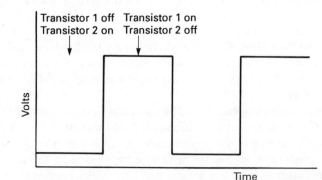

Fig. 3.9 Output from transistors shown in Figure 3.8.

General structure of electrical pulse generators

Pulse generators may be considered to have four functional parts:

1 A power source; this may be from the mains supply or a battery.
2 An oscillating circuit to provide a train of pulses, as described above.
3 A modulating circuit to alter the train of pulses, perhaps splitting it up into short bursts or surging it.
4 An amplifying circuit to increase the output voltage appropriately.

When power is drawn from the mains it will need to be modified. The voltage will have to be reduced to an appropriate level for the subsequent circuits and output. This is done with a transformer (see Appendix C), and rectified by means of a diode (semiconductor diodes are usually used). With a suitable controlling circuit these could be applied as diadynamic current to a patient. If the voltage-reduced rectified mains current is applied to a 'smoothing' circuit (a capacitor in parallel and a series inductance) it becomes an unvarying direct current and, if regulated with a potential divider could be applied to a patient (see Chapter 2).

Modern pulse generators go through the above steps to produce a smooth unidirectional current that can be applied to an oscillator to generate any type of current. For low-intensity TENS currents (used for patient-controlled pain modulation) the smooth DC can be supplied by a small battery. There is nearly always a light provided to indicate that the power circuit is on.

The oscillator to generate a train of pulses works, in principle, as a

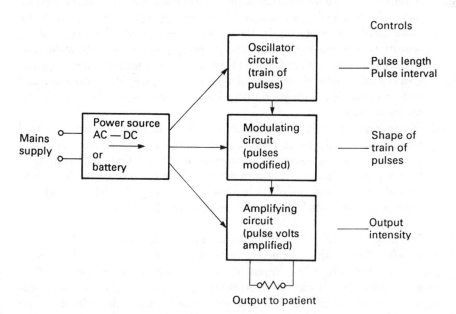

Fig. 3.10 Block diagram to illustrate electrical pulse generators.

multivibrator, as already described. Such circuits are usually manufactured all in one piece as an integrated circuit which can be fitted to appropriate resistors to give the desired pulse lengths and intervals. Where these are to be varied a switch on the panel of the machine connects the necessary resistance to give the pulse length required.

The train of pulses may then be modified, surged for example, by another integrated circuit which may also be controlled by a switch on the machine. A circuit may also make the DC pulses biphasic. Finally the output is amplified and applied to a potential divider to regulate the output to the patient. This is illustrated in Figure 3.10.

EFFECTS OF LOW-FREQUENCY ELECTRICAL PULSES ON THE TISSUES

When currents are passed through the tissues two groups of effects can be considered:

1 There are clear and well documented effects on excitable tissue, that is nerve and muscle, which lead to numerous indirect effects. For example, modifying pain perception in the central nervous system or causing muscle contraction is secondary to the stimulation of the nerve fibre. There is also evidence of direct effects on these tissues affecting their growth and metabolism (eutrophic electrotherapy is considered in this chapter).

   Peripheral nerves are composed of many fibres—nerve cell processes— both sensory (afferent) and motor (efferent). The motor fibres are the axons of cells in the anterior (ventral) horn of the spinal cord, hence called anterior horn cells, while the cell bodies of the sensory nerves are found in the posterior (dorsal) root ganglia. The motor nerves to skeletal muscles and the sensory nerves conveying touch and proprioception are all fast-conducting, of large diameter and myelinated (Table 3.1). The majority of fibres making up a typical peripheral nerve are of small diameter, are slow-conducting and non-myelinated; a high proportion are pain-carrying C fibres, while the others are autonomic.

2 Effects on non-excitable tissue at a cellular level are much less well recognized or understood. There is evidence that direct pulsed currents may accelerate healing in skin and other tissue, as noted in Chapter 2. It has also been suggested that pulsatile currents may affect cell metabolism leading to arterial, venous and lymphatic exchange at a microcirculatory level, but there is no substantial supporting evidence (Alon, 1987).

To apply electrical pulses to the tissues a complete circuit is needed so two electrodes with suitable conducting material are fixed to the skin. The effects will be evident where the current density is highest, i.e. in the superficial tissues under the smaller (active) electrode. Consequently the cutaneous sensory nerves are affected first and with greater current densities the more deeply placed motor nerves are stimulated. However, the sensory and motor

Table 3.1 Classification of peripheral nerve fibres

Type of sheath	Fibre diameter (μ)	Conduction speed (m/s)	Classification by letter — Efferent motor	Efferent autonomic	Afferent sensory	Classification by number — Afferent sensory
Myelinated	22	120	Aα: Extrafusal muscle fibres		Aα: Cutaneous, joint and muscle receptors; large interoceptors	Ia: Primary sensory fibres of muscle spindles Ib: Sensory fibres from Golgi tendon organs
		60	Aβ: Intrafusal muscle fibres		Aβ: Low-threshold mechanoreceptors Light pressure Rubbing Vibration	II: Secondary sensory fibres of muscle spindles
	2	30	Aγ: Intrafusal muscle fibres		Aδ: Fast pain high-threshold mechanoreceptors—strong pressure, pinch; thermoreceptors above 45°C	III: Nociceptors pressure-pain
		4		B: Preganglionic		
Non-myelinated	0.1	0.5		C: Postganglionic	C: Slow pain polymodal nociceptors; thermoreceptors; interoceptors	IV: Nociceptors

fibres are large-diameter, myelinated, fast-conducting fibres and thus more readily stimulated than the small-diameter pain fibres. If a low current density is applied to the skin the sensory nerves in the skin, which normally transmit touch, temperature and pressure, are the first to be stimulated. This causes a mild tapping sensation which may be due principally to rapidly repeated stimulation of touch receptors. Higher current densities will cause the current to affect more nerves leading to more intense tingling and eventually to spread to motor nerves causing muscle contraction. As still higher currents are applied more motor units will be affected resulting in both stronger and more widespread muscle contractions. Further increases of current will cause pain nerve fibres to be stimulated resulting in perceived pain. These three types of nerve fibres are affected in the same order with any form of stimulating pulse (see below). Clearly the positioning of the electrodes will determine the site of greatest current density and hence which nerves are affected; for example, in order to stimulate a normally innervated muscle effectively but painlessly the active electrode is applied to the motor point. This is a point on the skin surface at which maximum muscle contraction can be achieved because it is close to the point where the motor nerve trunk enters the muscle. Current applied at this point—often at the junction of the proximal third with the distal two-thirds of the muscle belly—will influence a large number of nerve fibres close together. Thus less current density will be needed than if the muscle belly were stimulated at some other place (Fig. 3.11). Notice that the phrase used above—'to stimulate a muscle'—is a convenience. The current is stimulating the motor nerves which convey nerve impulses to stimulate the muscle fibres.

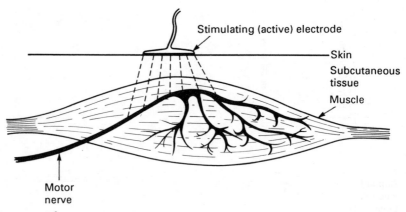

Fig. 3.11 The motor point.

Nerve stimulation by electrical pulses

Nerve fibres in a resting state have a potential difference of some 70 mV across the fibre membrane, the inside being negative and the outside positive. The nerve impulse is an electrochemical change that spreads along the fibre, as described in Chapter 1. The impulse can be set off by depolarizing the potential difference across the membrane with an electric pulse. The nerve impulse will travel in both directions but will only cause an effect in one direction (the orthodromic direction) because it is blocked by a synapse in the other direction; but see discussion on eutrophic electrotherapy below.

This occurs because the electrical pulse causes a movement of ions through the tissues and hence across the membrane. However it must be a sufficient disturbance—beyond the threshold value of about 10 mV—to fire the nerve impulse. Once the potential across the nerve membrane is altered beyond its threshold value the full nerve impulse occurs, thus it is an all-or-none response (Fig. 3.12). What the electrical pulse does is to trigger the nerve impulse but it needs a certain minimal amount of electrical charge to do so. This can be given by a small current for a relatively long duration or by a larger current for a short period (Fig. 3.13). There is, however, a certain minimum current needed to fire a nerve impulse at long durations; it is called the *rheobase*. This idea is demonstrated in the strength–duration curve shown in Figure 3.13—shorter pulse durations need larger currents to provoke a nerve impulse. It will be seen that as the curves are exponential an enormous current would be needed at very short pulse lengths so no practical muscle stimulation occurs. It must also be understood that pulses of greater current than is needed to trigger the nerve impulse have no further effect on that nerve fibre. No matter what the current intensity the same nerve impulse is triggered. As explained earlier,

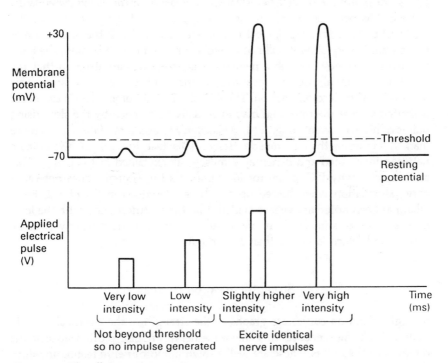

Fig. 3.12 The all-or-none response.

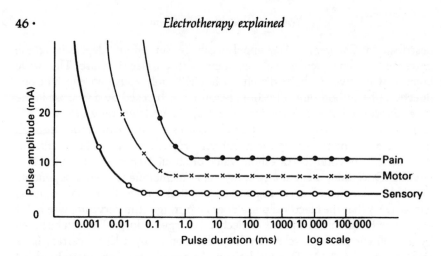

Fig. 3.13 Strength–duration curves.

increased sensory effects or stronger muscle contractions are due to a larger *number* of fibres being stimulated. Similarly if the electrical pulse has a longer duration no further effect occurs, as illustrated in the strength–duration curve in Figure 3.13, in which the same current triggers impulses at 1, 10 and 30 ms etc. It is the initial half-ms or so of the rheobase current which has sufficient charge to disturb the nerve fibre membrane beyond its threshold. Rather longer pulses of, say, 300 ms will provoke two nerve impulses, one when the current rises and the other when it falls. The reason for this is explained later.

What has been described so far is true provided the rate of rise of the electrical pulse is very rapid, i.e. it is a square wave pulse. If the rate of rise of the current is very slow it will not provoke a nerve impulse because the ionic balance across the nerve fibre membrane is able to adjust itself so that the threshold potential rises in response to the applied electric charge. This process is called accommodation. The rate at which accommodation can occur is limited so that the threshold may eventually be reached by the slow rising pulses of higher currents (Fig. 3.14). This ability to accommodate is much more marked in nerve than in muscle tissue. This fact is used to discriminate between innervated and denervated muscle, as explained in Chapter 4. This also explains why DC, given for iontophoresis for example, does not cause nerve stimulation when turned up slowly, as described in Chapter 2. From what has been noted above it is evident that the electrical pulse with the least charge that will stimulate a nerve impulse is one that rises rapidly—square wave—and which is of less than 1 ms duration.

Strength–duration curves

Strength–duration curves are graphs of the strength of the electrical pulse in volts or milliamps needed to generate a nerve impulse plotted against the duration of the pulses. These are well known in motor nerve testing in which the minimal muscle twitch is used, as described in Chapter 4. Similar curves

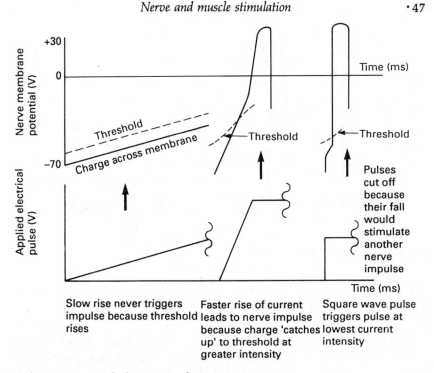

Fig. 3.14 Rate at which accommodation can occur.

have been produced for sensory nerves and pain responses (Fig. 3.13). It will be seen that greater currents are needed for pain fibres, less for motor nerves and less still for sensory nerves. The amplitude of current needed to stimulate a nerve fibre is inversely proportional to its diameter. Thus the small C fibres carrying pain impulses need the greatest current. It is not a difference in threshold but simply that the larger fibres have a lower electrical resistance (due to large cross-section and differing membrane characteristics), allowing a larger current for any given voltage (Ohm's law; see Appendix A). The difference in sensitivity between motor and sensory fibres is due to their different depths; sensory nerves in the skin receive a higher current density, as explained earlier.

It can also be seen from the strength–duration curves that this separation is greatest at short pulse widths. It is therefore easier selectively to excite motor or sensory nerves without eliciting pain by short-duration pulses, say around 0.05 ms.

The foregoing relates to single electrical pulses causing single nerve impulses. It will be recalled from Chapter 1 that once the nerve impulse has occurred, charging the membrane potential to $+30$ V, it returns to its resting value in about 1 ms. During this time, which is called the absolute refractory period, no stimulus, however large, will cause another nerve impulse. During the next 10–15 ms the nerve impulse can be triggered again but only by a larger stimulus than it normally needed. This is called the relative refractory period. After this the nerve is in its normal resting state (Fig. 3.15).

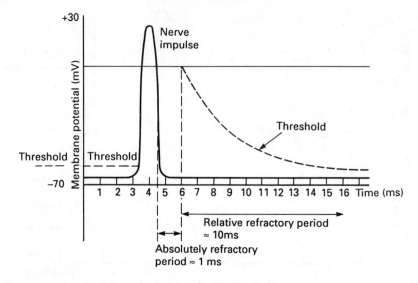

Fig. 3.15 The absolute and relative refractory periods.

These facts have important implications for the frequency of electrical pulses used to stimulate nerves. If a series of electrical pulses is applied to a motor nerve at one pulse per second (1 Hz), a corresponding series of muscle twitches will occur. Similarly, stimulation of a sensory nerve will lead to a series of separately recognized mild shocks. If the frequency is increased to, say, 10 Hz there is a corresponding tremor of the muscle, but if the frequency is increased to, say, 50 Hz the muscle contracts continuously—a tetanic contraction. Although the peak current remains the same the strength of the tetanic contraction increases with rising frequency up to about 100 Hz but not beyond. This is illustrated in Figure 3.16. Beyond 100 Hz the muscle

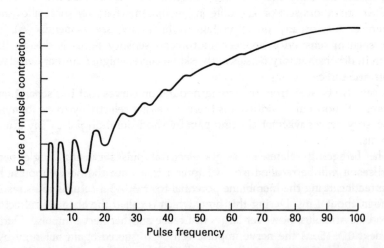

Fig. 3.16 Strength of tetanic contraction increasing with rising frequency up to 100 Hz.

contraction and sensory tingling do not increase with increased pulse frequency; in fact they may diminish unless the current intensity is increased. The reasons for this are obvious from what has been described already. Pulses of 1 ms at 100 Hz will have pulse intervals of 9 ms and at higher frequencies the interval would be shorter still; this means that each pulse is applied during the relative refractory period. In order to excite a nerve impulse during this time a greater current is needed. Thus higher peak currents are necessary to generate impulses at frequencies above 100 Hz. If shorter pulse durations are used, say 0.05 ms, to leave a slightly longer pulse interval, then the current must again be increased in order to provide sufficient charge to excite the nerve impulse (Fig. 3.13).

At higher frequencies above 500 Hz for 1 ms pulses, or about 1000 Hz (1 KHz) for 0.05 ms pulses, no increase in the number of nerve impulses can occur no matter how much current is applied, because succeeding electrical pulses would be given during the absolute refractory period.

Thus it can be seen that electrical pulses of 0.1–1 ms at 60–100 Hz would stimulate medium and large myelinated nerve fibres with the least possible current. It is notable that these parameters partly encompass both TENS (sensory) and faradic (motor) stimulation. However, the current density in the deeper tissues must also be considered.

Penetration of electrical pulses through the tissues

The impedance of the skin is very large for both direct current and the longer pulses—much greater than the rest of the tissues—but it is very much less for shorter pulses. Thus the skin may have an impedance of about 1000 Ω for a 10 ms pulse but only 50 Ω for a 0.1 ms pulse. This happens because the skin acts as a capacitor which offers much less impedance to short pulse lengths in the same way that it does for high-frequency currents.

The distribution of current through the tissues with shorter pulses is therefore more even, so that effectively the current penetrates further. Consequently the deeper nerves, e.g. motor nerves, are more easily stimulated with the shorter pulses. With longer pulses most of the current is 'used' in the skin, stimulating cutaneous nerves.

Electrical pulses for nerve stimulation

It can be seen that some of the currents used for stimulation and described earlier are more appropriate to excite a nerve impulse than others. Thus for stimulating motor and sensory nerves, i.e. large-diameter fast-conducting nerves, the pulses should be square wave and of short duration (0.5–0.1 ms). To achieve discrimination from pain nerves and greater depth even shorter pulses (0.05–0.02 ms) are appropriate. Evenly alternating pulses have the advantage of avoiding any risk of chemical damage. They are often referred to as depolarized pulses. Frequencies of around 80–100 Hz seem to be the best.

For other purposes, e.g. stimulating superficial pain nerves, longer pulses of around 10 ms would seem appropriate. Similarly if polar effects are needed to promote wound healing obviously direct current pulses are chosen. It must be understood that electrical stimulation has a multiplicity of effects which are not limited to stimulation of the alpha motor neurons and group 1A fibres only.

Secondary effects of nerve stimulation

Therapeutic electrical stimulation of both sensory and motor nerves has been widely used for many years. The principal purposes have been to cause contraction of healthy muscle by stimulating motor nerves and to control pain by stimulating sensory nerves. Various effects have also been claimed as a result of stimulating the autonomic nervous system.

PHYSIOLOGICAL EFFECTS AND THERAPEUTIC USES

Stimulation of innervated muscle

Electrical stimulation of normally innervated healthy muscle will have similar effects on the muscle and other body tissues and systems as an equivalent amount of active exercise. Where voluntary active exercise is restricted, electrical stimulation may be substituted. It is usually applied by surging (or ramping) a series of short pulses at frequencies around 50–100 Hz, i.e. a faradic-type current. If the surge of pulses is made to last for, say, 2 s and the interval between surges for 4 s then a slow physiological muscle contraction and joint motion will be mimicked. Obviously the surge length, rate of rise and fall and interval can be varied (Fig. 3.1e). In normal muscles at low force levels the main increase in muscle force is due to recruitment of motor units but as all units become involved further increases of muscle force are achieved by increased rates of nerve impulse firing (Milner-Brown and Stein, 1975). Clearly electrical stimulation at a fixed frequency can cause stronger muscle contractions only by recruiting more motor units with greater current densities. Electrical stimulation is used for a variety of therapeutic purposes which may be grouped as follows.

Muscle strengthening

The question of whether electrical stimulation of normal muscle can lead to an increase in muscle strength is not entirely resolved in spite of much research. The gist of this seems to be that electrical stimulation does increase muscle strength although not quite to the same extent as the equivalent voluntary exercise. In an extensive review Lloyd *et al.* (1986) concluded that in general electrical stimulation was not a satisfactory substitute for voluntary activity. However, a number of the studies showed that electrical stimulation (or electrical stimulation combined with voluntary activity) led to similar or in a few cases even greater strength gains than that due to voluntary exercise alone. Some studies showed marked differences in the response to electrical stimulation of different individuals but there is still much uncertainty, partly due to the variety of techniques and differing protocols adopted by the different studies.

In a recent well controlled study by Hon Sun Lai *et al.* (1988) it was shown that electrical stimulation of muscles over a 3-week period produced significant gains in muscle strength, being greater in the group treated with high-intensity electrical stimulation than in the group treated with lower intensities. The force of isometric contraction showed greater gains than that of concentric contraction. Eccentric contraction (isotonic lengthening) showed no significant gains. Although the gain in strength declined when treatment stopped it was still significant for the high-intensity group 3 weeks later. There was also a clear increase in isometric strength demonstrated in the opposite untreated limb, a cross-transfer effect which did not show a marked difference between the high- and low-intensity groups.

It is considered that the strength gain can be attributed to neural mechanisms, at least initially. This is suggested by several features: the speed with which the increase occurs—it can be demonstrated in about a week—and the speed with which it can decline, as well as the lack of evidence of any changes in muscle volume. Several neural mechanisms have been proposed. One is the increased activation of the spinal motor neuron pools, which regulate the force of muscle contraction due to stimulation of afferent neurons. This would account for the cross-transfer effect. Long-term potentiation has also been suggested. This involves increased sensitivity of synapses as a result of continuous stimulation of input fibres; the effect may last for some weeks. Synchronization of motor unit firing patterns is a further mechanism that has been proposed. The selective recruitment of large fast-twitch type II fibres over the slow-twitch, fatiguing type I fibres could also be implicated.

The force of voluntary muscle contraction is greater in most but not all subjects than the force that can be produced by electrical stimulation of the same musculature (De Domenico and Strauss, 1986; Strauss and De Domenico, 1986). This difference does not seem to be accounted for by the nature of the stimulating current since different stimulators did not produce significantly consistent differences in contraction force.

In weakened or weakening muscles the value of electrical stimulation is much clearer and significant gains have been reported with improvement of muscle function. Electrical stimulation at 30 Hz applied to the quadriceps of immobilized knees and given in 2 s on and 9 s off cycles for 1 h each day for 6 weeks has been shown to reduce muscle atrophy (Gibson *et al.*, 1988). In this study, cross-sectional area of the quadriceps was found to diminish by 17% in the untreated group, but there was no significant loss in those patients that were treated. The effect was considered to be due to the maintenance of protein synthesis in muscles rather than preventing protein breakdown. Similarly, improvement in muscle force over a 4-week period of electrical stimulation of chronically weakened quadriceps was found (Singer, 1986). In this study, however, no significant increase in muscle cross-sectional area was found but electromyograph changes suggested increased neuromuscular efficiency to account for the increased muscle force. Soo *et al.* (1988) have shown that stimulating the quadriceps at quite low intensities—50% of maximum voluntary contraction applied as eight contractions of 15 s duration twice a week for 5 weeks—led to a statistically significant increase in quadriceps torque. Thus surprisingly little electrical stimulation, a total of only 2 min stimulation in each of 10 sessions, has shown significant effect.

A faradic-type current has been used successfully in the treatment of chondromalacia patellae (Johnson *et al.*, 1977). Fifty patients given 19 treatments over a 6-week period showed considerable improvement; at least half became symptom-free. The quadriceps muscle was stimulated to produce 10 s isometric contractions with a 50 s rest period ten times every treatment. The current intensity was the maximum the patient could tolerate; in fact the authors concluded that the efficacy of treatment varies directly with the current intensity—highest currents give the best results. They also noted that the greater the initial atrophy the more effective the treatment and consequently felt that normal muscle would gain least from the technique.

The strengthening effect has been used to promote greater achievement in athletics but any advantage this might have over similar amounts of voluntary effort has not been unequivocally demonstrated. Its use for the prevention of disuse atrophy appears to be justified; for a full discussion see Currier (1987).

Facilitation of muscle control

Stimulation is extensively used therapeutically to initiate and facilitate voluntary contraction of muscle, although it is not possible to distinguish this effect from the strengthening effect already considered. This idea may be applied in several circumstances:

1 Where voluntary muscle contraction is inhibited by pain or injury. Stimulating the quadriceps, especially the vastus medialis, after knee surgery or knee injury, for example, is often utilized (Eriksson and Haggmark, 1979). Another example is stimulation of the calf and Achilles tendon in chronic and postsurgical cases of Achilles tendon injuries (Grisogono, 1989).
2 In situations where muscle action is not readily under voluntary control without practice. Education of the pelvic floor muscle in the control of incontinence, for instance, or the abductor hallucis for the management of early hallux valgus (see below for further discussion of both of these). Similarly, in circumstances such as postural flatfoot or metatarsalgia, where voluntary lumbrical control is desirable.
3 In circumstances in which a new muscle action has to be learned, for example, where a muscle or a motor nerve has been transplanted.
4 In the later stages of a recovering peripheral nerve lesion to encourage voluntary muscle contraction where reinnervation has only recently occurred.

5 In situations in which it is necessary to demonstrate to the patient that a particular muscle action or movement can occur normally, where hysterical paralysis is present, for example.

Maintenance or increase of range of joint motion

The motion may be limited by different tissues and from different causes. Electrical stimulation of muscle to stretch the shortened tissues has been used in:

1 Contractures of fibrous tissue and scarring. Limitation of joint motion due to shortening of soft tissues on one side of the joint has been treated by cyclical electrical stimulation of the muscles that stretch the contracture. This has been successful in increasing the range of movement in hemiplegic patients (Baker *et al.*, 1979).
2 Loss of motion due to spasticity of muscles in hemiplegia or other neurological conditions. To maintain the normal range of motion in such patients regular passive movements are recommended, often carried out at home by the patient's own family. Electrical stimulation has been applied as an alternative to manual passive movement to help prevent the loss of motion due to spasticity of the opposing muscles. This has been used successfully on the wrist and in finger movements of hemiplegic patients (Baker *et al.*, 1979).
3 Scoliosis. In the treatment of scoliosis the lateral trunk muscles on the convexity of the curve are stimulated electrically. Surface electrodes (carbon rubber) are attached to the patient's back and muscle contraction is provoked in short cycles at a level that allows the patient to sleep during the treatment (Eckerson and Axelgaard, 1984). In moderate scoliosis (20–45°) it has been shown that a progression of the curve can be halted in over 80% of patients (Axelgaard and Brown, 1983).

Effects on muscle metabolism and blood flow

Electrical stimulation will have the same effect as normal voluntary muscle contraction in causing a temporary increase in muscle metabolism. There will be the associated consequences of increased oxygen uptake and carbon dioxide, lactic acid and other metabolite production, as well as raised local temperature and greater local blood flow. Many studies have demonstrated an increased blood flow, for example Currier *et al.* (1986). Using 10 and 30% of maximum voluntary contraction these authors quantified a 20% blood flow increase which occurred about 1 min after electrical stimulation had started and continued for some 5 min after it had finished.

Not only is the intramuscular blood flow increased but as a consequence of regular muscle contraction and relaxation the flow in adjacent soft-walled veins will be increased—the muscle pumping action. This effect is used therapeutically to help control limb oedema by raising the rate of flow in venous and lymphatic vessels. It has been found that stimulating parts of the quadriceps with 0.4 ms pulses at 50 Hz in 4 s on/4 s off cycles leads to an 18.5% increase in blood flow in the femoral artery (Tracy *et al.*, 1988). This study used sufficient current to stimulate the muscle to 15% of its maximum voluntary contraction and measured the blood flow in the femoral artery with an ultrasonic Doppler device. The increased blood flow was noted within 5 min of the start of electrical stimulation and fell to normal levels within 1 min of cessation of stimulation.

Changes in structure—eutrophic electrotherapy

The structure of muscles, like all other tissue, does not remain fixed. There is, for example, a constant exchange of muscle proteins being synthesized while existing ones are catabolized. The rate of protein turnover varies but can be 5–10% of skeletal muscle protein per day. Turnover in the 'red' slow twitch muscle is higher than in 'white' fast twitch muscle. Further, the molecular form of the muscle can change as an adaptation to function. An example is the hypertrophy that occurs in response to increased muscle work which is due to increased quantities of muscle and collagen tissue.

It has been shown in animal experiments that fast twitch muscle can be converted to the slow twitch type by electrically stimulating the muscle at a slow twitch frequency (Salmons and Vbrova, 1969). This has also been applied successfully to human muscle (Scott *et al.*, 1985). It is believed that the plastic adaptation of skeletal muscle is under both hormonal and neuronal control— the latter being evinced by means of the action potentials in the motor nerve. The frequencies of motor unit action potentials have been recorded electro-myographically and used to select the frequency of electrical stimulation of muscle (Kidd and Oldham 1988a and b). This form of stimulation has been referred to as eutrophic electrotherapy. Kidd *et al.* (1989) compared uniform and eutrophic electrotherapy in the clinical rehabilitation of hand movements in arthritics and found that after six weeks both force and endurance had improved with eutrophic but that force had deteriorated with uniform electrotherapy. Eutrophic electrotherapy has also been effectively applied therapeutically to cases of non-recovering Bell's palsy (Farragher *et al.* 1987). The mean frequency of motor unit firing, in particular facial muscles, was used to dictate the frequency of 5–8 pps at a rectangular pulse width of 0.08 ms. This was applied for 2 s on and 2 s off for up to 8 h each day over several weeks and led to a very considerable improvement objectively assessed. Incontinence has also been treated using eutrophic electrotherapy.

It is theorized that by applying the precise motor unit action potential as a stimulus train there is an antidromic flow via the axoplasm to the motor unit. This stress leads to plastic adaptation of the phenotype by the expression of different genes.

Other therapeutic uses of electrical stimulation of muscle

1 Electrical stimulation to replace splinting. The concept of stimulating

inactive muscles at appropriate times to enable them to contribute to their normal functional activities is not new. Technical advances have recently made this a more realistic possibility. Electrical stimulation of the dorsiflexors in hemiplegic patients triggered by a switch in the shoe has been used. Similarly stimulation of the deltoid has been used to prevent glenohumeral subluxation in hemiplegic patients (Baker, 1987). Rather more complex systems are being devised to enable paraplegic patients to gain control of standing and walking.

2 Electrical stimulation for the control of spasticity. The effects of electrical muscle stimulation on spasticity are not clearly established and reported results are variable. This is partly due to the difficulty of measuring and defining spasticity. In general there have been two approaches: firstly, stimulation of antagonists to utilize the effect of reciprocal inhibition and secondly, stimulation of the spastic muscles themselves. Although some success has been claimed it has often been inconsistent. Those studies which have been done did not support the opinion, sometimes expressed that spasticity may be increased by such treatment (Baker, 1987). Lagassé and Roy (1989) studied the effects of a functional electrical stimulation training programme on the co-contraction level of spastic hemiparetic patients during a maximal speed forearm extension movement. The pattern of electrical stimulation was adjusted individually from electromyograph parameters of the non-affected limb. This treatment reduced the antagonist co-contraction level associated with spasticity. Stokes and Cooper (1989) sound a cautionary note against the indiscriminate use of functional electrical stimulation until more work has been done on the beneficial and adverse long- and short-term effects of electrical stimulation on muscle, including fatigue mechanisms.

Stimulation of denervated muscle

Denervated muscle is different in many respects from innervated muscle, including its response to electrical stimuli. Without a functional nerve supply muscle can only be caused to contract by direct stimulation of the muscle fibre. There are therefore differences between stimulating muscle via its nerve and direct denervated muscle stimulation.

1 Muscle tissue is less excitable than nerve so that a greater electric charge is needed. This is evident from the strength–duration curve for denervated muscle (Fig. 4.4). Thus a square wave pulse of suitable current intensity will stimulate denervated muscle to contract provided the pulse is of sufficient duration, i.e. more than 30 ms. Greater currents will be needed for shorter pulses to provoke a muscle contraction.

2 When a bundle of motor nerves is stimulated at the motor point it causes the simultaneous stimulation of many motor units, each of which activates many muscle fibres thus causing the synchronous contraction of a large part of the muscle. This is evident as a brisk twitch, or a series of twitches, or a

tetanic contraction if the frequency is high enough. If there is no nerve the individual muscle fibres are stimulated when the current density across them reaches sufficient intensity so that the contraction spreads slowly through the muscle. Furthermore, the rate of contraction and relaxation of denervated muscle fibres is slower than that of normal muscle. Both these effects contribute to the different quality of contraction which is sometimes called a 'worm-like' contraction.

3 It has already been noted that nerve is able to accommodate to ionic changes across its membrane provided those changes are not too rapid. Muscle tissues have less ability to accommodate than nerve so that quite slow changes can stimulate the muscle fibre, as described below. This property provides a means of selectively stimulating muscle, as opposed to nerve tissue, by means of slow-rising triangular pulses.

The term 'rheobase' is defined as the minimum current needed to stimulate a nerve or muscle using a pulse of infinite duration. The rate of rise of an electrical pulse can be described in terms of the time that it takes to reach the rheobase current for a square wave pulse. (Square wave pulses rise very rapidly and hence reach the rheobase almost instantly.) If a square wave pulse is applied to a nerve fibre an impulse is evoked at a certain current intensity, the rheobase. If a triangular pulse is applied, taking 10 ms to reach the same current intensity, a very slight increase in current is needed to cause the nerve impulse because the nerve impulse threshold has had little time to change. A pulse taking 20 ms to reach the rheobase would need a greater intensity to evoke the impulse and one taking 30 ms would need a current nearly twice the rheobase before it 'caught up' with the threshold to trigger an impulse. Clearly, if the rate of rise is made just a little longer (33 ms to rheobase) the current can rise to a very high intensity without catching the rising threshold and hence without stimulating the nerve (Stephens, 1965). This rate of rise has been called the 'liminal current gradient'. Slower rates of rise will be unable to stimulate nerve. The idea is shown in Figure 3.17 (see also Fig. 3.14).

The liminal current gradient typical of a nerve is thus described as taking about 33 ms to rheobase (or rising at 30 rheobases per second). The gradient for normal innervated muscle tissue is less steep, about 100 ms to rheobase, and that for denervated muscle is very much less steep, being about 330 ms to rheobase (Fig. 3.18).

Thus triangular pulses with rise times of about 50 ms will selectively stimulate both innervated and denervated muscle and those with rise times longer than 100 ms—300 or 500 ms are often used—will selectively stimulate denervated muscle only.

From the above it is evident that denervated muscle can be made to contract with square wave pulses of sufficient duration (30 ms or more) or triangular wave pulses of long duration (rise times of 100–500 ms). In both cases the current needs to be applied through the muscle tissue itself, because there is no motor point. The current is usually most successfully applied in the long axis of the muscle fibres, that is with the stimulating electrodes at each end of the muscle belly.

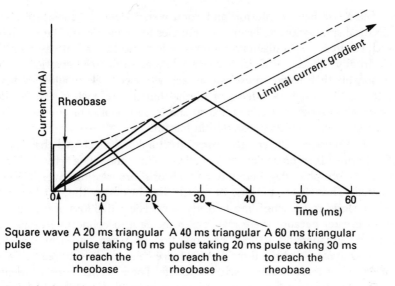

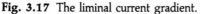

Fig. 3.17 The liminal current gradient.

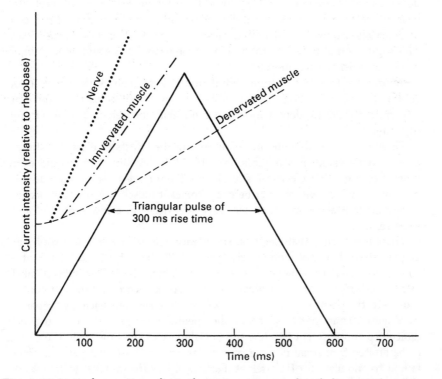

Fig. 3.18 Liminal current gradients for nerve, innervated and denervated muscle showing how a pulse of 300 ms rise time will stimulate denervated muscle only.

There has been confusion and controversy over the therapeutic use of electrical stimulation of denervated muscles for many years. The rationale for such treatment is to maintain the muscle in as healthy a state as possible by electrically induced artificial exercise while awaiting reinnervation. It seems reasonable that making muscles contract with electrical stimuli would substitute for the beneficial effects of normal muscle contraction. The evidence, however, is somewhat contradictory and in particular clinical benefit has not been unequivocally demonstrated in humans.

When muscle is denervated many structural and functional changes occur. Firstly there is an immediate loss of all voluntary and reflex activity. Secondly there is atrophy, degeneration and fibrosis progressing over weeks and months. There is a rapid loss of muscle weight during the first few months which slows to become almost steady later. The actual loss of muscle fibre is even greater because there may be an increase in connective tissue during atrophy (Sunderland, 1978). The question of when and why denervated muscles fibrose is of the utmost importance because ultimate reinnervation is of no use if there is no muscle tissue left. There seems to be no definitive answer but in humans degeneration of muscle does not seem to be complete for some 3 years after the nerve lesion. It has been suggested that prolonged intramuscular stasis and perhaps thrombosis due to vasoconstriction paralysis and loss of muscle pumping action lead to deficient muscle nutrition and hence degeneration (Sunderland, 1978). In addition, trauma—excessive stretching, heat and cold—has been implicated in accelerating the degenerative processes of denervated muscle. (Innervated muscle seems better able to repair itself.) This suggests that measures to diminish oedema and stasis and prevent injury will benefit denervated muscles.

In addition to these changes fibrillation occurs. This is the spontaneous contraction of individual muscle fibres in an irregular pattern. It occurs intermittently during denervation and can usually be detected by electromyography.

There is considerable literature concerning the effects of electrical stimulation on denervated muscle (Spielholz, 1987). In humans there would be no point treating with electrical stimulation the muscles paralysed due to a neurapraxia which will recover before significant muscle atrophy can occur or in any circumstances in which recovery will occur in a few months for the same reason.

There is evidence that electrical stimulation will retard muscle atrophy and degeneration but not completely prevent it. The type and amount of stimulation used to achieve this is very variable. The best results (Hnik P., 1962) seem to have been achieved with vigorous isometric muscle contractions—to the point of fatigue—for two or three sessions each day separated by at least 10 min intervals. From a therapeutic point of view such a regime is difficult to apply except to a few superficial muscles at a time. This, then, tends to be limited to a small number of muscles and to those that patients can be taught to stimulate for themselves. Further, if this treatment is to be useful it will require considerable compliance and tolerance on the part of the patient to continue treatment over a long period of, perhaps, 1 or 2 years. Some clinical studies have been unable to demonstrate any benefits due to the application of electrical stimulation over long periods provided other appropriate care is given to the paralysed muscles. In summary, the value of electrical stimulation for denervated muscle is not proven and its application to gain what may be only a small benefit is often not justified.

The contradictory experimental findings may be due to variations in the type of electrical stimulation—the parameters of frequency, rise time, intensity and so forth—or the varying amounts of stimulation given or, perhaps, it is the trophic effects that are important. In view of this and the availability of conveniently small muscle stimulators that can be used by the patient, the benefit of denervated muscle stimulation may well be demonstrated in the future; see also eutrophic electrotherapy.

Stimulation of afferent nerves

Electrical stimulation is extensively used for the control of pain. Although the idea had been proposed for many years the rationale was provided by the gate control theory of pain proposed in the mid 1960s by Melzack and Wall (1965). To account for the effects of electrical stimulation it is necessary to consider pain mechanisms first.

Pain

All sensations recognized at a conscious level can be altered or modulated by the central nervous system. This is true of pain. Two distinct kinds of pain may be described. *Fast* pain is usually equated with acute pain. Receptors, present in the skin all over the body surface, respond to the noxious stimulus and the impulse is carried by small myelinated A delta fibres (Table 3.1). Fast pain seems to be functionally concerned with helping the body avoid tissue damage since it provokes an immediate flexor withdrawal reflex and evokes rapid well localized conscious awareness. *Slow* pain, or second pain, on the other hand is equated with chronic pain and results from tissue damage. It is carried by unmyelinated C fibres (Table 3.1), whose free nerve endings are found in all innervated body tissue except the central nervous system. Functionally it appears to enforce inactivity of damaged tissue in order to allow healing to occur. It is thus associated with muscle spasm. Both these types of pain are due to stimulation of peripheral receptors and seem to have clear physiological functions. Neurogenic pain is entirely different in quality— often a burning sensation—and may be associated with autonomic disturbance. It is due to some form of neuronal damage; causalgia and postherpetic neuralgia are examples.

What has been said is somewhat simplified. The nature of chronic pain is not completely understood; some low-level prolonged pain seems to occur unrelated to tissue damage and evident damage occurs with little or no pain. Pain is also influenced by hormones and, markedly, by psychological factors. So much so that types of pain are often classified as neurogenic, somatogenic (acute or chronic) or psychogenic.

Pain receptors

The A delta receptors respond to strong mechanical stimulation and some to damaging heat, i.e. above 45°C. When these fibres are stimulated experimentally they cause a pricking or stinging sensation. The C fibre receptors appear to be sensitive to many kinds of stimuli—mechanical, chemical and heat (hence they are called polymodal receptors)—but probably they are sensitive to a chemical released from tissue damaged by any stimulus.

Pain pathways

The cell bodies of these neurons are found in the dorsal root ganglia and their central connections enter the spinal cord via the dorsal root, except for some 30% of the C fibres which return to the peripheral nerve and enter the cord via the ventral root (Fig. 3.19). C fibres synapse in lamina II (substantia gelatinosa) with interneurons and neurons which ascend in the anterolateral funiculus on the opposite side of the cord via, and with connections to, the reticular formation and thence to the intralaminar nuclei of the thalamus. Here they synapse with further neurons passing to all parts of the cerebral cortex but especially to the prefrontal region. The A delta fibres synapse in the outer part of the posterior horn, lamina I and some in lamina V. The next neuron crosses to the opposite side to ascend in the spinothalamic tract to the ventrobasal thalamus. A further neuron passes to the postcentral gyrus, the sensory area of the cerebral cortex (Bowsher, 1988; Fig. 3.19).

Control of pain

The gate control theory of pain was suggested in 1965 by Melzack and Wall and has been expanded and modified since. The essence of it is that pain perception is regulated by a 'gate' which may be opened or closed, thus increasing or decreasing the pain perceived by means of other inputs from peripheral nerves or from the central nervous system. Specifically it is believed that the low-threshold mechanoreceptors in the skin (and elsewhere)—the A beta fibres—which pass without synapsing up the posterior columns of the spinal cord give off collateral branches in the posterior horn. These collaterals impinge on nociceptor cells of the A delta and C pain fibres in laminae I and II of the posterior horn. The input of the mechanoreceptors effectively reduces the excitability of these cells to pain-generated stimuli; it is referred to as presynaptic inhibition.

Thus electrical pulses which stimulate these A beta mechanoreceptor fibres are effective in reducing pain perception. As noted already, these relatively large-diameter nerves are capable of being stimulated at low current intensities (Fig. 3.13) and will convey impulses at quite high frequencies. Therefore low-intensity (i.e. just perceptible), high-frequency (100–200 Hz) TENS is appropriate and effective.

Morphine acts on the C fibre system and hence controls tissue-damage pain but not other types of pain. This occurs because morphine imitates naturally

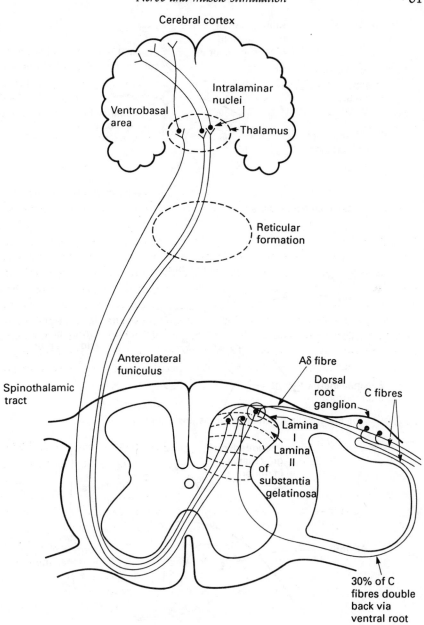

Fig. 3.19 Diagrammatic representation of pain pathways.

occurring neurotransmitters, encephalin and endorphin. In the substantia gelatinosa (lamina II) there are interneurons which can produce encephalin to inhibit the C system cells in this region. Collateral branches of A delta fibres in the posterior horn connect with these interneurons and stimulate them. Thus stimulation of the A delta fibre by electrical pulses—high intensity and low frequencies (about 2–10 Hz) are needed—will damp down C fibre system-

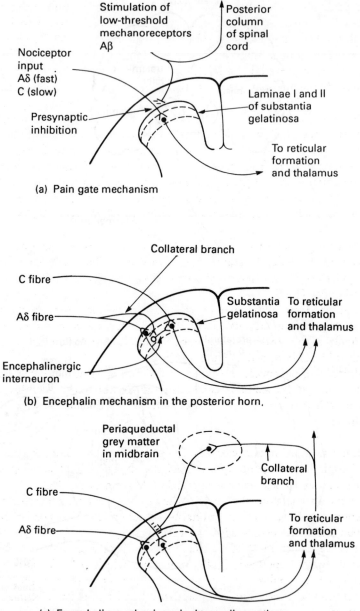

(a) Pain gate mechanism

(b) Encephalin mechanism in the posterior horn.

(c) Encephalin mechanism via descending pathway

Fig. 3.20 Control of pain.

type pain. This accounts for the effect of acupuncture since these A delta nerves are stimulated by pinprick. (Acupuncture points seem to be where bundles of these nerves pierce the deep fascia (Bowsher, 1988). The stimulation must be done in the same neural segment.)

It is also recognized that activation of these A delta pain fibres may provoke impulses in the midbrain that then travel back down the spinal cord to inhibit nociceptor neurons at the original level: a descending pain suppression system (De Domenico, 1982; Bowsher, 1988). This system also generates encephalin in the substantia gelatinosa. The A delta nociceptors in the spinothalamic tract give off collateral branches to the periaqueductal grey matter in the midbrain. Descending neurons from this region use serotonin (5-hydroxytryptamine) as the neurotransmitter. Other descending pain-inhibiting pathways are also known that involve noradrenaline as the neurotransmitter (Bowsher, 1988).

The mechanisms so far described are summarized in Figure 3.20 and below:

1 The pain gate effect on both A delta (fast) and C (slow) pain fibres in the posterior horn due to stimulation of mechanoreceptors (A beta) fibres by high-frequency, low-intensity electric pulses, sometimes called hi-TENS or traditional TENS.
2 Morphine-type (encephalin) effect on C fibre system by encephalin producing interneurons stimulated by the A delta pain receptor fibres being stimulated by low-frequency, high-intensity electrical pulses, sometimes called lo-TENS or acupuncture TENS.
3 Morphine-type (encephalin) effect on C fibre system as in point 2 above but via centres in the midbrain and involving serotonin as a neurotransmitter; also activated by A delta stimulation by low-frequency, high-intensity stimuli.

Stimulation at frequencies above 50 Hz may be able to produce a physiological block in both types of peripheral pain fibres. This effect is rather unclear and its clinical value is uncertain (De Domenico, 1982).

Electrical stimulation also reaches the cerebral cortex in the sense that the patient is aware of a prickling or tingling sensation. This may contribute to the placebo effect that occurs with all treatments.

As noted earlier, most of the treatments for pain relief are given by means of small battery-operated TENS stimulators which provide fairly short—around 0.2 ms—pulses of low intensity and variable frequency—up to 200 Hz. Similar effects are, of course, produced by similar electrical pulses. Many different sources of electrical stimulation, e.g. diadynamic, interferential and faradic-type currents, can lead to pain relief, which may be due to one or more of these mechanisms.

The effectiveness of TENS for pain relief is well supported in quite a large number of clinical studies and trials (for a review see Thorsteinsson, 1983). In general when treating acute pain and some neurogenic pain the results appear to be better than those achieved in the treatment of chronic pain. Successful treatment of neurogenic pain has been reported (Meyer and Fields, 1972).

Perhaps not surprisingly, postoperative and obstetric pain have been quite successfully treated (Santiesteban, 1981). In a double-blind trial the efficacy of TENS has been found to be much greater than would be accounted for by the placebo effect. Pain was relieved in 48% of instances due to TENS and in 32% of instances due to placebo treatment (Thorsteinsson *et al.*, 1977).

There is a definite difference in the mode of action of high-frequency, low-intensity TENS compared to that of the low-frequency, high-intensity type which acts by the release of morphine-like neurotransmitters, shown by the fact that it can be blocked by a morphine inhibitor (Sjölund and Eriksson, 1979). This difference does not seem to be reflected in any differences in clinical use; both types were reported to be successful in similar conditions. It has been suggested (Thorsteinsson, 1983) that high-intensity, low-frequency TENS gives somewhat better results but is less well tolerated.

The duration of pain relief due to TENS is very variable. One study (Thorsteinsson *et al.*, 1977) found a mean of 4–7 hours, but it is not clear why pain should be relieved for such long periods due to any of the described mechanisms.

The effects of other types of current on pain have not been nearly so extensively researched. Although it is widely agreed that interferential currents have a pain-relieving effect, there seems to be a dearth of objective studies. It has been shown that a rise in the pain threshold may occur after interferential treatment (Pärtan *et al.*, 1953), but a more recent study could find no significant difference between interferential and placebo treatments. Quirk *et al.* (1985) found that the symptoms of osteoarthritis of the knee were significantly relieved by treatment using interferential therapy and exercises, shortwave diathermy and exercises, or exercises alone. Overall analysis revealed no significant difference between the three regimes except that the only patients to deteriorate during treatment were those in the exercise-only group. For a full discussion of the way interferential currents may relieve pain see De Domenico (1982).

There is, of course, good reason to suppose that many types of electrical currents which are not customarily regarded as TENS, such as interrupted direct currents, faradic-type currents, sinusoidal currents and diadynamic currents, could all relieve pain by the mechanisms described above. Indeed other modalities such as mechanical vibration and heat will also act in the same way.

Other effects

Vasodilation

Cutaneous vasodilation occurs in the area of application of some electrical stimulation, often observed with faradic-type currents and sinusoidal or diadynamic currents of sufficient intensity. This is considered to be due to stimulation of sensory nerves causing arteriolar vasodilation by means of the axon reflex at first and subsequently due to the release of histamine-like substances causing capillary dilation (Wadsworth and Chanmugan, 1980). The effect can be quantified by recording the change in skin temperature. With monophasic (unidirectional) currents the pH and other chemical changes seem to cause the vasodilation, as described in Chapter 2.

Effects on the autonomic nervous system

It is to be expected that some autonomic nerves would be stimulated by electrical pulses of suitable intensities since somatic nerves of similar size are stimulated. Such effects are frequently postulated as an explanation for therapeutic benefit, particularly in connection with interferential currents. The evidence for these effects, such as it is, seems to be inconsistent.

Altering the ionic distribution around the cell

Altering the ionic balance around the cell—as electrical stimulation inevitably does—would be expected to lead to some effects, but clear evidence and clinical correlation are lacking at present. It has been indicated in Chapter 2 that monophasic currents can accelerate the healing of cutaneous wounds and bone. Remodelling of bone and fibrous tissue have also been proposed. Many other effects have been considered to occur, such as increases in cell metabolism and exchange across the cell membrane, both being associated with increased microcirculation (Alon, 1987); see also Chapter 1.

Summary

The effects of electrical stimulation have sometimes been described in a confusing and illogical manner with no distinction being made between the direct and indirect effects. A more rational approach has been proposed (Alon, 1987) in which the physiological responses to electrical stimulation are organized into cellular, tissue, segmental and systemic levels. Thus nerve excitation occurs at a cellular level and the muscle contraction it induces is an effect at the tissue level. Muscle group contraction and its effect on venous and lymphatic flow occur at a segmental level whilst the analgesic effects due to the release of endorphins and encephalins is an effect at the systemic level.

A rather simplified summary of some of the major effects is given in Table 3.2, but it must be understood that neither the magnitude nor the therapeutic importance is taken into account in this table.

PRINCIPLES OF APPLICATION

Electrical energy for therapy must be applied to the body tissues with at least two electrodes to form a complete circuit. The transition of an electric current of conduction in the wires (electron movement) to a convection current in the tissues (ionic movement) is complex and very important in determining the resulting effects.

Table 3.2 Outline of effects of pulsed electric currents on excitable cells

Effects on excitable cells

Nerve

Peripheral nerves

- Sensory nerves →
  - Prickling sensation
  - Vasodilation—due to axon reflex
  - Pain relief—due to pain gate mechanism

- Motor nerves →
  - Skeletal muscle contraction →
    - Re-education of movement
    - Increase in strength and endurance
    - Increase in intramuscular blood flow
    - Pumping action on veins, lymphatics leading to increased blood flow in tissues
    - Trophic changes (eutrophic effects)
  - Visceral muscle →
    - Altered vessel diameter resulting in possible altered blood flow

- Myelinated Aδ pain fibres →
  - Pain sensation
  - Pain relief via encephalins, endorphins and other central nervous system mechanisms

- Non-myelinated C pain fibres →
  - Pain perception

Muscle

- Innervated muscle → Muscle contraction
- Denervated muscle → Muscle contraction

Electrode–tissue interface

The changes that occur between the conducting metal and conducting fluid on and within the tissues consist of complex dynamic electrochemical interactions. The simple consequences of these have been described in Chapter 2 and Appendix B. If the applied current is evenly alternating (biphasic) there are no significant chemical changes; also if the total current, although unidirectional, is very small (low intensity and/or very short pulses) the chemical effects will be negligible.

A layer of ion-containing fluid is needed to pass current from the metal electrode to the tissues, normally skin. This is usually water or conducting gel. This serves to ensure a uniform conducting pathway between the metal electrode and the epidermis and secondly to make the electrochemical changes occur outside the epidermis. Since the epidermal surface is very irregular a flat metal electrode pressed on to it would be in contact at only a few points, leading to a high current density at these points. Further, the epidermal surface has a high electrical resistance because it is largely dry keratin, and because of the presence of oily sebum. This resistance is lowered by wetting the skin surface.

Types of electrode

There are three basic electrode systems:

1 A malleable metal electrode such as tinplate or aluminium coupled to the skin with water retained in a pad of lint, cotton gauze or some form of sponge material, e.g. Spontex (Fig. 3.21). The water provides the uniform ion-containing low-resistance pathway for the current while the absorbant material simply serves to keep the water in place. Ordinary tapwater is suitable in most instances but in some soft-water areas a little salt or bicarbonate of soda may need to be added. The whole assembly is fixed in place by a strap, bandage or by suction. The thickness of the pad needed, and hence the quantity of water, depends on the irregularity of the skin surface and on whether significant chemical changes will occur. If the latter is the case then about 1.25 cm (16 thicknesses of lint) is considered an

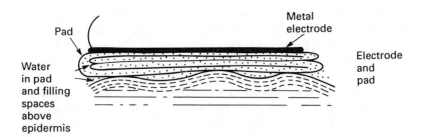

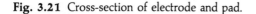

Fig. 3.21 Cross-section of electrode and pad.

appropriate thickness. Otherwise rather thinner (0.5–1 cm) wet thickness seems to be sufficient for most treatments.

In a system in which current passes through the body the total current at each of the two electrodes must be equal but the important factor is the current density, i.e. current per unit area. Thus if two pads are of unequal size, most effect will occur close to the smaller one, which is called the active electrode. The other electrode is called the indifferent or dispersive electrode. In order to limit the effects to an area such as the motor point of a muscle, the active electrode can be a small metal disc covered with lint or other suitable material and attached to a handle. This is often called a button electrode.

2 The second system involves electrodes that will conform to the body surface more easily than the metal electrodes described above. These are made of carbon-impregnated silicone rubber. They may be used with sponge pads or coupled to the skin by a thin layer of conducting gel and fixed in place either with a strap or adhesive tape. The latter electrodes are usually small and are used for low-intensity TENS to give pain relief. A somewhat similar system for more lengthy application of TENS involves karaya gum (obtained from a particular kind of tree in India) which when wetted is both conductive and adhesive. Some synthetically produced polymers act in the same way (Paterson, 1983). In general, the carbonized rubber and similar electrodes are convenient for long-term use and repeated self-application by the patient, whereas the water pad conduction methods are appropriate for treating larger areas with higher currents and are usually used in the physiotherapy department. They are somewhat more efficient in passing current to the tissues than carbonized rubber and other similar types in that they have a lower impedance (Nelson *et al.*, 1980). Further, it has been noted that carbonized rubber electrodes have significant resistance compared to the electrode–tissue junction so that most current will take the shortest pathway and thus the current density is likely to be higher near where the metal wire enters the electrode (Paterson, 1983).

3 The third system is by means of a water bath (or baths) in which the body part is immersed with an electrode. Current is passed from electrode to tissues through the water. This system is considered later.

Current flow in the tissues

The quantity of current that flows in the tissues and the path it follows will depend on the impedance of that pathway. The impedance includes the ohmic resistance, capacitive resistance (or reactance) and the inductive resistance. The latter is negligible in the tissues but the two former have an important influence on the effects of the electrical stimulation. Generally, watery tissue such as blood, muscle and nerve have low ohmic resistance; bone and fat are rather higher and epidermis is the highest of all. Where two low-resistance regions are separated by a high-resistance region, i.e. a near insulator, a capacitor is formed and capacitive effects occur. Thus where an electrode is separated from nerve and muscle by skin and fat there is a capacitor. The concept of these electrical pathways is illustrated in Figure 3.22.

For direct current (unidirectional current) and slowly changing pulses of current the skin resistance is high and thus most of the electrical energy is released in the skin and subcutaneous tissues, hence cutaneous nerves are affected. As the current spreads through the low-resistance pathway of the deeper tissues it can have less effect. However, capacitive resistance diminishes for short pulses of current or alternating (biphasic) currents of higher frequencies, thus the current can pass through the skin more easily and more energy is released in the deeper tissues. It is also the reason why particular currents—interferential, for example—can penetrate the tissues more deeply. Thus the shorter the pulse length, the lower the capacitive resistance of the skin and subcutaneous tissues and therefore the more easily it will penetrate the tissues. This is the same for pulses separated by long intervals as for continuously alternating pulses of the same pulse (phase) length. Thus single pulses of 0.125 ms will penetrate tissue in the same way as 4000 Hz medium-frequency current, because if the current alternates at 4000 cycles per second each full cycle lasts 0.25 ms, therefore each phase lasts 0.125 ms. Two medium-frequency currents, i.e. interferential currents, can be used to produce electrical stimulation in the deeper tissues.

Taken together the effects described above suggest that some deeply placed low-threshold nerves, such as motor nerves, would be more efficiently stimulated by shorter pulses, say about 1/20th of a millisecond (0.05 ms) because of the skin capacitance. On the other hand to stimulate high-threshold unmyelinated pain fibres (C fibres) in the skin it would seem sensible to use longer pulses of a few milliseconds.

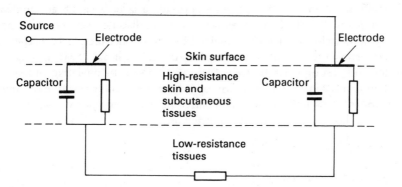

Fig. 3.22 Electrical pathways of current applied to the tissues.

Arrangements of electrodes

It has been noted already that what matters for producing an effect in the tissues is the current density. Adding to the size of the electrodes will decrease the current density. This occurs whether the greater size is due to a single larger electrode or to one or more additional parallel connected electrodes. Since the water in the pad has a very low ohmic resistance the effective area of application is that of the pad.

With carbon-rubber electrodes there may be a slightly higher current through the region where the wire enters the electrode but since these electrodes are usually small the effect is not great.

The position of the electrodes will obviously determine the path that the current will follow in the tissues. In many situations a small electrode is used to give a high localized current density, such as to stimulate the motor point of a muscle or an acupuncture point. In these circumstances the dispersive (or indifferent) electrode can be placed on any convenient area of skin that is reasonably close. The further away it is placed the more current will be needed and less effective localization will occur. If the two electrodes are of similar size the current density under each will be similar and therefore effects such as sensory stimulation will occur under both. If the electrodes are placed close together the effects will be localized to the region between them, e.g. placing electrodes at either end of the long axis of the belly of a muscle will cause local stimulation of that muscle, or stimulating sensory nerves in a local area of skin will give pain relief. If the electrodes are placed too close together current will be localized to the adjacent edges and to the intervening small area of skin rather than passing through the whole area of electrode and epidermis in contact.

Water baths

The hand, forearm, foot and leg can conveniently be put into baths or bowls of water with electrodes to provide a means of passing current to the tissues. Such an arrangement can be used to provide a large area for an indifferent electrode, as described in Chapter 2. They can also be used as a method of applying muscle-stimulating currents. If two electrodes are placed in the same water bath with the part to be treated, current will pass both through the water and through the tissues—two pathways in parallel (Fig. 3.23). The current density in the tissues is critically dependent on the position of the two electrodes in the bath and on the relative resistance of the two paths. Such a system, called a faradic foot bath, is often used to stimulate the intrinsic muscle of the foot for re-education.

Unipolar and bipolar

The system described above, with both electrodes in the same bath, is referred to as 'bipolar' whereas if one electrode is in the bath and the circuit is completed by a pad electrode or an electrode in another bath it is called 'unipolar'. It may be noted that adding salt to a unipolar bath results in a greater current passing through the tissues because it lowers the resistance in series thus reducing the total resistance. Adding salt to a bipolar bath will decrease the current through the tissues since greater current will now pass in

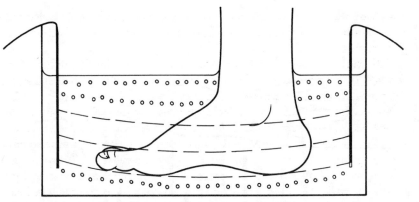

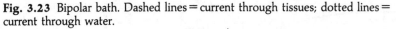

Fig. 3.23 Bipolar bath. Dashed lines = current through tissues; dotted lines = current through water.

the parallel water pathway due to its lowered resistance. In some publications (Alon, 1987) bipolar treatments are described as those in which both electrodes or pads are applied to the area being treated, whereas unipolar are those involving a (usually) larger indifferent electrode applied at some distance from the active electrode which is sited over the target tissue. However, it must be emphasized that all these treatments involving a flow of current in the tissues are essentially bipolar in the sense that there must be two connections to the tissues. The use of the terms 'unipolar' and 'bipolar' sometimes creates confusion.

Lowering the electrical resistance at the skin surface

As has been noted already, the electrical resistance of the epidermis is high. It can be reduced by washing the surface to remove some of the keratin and sebum and leaving the skin wet. Warming the skin also helps to lower its resistance by increasing the rate of particle and ionic movement; also perhaps increasing the activity of the sweat glands and blood flow. Thus warming, washing and wetting the skin will allow larger currents to flow for the same applied voltage.

To record small currents generated by the tissues, such as the electrocardiogram or surface electromyogram, it is sometimes necessary to reduce the skin surface resistance still further by gently scraping or sandpapering some of the surface epidermis off—removing some of the dead cells that form the outer epidermis—before fixing the electrodes.

In all cases it must be realized that maintaining the same skin–electrode junction throughout treatment is essential. If the adhesion of the electrode to the skin surface alters, or the pressure of sponge or pad decreases, this can lead to a higher resistance; consequently the fixation of the electrodes to the body surface is very important in keeping a constant uniform low resistance at this junction.

Fig. 3.24 Guide to motor points.

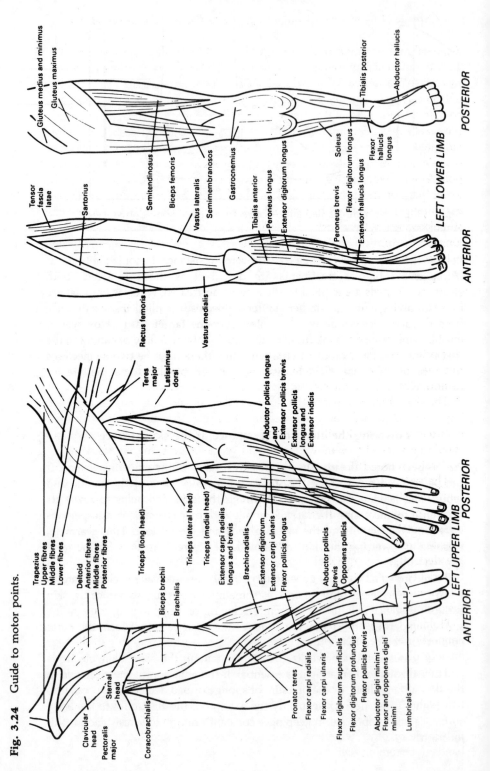

Application of low-frequency currents for muscle stimulation

Electrical muscle stimulation is usually achieved by faradic-type currents (0.1–1 ms duration at any frequency between 30 and 100 Hz). In order to localize the current to individual muscles a small active electrode, i.e. a small pad or button electrode, is applied to the motor point of the muscle, the circuit being completed with a larger dispersive electrode sited in some convenient, usually proximal, area. The motor points of some superficial muscles are often indicated on charts (Fig. 3.24). Such charts act as a guide but a knowledge of the relevant anatomy coupled with a little trial and error will locate the precise point at which the muscle is most effectively stimulated. The usual site is in the lower part of the proximal third of the muscle belly but there are many exceptions. It is obvious that deeply placed muscles can only be successfully stimulated where their fleshy belly emerges, for example, the extensor hallucis longus emerging in the lower part of the leg between tibialis anterior and extensor digitorum longus (Fig. 3.24).

Technique of application

The patient is positioned so that the part to be treated is comfortably supported with the muscles to be stimulated in a shortened position, although this may be modified when movement is to be produced, e.g. slight knee flexion allowing quadriceps stimulation to cause extension.

The skin surfaces to which the current will be applied must be examined and any cuts, abrasions, or other lesions that might cause uneven current distribution insulated (with a dab of petroleum jelly) or avoided. These areas should be washed to remove sebum and epithelial cells and left damp; using hot water warms the skin and helps to lower the resistance further.

The size of the active electrode, which may be a small plate and pad or a button electrode, is chosen by considering the size of the area to be treated; the motor point of a small muscle close to others is clearly best stimulated with a small button electrode. In all cases the dispersive or indifferent pad should be two or three times larger. Leads are connected to the machine and attached to the electrodes. The metal electrode should be smaller than the pad or sponge material to prevent the edge of the electrode being bent down on to the skin which could lead to high current density at that point and would be very uncomfortable.

Holding the two electrodes, separated, in one hand allows the machine and connections to be tested by the therapist. Observing this may help to allay the anxiety of a patient experiencing this treatment for the first time.

The pads or sponges should be soaked in warm tap water, saline or sodium bicarbonate solution, which are somewhat better conductors, particularly in soft water areas, and applied to the skin. Fixation is achieved with a rubber strap, a crêpe or similar bandage, or simply by body weight. A piece of polythene or other waterproof material is placed on the pad to prevent the bandage becoming wet.

The nature of the treatment and the sensations to be expected—a tingling sensation and muscle contraction—should be explained to the patient with reassurance that there is no way that any damage can be caused by this treatment.

When a single muscle is to be stimulated the active electrode is placed firmly over the approximate motor point, indicated in Figure 3.24, and a small current is applied. Small adjustments of the position of the active electrode will allow the best position to be found; the current may need to be increased and then decreased as the exact motor point is found and good contractions can be obtained with less current.

When a muscle group is to be stimulated the active pad can be made to straddle all the motor points or the two pads may be of approximately the same size, placed at either end of the muscle group so that current spreads through the whole group: this happens in the faradic foot bath, shown in Figure 3.23.

The stimulation of individual muscles is often done to re-educate the activity. In this case the patient attempts a voluntary contraction at the same time as the current causes the muscle to contract. To enable the patient to co-operate, the length of the contractions and the intervals between them should be suitably long. This allows patients time to match their efforts with the stimulated contractions and an adequate rest between each one.

As an example of re-education, the stimulation of the abductor hallucis will be considered. This muscle in the sole of the foot contributes to the stability of the first metatarsophalangeal joint in walking and running. If the joint is free it will act to flex the toe and abduct it. In those people who have worn shoes throughout childhood the ability to abduct the big toe when the foot is supported on a smooth surface is often absent. However, at least in young adults, a little re-education and practice will restore this ability to some degree. The abductor hallucis may be stimulated in a bipolar bath with two electrodes, one under the heel and the other close to the belly of the muscle; a modification of the arrangement shown in Figure 3.23. Alternatively the indifferent electrode may be a pad fixed behind the medial malleolus while a small button electrode is used over the muscle belly.

The patient is instructed first to feel the movement of the big toe brought about by the faradic current. When he or she is able to appreciate this movement he or she is asked to attempt to join in voluntarily so that the action becomes, in effect, active-assisted. As the patient's ability increases the intensity of the current is progressively reduced and he or she is asked to hold the contraction at the end of the surge. When he or she can initiate a contraction actively without the assistance of the current, re-education continues by other means (see discussion in Chapter 4).

Re-educating the pelvic floor musculature for the treatment of stress incontinence requires a special technique to stimulate the sphincter muscles of the urethra. This can be done with a large dispersive over the lumbosacral region and a rectal electrode as the active with the patient lying on one side or in crook half-lying. In females a vaginal electrode can be used; a button electrode placed over the perineal body can be used as the active electrode in either sex (Wadsworth and Chanmugan, 1980). Voluntary contraction is attempted with the electrical stimulation. Faradic-type currents have been used in the successful treatment of this condition (Montgomery and Shepherd, 1983) as well as interferential currents (see p. 85).

Muscle groups in the limbs can be stimulated rhythmically to effect a muscle-pumping action, enhancing the venous and lymphatic flow to assist the reduction of oedema. This is combined with elevation of the limb and the application of a pressure bandage. The largest volume of muscle that can be stimulated is required, so the quadriceps and plantarflexors of the lower limb and flexors of the elbow and hand in the upper limb are usually chosen. Large pads are applied over these muscle groups, or on the sole of the foot and quadriceps; there are numerous other pad positions to achieve the strong generalized muscle contractions needed. The compression bandage, applied over the pads should give firm pressure against which the contracting musculature can press but should not be constrictive. Strong slow muscle contractions should be produced with a long period of relaxation (several seconds) to allow vessel filling.

Application of TENS for pain relief

It is customary, as already noted, to limit the acronym 'TENS' to low-intensity, short impulses produced by battery-operated sources specifically for pain relief. As local areas are usually treated and self-treatment is common, small carbon-rubber electrodes are usually employed. Since both the intention and effect of the treatment are to relieve pain it is important to be certain that this is appropriate and does not lead to the neglect of the underlying causes of the pain. It is also very important that the pain should be evaluated both initially and during the course of the treatment. This serves both to monitor the effectiveness of the particular treatment parameters used, such as the position of the electrodes, and to measure the progress of the treatment. Any objective methods that are appropriate, such as measuring the range of movement, should be used but often subjective pain assessment is the principal means used. A 10 cm horizontal visual analogue scale (on which the patient marks the intensity of pain between one end marked 'no pain' and the other end 'worst pain ever') and pain behaviour analysis have been recommended (Frampton, 1988).

The application of TENS requires decisions about where to place the electrodes and what current parameters to use.

Electrode placement

There are four approaches to be considered. Firstly, the most usual is to site electrodes close to where the pain is perceived to be; often one electrode is sited over the place where the most intense pain is felt or the greatest tenderness elicited. Secondly, the electrodes may be placed within the same dermatome, myotome or sclerotome. They may be placed to pass current through the long axis of the dermatome. In many, but not all, circumstances the dermatome, myotome and sclerotome overlap. Thirdly, trigger or acupuncture points may be the preferred sites of current application. It is considered (Klein and Pariser, 1987) that acupuncture points can be located by their lower resistance compared with the surrounding skin (due to active sweat glands and/or local vasodilation); they can be found by using an electronic probe. Fourthly, stimulation of peripheral nerves is used. Electrodes are placed in the line of the nerve and where it is particularly superficial. This method is used principally for the treatment of neurogenic pain such as postherpetic neuralgia.

It is evident from a clinical point of view that these four approaches are by no means mutually exclusive. Thus trigger points, peripheral nerves and the painful area all lie in a dermatome. The choice of electrode position is often dictated by an effective result, i.e. relief of pain. Several positions may be tried before success is achieved.

Current parameters

TENS is most often applied as short pulses of around 0.05 ms at 50–100 Hz; this is called conventional TENS. The intensity is turned up gradually until a prickling or tingling sensation is felt. It should be neither painful nor should it cause a muscle contraction. It is presumed that these low-intensity short pulses will selectively stimulate the large low-threshold A beta fibres to produce pain inhibition by the pain gate mechanism, as described on p. 60. This conventional mode is the most usual method for self-treatment. The recommended duration and timing of such treatments varies from 30 to 60 min sessions once or twice a day (Klein and Pariser, 1987) to continuous TENS for a minimum of 8 h/day or even a full 24 h/day (Frampton, 1988).

High-intensity, low-frequency (acupuncture-like) TENS is another frequently used approach. Pulses of around 0.2 ms at about 2 Hz are given at intensities close to the maximum that the patient can tolerate. This stimulates the high-threshold A delta and C fibres which leads to the release of endorphins and encephalins, as described on p. 61. This kind of stimulation is often applied to acupuncture points which, it is considered, are places where small bundles of A delta and sympathetic efferent fibres pierce the deep fascia to become more superficial (Bowsher, 1988). It is also sometimes applied to the motor points of muscle in the segmentally related myotome. In contrast with conventional TENS it is usually applied once per day for 20 or 30 min (Klein and Pariser, 1987).

Another method referred to as 'brief intense TENS' involves the application of high-frequency, relatively long trains given at high intensity. 'Burst TENS' is simply a series of trains of pulses repeated at 2 or 3 Hz with a few tenths of a second intervals; each train or burst consists of high-frequency pulses at between 70 and 100 Hz. The benefit claimed for this latter method is that it combines both the conventional and acupuncture-like TENS and therefore provides pain relief by both routes. These modes of stimulation are illustrated in Figure 3.25.

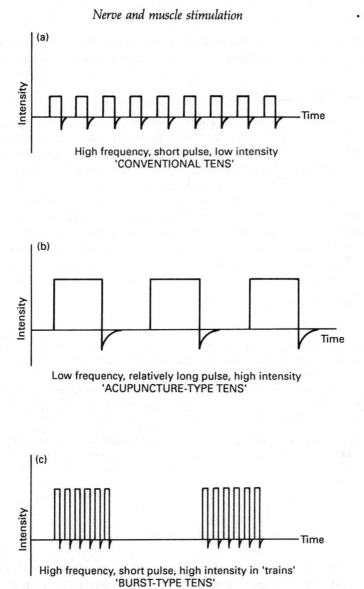

Fig. 3.25 Different forms of TENS. (a) High-frequency, short-pulse, low-intensity conventional TENS; (b) low-frequency, relatively long-pulse, high-intensity acupuncture-type TENS; high-frequency, short-pulse, high-intensity burst-type TENS.

In 'modulated TENS' the pulse width, frequency and intensity are all constantly and automatically varied. As well as the benefits of delivering both the conventional and acupuncture-like modes it is also believed to prevent adaptation of the nerves to the current. It has already been noted (p. 63) that TENS has been widely used for the relief of acute pain, including postoperative and obstetric pain, as well as chronic and neurogenic pain. Electrodes are fixed to the skin with adhesive tape or bandaged into place. A conducting gel is applied between electrode and skin. The leads from the TENS unit are

Electrotherapy explained

concealed and fixed in the clothing if continuous home treatment is being given. Convenient ready-gelled adhesive electrodes are available.

Contraindications to TENS

TENS should not be used for patients with demand-type cardiac pacemakers. However, it is apparently safe with fixed-rate pacemakers (Eriksson and Schuller, 1978). Electrodes should not be placed over the carotid sinus as this could lead to cardiac arrhythmias. Similarly placement over the pharyngeal region could interfere with normal breathing and swallowing co-ordination. In any circumstances in which the skin is devoid of sensation, uniphasic (unidirectional) TENS should not be used because of the risk of unnoticed chemical change. Electrodes should not be placed over skin lesions or open wounds because of the different resistance and the risk of infection. Placing electrodes over or close to the pregnant uterus is contraindicated but there is no evidence of any damage; avoidance is usually recommended for medico-legal reasons.

Table 3.3 Summary of TENS

Electrode placement	Stimulus parameters
1 Site of pain	1 High-frequency, short pulse length, low-intensity conventional TENS
2 Dermatome, myotome sclerotome	2 Low-frequency, wider pulse, high-intensity acupuncture TENS
3 Trigger point, acupuncture point, motor point	3 1 and 2 mixed; burst TENS
4 Peripheral nerve	4 1 and 2 varied; modulated TENS

Electroacupuncture

Electroacupuncture consists of two aspects. First, the acupuncture point may be found on the surface by testing the electrical resistance. Second, stimulation of the point may be given with an electric pulse rather than the traditional needle penetrating the skin. Some machines allow both testing and stimulation through the same electrode. Acupuncture points and trigger points (which appear to correspond to each other (Melzack *et al.*, 1977)), apparently have a lower electrical impedance than the surrounding area, as noted above (Klein and Pariser, 1987). These points are located with a point electrode (probe) on the skin and a small applied current is then measured; thus the circuit impedance (or conductance) can be displayed on a meter. The electric pulses used for treatment are usually some form of low-frequency, high-intensity TENS stimulating A delta nerve fibres to achieve encephalinergic pain relief (see p. 60).

Ryodu-Raku (from Japan) is an example of such a system. The device is called a neurometer and can be used to test the tissue resistance between a point electrode applied to the skin and a dispersive held in the hand. Where large differences of conductivity are found treatment is applied. This consists of a few seconds of direct current from the same device given either by means of a small surface electrode or a fine needle into the skin.

The Rebox is a device that is applied in a similar way but involves a different current form; it was developed in Czechoslovakia in the 1970s. There is a hand-held dispersive and current is delivered by a point-type electrode. The point electrode is made the negative pole. The current consists of unipolar rectangular pulses of between 0.05 and 0.25 ms at 3000 Hz; thus it is a medium-frequency current. The circuit also contains a microammeter and an earphone and can be linked to a small computer and printer to display a graph of current and other parameters. When applied to normal tissue the current rises over a period of about 1 s giving a characteristic displacement of the meter, of sound in the earphone, and of the shape of the graph. When applied to damaged or abnormal tissue a different pattern is said to occur in which the rise of current is slower, taking 3 or 4 s, and may occur in a series of steps. These differences do not seem to have supporting experimental evidence nor is there a clear theoretical basis for them.

Repeated application of this current for a few seconds at a time (up to 20 V leading to a maximum current of 0.3 mA proximal to the injured area), using the device as a treatment is claimed to lead to a normal response when the same area is subsequently tested, and to therapeutic benefit. It has been used in the treatment of musculoskeletal pains, recent trauma and a number of other conditions. The benefits have been accounted for by postulating that the current causes increased ionic movement in the tissue fluid, and that monitoring rate of change of current in the tissues helps to localize the area of abnormality (Hervik, 1989).

High-voltage pulsed galvanic stimulation

This form of current was originally developed in 1945 by Haslip in the USA and called 'Dyna-wave neuromuscular stimulation'. Later, in the mid 1970s, there was increased interest in this type of current when it became known as 'high-voltage electrogalvanic stimulation' or 'high-voltage pulsed galvanic stimulation' (HVPGS). The latter is considered the preferred name since it obviates the mistaken idea that this is a constant direct current (Newton, 1987).

The twin pulse waveform, described on p. 36 (Fig. 3.5), has almost instantaneous rises with exponential falls. The pair of pulses lasts for only 0.1 ms and each peak lasts for only a few microseconds; the shape and duration are normally fixed. The frequency of the double pulse can be varied, usually from 2 to 100 Hz. With such short peaks very high voltages are needed (hence the name) to provide high enough currents to stimulate nerve fibres (see Fig. 3.13). Peak currents of 2–2.5 A (Alon, 1987) may be generated during the few microseconds of peak voltage but, of course, the total average current is very low—around 1.2–1.5 mA. Such currents will pass easily through the tissues because they are so brief (see p. 69) and will be relatively comfortable due to their wide discrimination between sensory, motor and pain nerve fibres (see Fig. 3.13).

As well as the frequency the intensity can be varied (0–500 V) and the polarity altered. The pattern of current can be changed by a mode switch. In continuous mode the train of twin pulses is delivered continuously. Reciprocate mode refers to the alternate application of trains of pulses to one or other of two active pads and does not mean that the current direction is reversed. Surge mode gives a train of pulses whose intensity is gradually increased, as indicated with square wave pulses in Figure 3.1e. A meter to indicate peak current may be provided. On some machines the interval between the two peaks may be altered; this is called the intrapulse interval. The current is applied by flexible electrodes and sponges. The electrodes are usually small and sometimes are mounted on a handle. Various special electrodes are available.

Uses of HVPGS

Wound healing

Since a direct current, albeit of very low total intensity, is being applied, the discussion on this subject in Chapter 2 is relevant. There seems to be evidence that low-intensity currents lead to tissue healing (Newton, 1987; see references, Chapter 2) but those treatment parameters that work best are uncertain. Further, the specific use of HVPGS for wound healing has had only a few assessments so far (Kloth and Feedar, 1988). It has been suggested (Newton, 1987) that the cathode (negative pole) appears to retard bacterial activity while the anode (positive pole) seems to promote cell migration and perhaps proliferation; see also the research cited in Chapter 2.

A suggested procedure is to apply the active electrode, encased in gauze and soaked in sterile saline, directly over the wound. The dispersive is placed proximally and arranged so that current passes through the wound. Current at an intensity just insufficient to cause muscle contraction is applied at a frequency of around 100 Hz. Negative polarity of the active electrode is used if the wound is infected, changing to positive if or when the wound is clean. This treatment is given for fairly long periods (> 30 min) daily or three times per week.

Pain modulation

How pain may be controlled by electrical stimulation has already been discussed (p. 60). Since both the frequency and intensity of HVPGS can be controlled it is possible to apply both high-frequency, low-intensity stimulation for pain gate control and low-frequency, high-intensity stimulation for encephalin-type pain control. HVPGS has been recommended for controlling all kinds of pain—acute, chronic, neurogenic and pain from many sources (Newton, 1987).

Muscle stimulation

HVPGS is used for the stimulation of innervated muscle and, due to the short pulses and hence good transmission in the tissues, it is an efficient way of doing so. Consider the strength–duration curve (Fig. 3.13) which shows that short pulses at high intensities will be more selective in stimulating motor rather than pain nerves. HVPGS has therefore been used for muscle strengthening and the reduction of disuse atrophy of innervated muscle. A frequency of around 30 Hz has been suggested with long intervals between bouts of tetanic contraction as the optimum schedule.

Other uses

Effects on the vascular system are claimed in that rhythmical muscle contraction and relaxation due to HVPGS of motor nerves will have a pumping effect, increasing blood flow in muscle and surrounding tissues, as considered on p. 53. This effect can aid in the reduction of tissue oedema. Direct effects on autonomic nerves leading to local vasodilation, increased fluid exchange in the tissues and other beneficial effects have been claimed without supporting evidence (Wadsworth and Chanmugan, 1980). Due to the fact that it is a direct (unipolar) current the anaphoretic effect (see Chapter 2) has been invoked as the reason for a beneficial effect on oedema. Consequent upon its ability to stimulate innervated muscle HVPGS has been recommended in the treatment of muscle spasm and to increase joint mobility (Newton, 1987).

Some uncertainty exists over the advantages of the twin peaks wave form, which is what makes this current unique. It has been suggested that a single pulse could be just as effective (Alon, 1987).

Sinusoidal currents

An evenly alternating 50 Hz sine wave current—the form of the mains current—is called 'sinusoidal current' when it is used therapeutically (p. 36). Since it gives 100 phases in each second it is able to stimulate nerves but because of the sine wave form of each phase (lasting 10 ms; see Fig. 3.5) it is less efficient than a similar square wave pulse. It can be produced from the mains by simply reducing the voltage to 60 or 80 V with a step-down transformer. The 10 ms sine wave phases are the same as those of diadynamic currents, but sinusoidal current is alternating.

Effects

If it is applied continuously it will cause a tetanic muscle contraction and a tingling sensation due to stimulation of motor and sensory nerves. It is usually surged to cause rhythmical muscle contractions. The sensory stimulations can lead to pain relief by some of the mechanisms described in connection with TENS. The rhythmical muscle contractions induced can help reduction of oedema by muscle pumping action and other consequences, discussed on p. 53. Various specific effects have been claimed, such as increased blood flow in the treated region suggested by the marked cutaneous erythema that can develop. Similarly it is claimed that unsurged sinusoidal current will help the absorption of oedema or inflammatory exudate (Wadsworth and Chanmugan, 1980). There seems to be no clear evidence to support these latter claims.

Application

Sinusoidal current can be applied in the same way as other low-frequency currents by means of electrodes and pads. However, because of the marked sensory stimulation this current is often applied to large areas and rarely used for local muscle stimulation. Thus it is applied either through large pads or water baths (see p. 67) or both. For pain control continuous sinusoidal current at intensities close to the limit of tolerance are recommended, increasing the current as the patient accommodates. This is applied for about 5 min and repeated if there is insufficient immediate effect. For reduction of oedema and to increase the limb circulation surged sinusoidal current is suggested, causing regular rhythmical muscle pumping actions.

Sinusoidal current is rarely used in modern physiotherapy departments. It is interesting, however, to note that the series of 10 ms phases gives marked sensory nerve stimulation in the skin, acting in part like modern TENS stimulators. Recent understanding of pain control (see p. 60) may account for some of the benefits that were claimed for this treatment (Wadsworth and Chanmugan, 1980).

Diadynamic currents

Diadynamic currents were introduced by Pierre Bernard nearly 60 years ago. They are monophasic sinusoidal currents, being rectified mains-type current. Diadynamic currents have two basic forms:

1 Half-wave rectified sinusoidal current known as MF (*monophase fixe*). This consists of a series of 10 ms half sine wave-shaped pulses with 10 ms pulse intervals.
2 Full-wave rectified sinusoidal current known as DF (*diphase fixe*). This is a continuous series of 10 ms sinusoidal pulses resulting in a frequency of 100 Hz (Fig. 3.26). (Note that the above refers to rectified 50 Hz mains current. If 60 Hz mains, as in the USA, is used then the pulse lengths and intervals will be 8.333 ms.)

If these two current forms—MF and DF—are applied alternately for 1 s

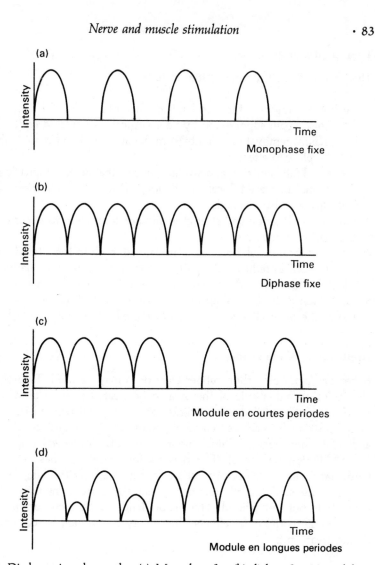

Fig. 3.26 Diadynamic pulse modes. (a) *Monophase fixe*; (b) *diphase fixe*; (c) *module en courtes périodes*; (d) *module en longues périodes*.

each the resulting current is called CP module (*module en courtes périodes*). If two MF currents are applied so that one series of pulses occupies the pulse intervals of the other and one is of constant intensity while the other is surged, the result is called LP module (*module en longues périodes*). The length of each surge and surge interval varies with different sources but is usually 5 or 6 s (Fig. 3.26).

The physiological effects of such currents have already been considered and will obviously cause sensory and motor nerve stimulation and thus muscle contraction, as well as chemical changes due to the unidirectional current.

Therapeutic effects

The effects claimed (Rennie, 1988) include:

1 Pain relief due to the mechanisms described already, i.e. pain gate mechanism, pain suppression by neurologically stimulated endorphins and encephalins, removal of irritants from the area by the increased circulation, and the placebo effect.
2 Decreased inflammation and swelling due to the increased muscle pumping action and increased local circulation; changes in cell membrane per-meability are also claimed.
3 Muscle re-education and strengthening are considered to occur due to the stimulation of muscles.
4 Increased local circulation due, it is claimed, both to the altered autonomic activity such as reduced sympathetic tone leading to vasodilation and the release of histamine-like substances due to the unidirectional effects.
5 Facilitation of tissue-healing due to local circulatory changes noted above and to the polar effects leading to increased cell activity (see Chapter 2).

Application of electrodes

Either pad/plate or carbon rubber electrodes may be used. Two equal-sized electrodes on either side of the area to be treated may be used or a small electrode may be placed over a trigger or motor point with a larger electrode placed proximally. Various treatment parameters are suggested. For pain relief and most other effects, an initial minute or so of DF followed by up to 5 min of CP or LP (Rennie, 1988). The reasons for preferring these or any other particular regimes are not provided in commentary on this subject.

It is suggested for all treatments that the current intensity should be perceptible but not painful. The major danger with such currents is tissue damage due to the polar effects. These may be avoided by current reversal during treatment.

Russian currents

In the 1970s claims were published that the 2500 Hz medium frequency interrupted current could be used to generate greater muscle force than a maximal voluntary muscle contraction. This current has been described on p. 36. It is called 'Russian' because its use was first described by Dr K. M. Kots in the Russian literature. It provoked much interest because the very successful Russian Olympic team were using it in addition to their usual training methods and it was suggested that its use led to significant (30–40%) gains in muscle strength.

Although it is a medium-frequency current the nerves are stimulated because it is interrupted to give a low-frequency stimulation of 50 Hz. Due to the short pulses (of 0.2 ms phase) it will pass fairly easily through the skin and be effective in stimulating motor nerves (p. 42) but the stimulus is due to the initial electrical pulse, thus the purpose of the rest of the 10 ms train is not clear. It is, in fact, like a short-duration faradic-type pulse at 50 Hz.

The theoretical basis for its use is that maximum electrical stimulation can cause nearly all the motor units in a muscle to contract synchronously: something that cannot be achieved in voluntary contraction, it was claimed. This would allow stronger muscle contractions to occur with electrical stimulation and hence greater muscle hypertrophy. This has not been found to occur in the subsequent research. Many investigations have determined that electrical muscle stimulation leads to muscle hypertrophy but not to any greater degree than voluntary activity (Currier, 1987)—see p. 50.

Not only was it claimed that the electrically generated force was greater than that generated voluntarily but also that this occurred without producing pain. This claim has not been entirely supported either; in one careful study which assessed torque values and pain scores (Gilles and Bélanger, 1987) the assertions were definitely refuted.

This current can be applied in the usual way with electrodes applied over the muscle belly. To achieve muscle hypertrophy, which is the usual purpose, currents of high intensity producing maximum tolerable muscle contraction are given in spells of a few seconds separated by somewhat longer rest periods.

Interferential currents

The principle of interferential therapy is to pass two medium-frequency alternating currents which are slightly out of phase through the tissues. Where the currents intersect a new current is set up (Fig. 3.27a). The resultant amplitude of this new current is the sum of the individual current amplitudes at any given point. Thus when two peaks of amplitude in the same direction coincide the resultant amplitude is at a maximum. When the peaks are in opposite directions there will be no current. Providing the amplitudes of the two currents are the same the resultant carrying frequency will be the average of the two individual frequencies. If the frequency of the first current is 4000 Hz and the second 4100 Hz, the resultant carrying frequency is 4050 Hz. This resultant current varies in amplitude, i.e. it is amplitude-modulated. The frequency with which the amplitude varies is called the amplitude modulation frequency or beat frequency, and is equal to the difference in frequency between the two interference currents—in the above instance, 100 Hz.

That the two currents will be equal in amplitude is unlikely in the body as the pathways of the two currents will have different resistances. If they are not equal the modulation depth will not be 100%, i.e. there will be partial beating only (Fig. 3.27b).

These medium-frequency currents will pass much more easily through the skin than low-frequency currents due to the lower impedance offered to very short electrical pulses (p. 49). With a 4000 Hz current each individual phase is 0.125 ms long which would require a very high current intensity to stimulate

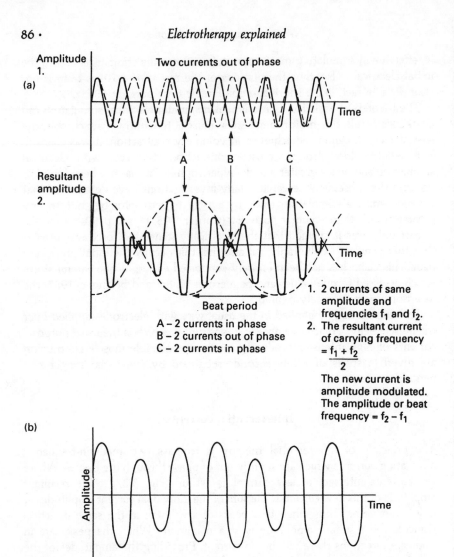

Fig. 3.27 (a) Interference of two medium-frequency currents. A = Two currents in phase; B = two currents out of phase; C = two currents in phase. 1 = two currents of same amplitude and frequency: f_1 and f_2. 2 = The resultant current of carrying frequency = $f_1 + f_2/2$. This new current is amplitude-modulated. The amplitude modulation or beat frequency = $f_2 - f_1$. (b) Partial beating.

nerves. It is the beat effect that acts like any other low-frequency current and stimulates nerves. Thus, such currents will pass easily through the tissues because they are medium-frequency but stimulate nerves because of the amplitude modulation.

Although the spread of medium-frequency current in the tissues is more uniform than a low-frequency current it is still at greater intensity close to the electrodes (Fig. 3.28a and b). The great advantage of true interferential currents is that the low-frequency modulation is made to occur deep in the tissues.

About 40 years ago this idea was developed by Hans Nemec in Vienna and

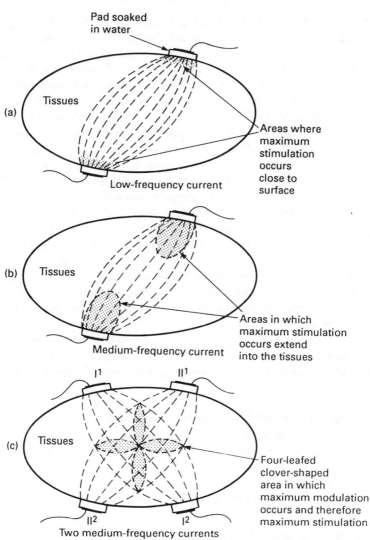

Fig. 3.28 Areas of maximum stimulation.

although used quite widely in the intervening years, it has become much better known recently with the development of cheaper electronic circuitry. A later development involves the use of a third current in a path at right angles to the other two; this is called stereodynamic interference current (Kloth, 1987). Thus the tissues are stimulated in a three-dimensional system; however, the usefulness of such a system is not clearly established.

Most interferential machines allow a constant beat frequency to be selected, e.g. 10, 50 or 100 Hz—in fact any frequency from 1 to 250 Hz—called the constant or static mode. They also have an arrangement that allows the beat frequency to change automatically and regularly between some pre-set pair of frequencies over a specified time period. This is called a frequency swing or sweep. Thus the machine could be set to sweep, for example, between 20 and

80 Hz over a period of 6 s and back over the next 6 s. Such an arrangement is useful to prevent nerve habituation and extend the range of nerve types that can be stimulated. The higher frequency and hence shorter pulse length will stimulate the low-threshold large nerve fibres, as already explained. Since the pulse is sinusoidal, not square wave, it is not easy to define the pulse length.

Figure 3.28c shows the theoretical distribution of current in a homogeneous medium. The clover leaf shape of maximum current modulation is due to the fact that both the current amplitudes and their directions need to be summated, i.e. vector addition. The distribution shown for four equally spaced electrodes is unlikely to be realized in real tissue, since variations in tissue resistance and electrode distances would prevent this neat uniformity. The real pattern is likely to be much more irregular and diffuse in all tissues between and around the electrodes. None the less the pattern shown is a valid concept and a useful guide. This is a static pattern but by varying the current intensity in a suitable manner it is possible to move the clover leaf pattern of maximum modulation to and fro through 45°, thus giving a more uniform total distribution of the interferential current in the tissues. There are various names for such a mechanism, including 'vector sweep', 'scanning', 'rotating vector system' or 'dynamic interference field system'. It serves to increase the area of effective treatment.

Control of the current intensity is provided to allow more or less stimulation as needed. There is also usually automatic timing control for the timing of treatment. Thus, in summary, controls on the interferential machine are:

1 Settings for constant beat frequency, e.g. 80 Hz.
2 Settings for variable beat frequencies, e.g. 20–80 Hz.
3 Control for time of variable beat frequencies cycle, e.g. 6 s.
4 Intensity control.
5 Control for using rotating vector mechanisms, e.g. on or off.
6 Control for total treatment time, e.g. 10 min.

Application of interferential therapy

Currents are applied by metal or carbon rubber electrodes with water-soaked sponges or lint. Carbon-rubber electrodes may be used with conducting gel, as already described. Since two circuits are involved, four electrodes, i.e. a quadripolar technique, are usually used. These electrodes may be secured by rubber straps or bandages; alternatively they may be secured by suction. Suction units can be connected to the interferential machine. Flexible rubber cups are connected by tubes to a pump that can provide a negative pressure. This suction may be continuous or variable. Metal electrodes mounted inside the cups are connected by wires carried within the tubes to the interferential source. Contact is made by moistened sponges placed inside the cups between the metal electrode and the skin. The negative pressure is set to vary rhythmically during treatment, which diminishes the risk of skin damage. It should be adjusted to maintain good electrical contact without causing discomfort. As well as maintaining electrical contact the suction has a mild massaging effect on the skin, stimulating cutaneous sensory nerves and causing slight vasodilation, both of which may contribute to the effectiveness of treatment.

The electrodes must be placed so that the currents cross one another in the target tissue. In Figure 3.29 the current of the first circuit is carried via electrodes I^1 and I^2 and that of the second circuit by electrodes II^1 and II^2, thus generating the interferential field in the deep tissue. The electrodes are positioned in a coplanar arrangement to treat a flat surface such as the back. It is normally recommended to use the largest electrode sizes that can conveniently be applied (Savage, 1984) in order to ensure a comfortable current of sufficient intensity throughout the treated area. The leads (and suction tubes) are colour-coded to ensure correct arrangement of the circuit.

It is also possible to use only two electrodes; this is called the bipolar mode. In this case the two medium-frequency currents are superimposed at the electrode level with the result that interference occurs throughout the region between the two electrodes. The modulation is always 100%. This method is occasionally referred to as 'electrokinesy'. For this type of application the two electrodes should be placed opposite one another so that the part to be treated lies between them. Because the current modulation occurs throughout the area, including the superficial tissues and skin, there tends to be more sensory stimulation than with the four-pole technique.

Precautions

It would seem wise to wash the skin before treatment to reduce skin impedance and to use large enough (sponge) pads to ensure that neither the metal electrodes nor their connections touch the patient's skin. This obviates the risk of damage which could occur with high current densities.

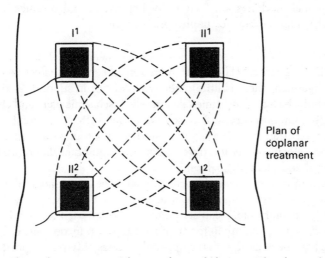

Fig. 3.29 Electrode arrangement for interferential therapy. Plan for coplanar treatment.

It has been estimated that interferential currents of 50 mA applied to the thorax could induce currents of sufficient intensity to cause ventricular fibrillation (Health Protection Board of Health and Welfare Canada, 1988). It is considered inadvisable, therefore, to apply high-intensity interferential currents to the thorax.

Comments on the effects

Different frequencies and ranges of frequencies are recommended, often for the treatment of similar problems. The appropriate dosage parameters are not universally agreed.

Interferential currents are frequently employed for pain relief by means of mechanisms already described and summarized below:

1 Activation of the pain gate mechanism due to stimulation of large-diameter, low-threshold nerve fibres with high-beat frequencies — around 100 Hz.
2 Activation of A delta and C fibres causing encephalin and endorphin release, probably activated by low frequency (10–25 Hz).
3 It is possible that high-frequency (above 50 Hz) stimulation may lead to temporary physiological block of finely myelinated and non-myelinated nociceptive fibres.
4 The local increased fluid flow and fluid exchange consequent on mild muscle contraction and possibly stimulation of autonomic nerves may help to remove chemical irritants affecting pain nerve endings and reduce local tissue pressure. When interferential therapy is applied in this way, the varying suction could also contribute to this effect. Savage (1984) states that frequencies of 10–150 Hz stimulate the parasympathetic nerves increasing blood flow through the area, and 0–5 Hz the sympathetic nerves.
5 A placebo effect, which occurs in all treatments, is likely, especially since interferential machines are technically impressive and produce a distinct, somewhat unusual but not unpleasant sensation.

For fuller discussion of these points see De Domenico (1982).

While there are many claims that interferential current is effective as a pain-relieving treatment there is little objective evidence in support. A rise in the pain threshold, based on the time taken to elicit ischaemic pain, and changes in the strength–duration curves of muscle were found after interferential therapy in one study (Pärtan *et al.*, 1953). Other studies have found no change in nerve conduction velocities after interferential and no significant difference between interferential and placebo treatments.

Muscle contraction can also be achieved with the lower range of interferential frequencies. Strong muscle contractions can be achieved without any significantly uncomfortable skin sensation. It is often used for re-education of the pelvic floor musculature in the treatment of stress incontinence. Swings of 0–100 Hz have been used with the upper electrodes of two pads positioned on the lower abdomen and the lower ones on the upper medial aspect of the thighs. Such treatment combined with pelvic floor exercises has produced very convincing improvement (McQuire, 1975). Laycock and Green (1988) recommended a bipolar method. For female patients the posterior electrode is placed under the ischial tuberosities and the anterior inferior to the symphysis pubis. Male patients are treated with two electrodes either side of the gluteal cleft under the ischial tuberosities, anterior to the anus.

Savage (1984) states that frequencies of 10–50 Hz stimulate motor nerves and 0–10 Hz unstriped muscle.

SAFETY WITH ELECTRICAL CURRENTS

Primum non nocere—firstly do no harm—is a central tenet of every therapy but is especially applicable where damage can easily occur. Damage to the tissues as a result of the passage of electrical currents can occur in three ways:

1 Direct or uniphasic currents can cause electrochemical damage, often called a chemical burn (see Chapter 2).
2 Currents varying at rates that will stimulate nerve or muscle, that is, all those currents discussed in this chapter, could cause damage by provoking excessively powerful or prolonged muscle contractions or more seriously, the heart muscle, thus stopping the circulation.
3 Currents of sufficient intensity can cause heating in the tissues leading to a heat burn.

All these kinds of damage could occur together but serious shocks or fatalities are usually confined to the last two points. If large currents are passed it is called an electric shock. In all cases what matters is the electric charge, that is, the current intensity and the length of time for which it flows.

Damage due to the therapeutic use of electricity is, in fact, extremely rare and most damage that does occur is due to the mains current and is of the kind that may equally well take place in the home with ordinary domestic equipment.

It is usual to distinguish *macroshock*, in which current passes through the skin, from *microshock* which refers to the very small currents which are applied directly to, say, the heart as an external pacemaker; in this situation quite small current increases can be fatal. This latter will not be considered further.

It will be apparent from what has been described earlier in this chapter that quite high currents can be passed through the body without ill effects provided they are applied as very short pulses (Fig. 3.13). As a general observation electrotherapeutic equipment is designed so that it cannot deliver pulses of sufficient intensity to be seriously damaging to the tissues, except as considered below.

Electric shock due to mains-type current

If an electric current is passed through the whole body it tends to spread throughout the low-resistance subcutaneous tissues. It will be recalled that the skin resistance here is very much greater than that of the internal tissues. Normal skin resistance is many thousands of Ω, but wet skin can be as little as 1000 Ω; the internal tissues have resistances of only a few hundred Ω; for instance, the resistance between hand and foot excluding the skin resistance is about 500 Ω (Ward, 1980).

The current through the body—it is the current which is the critical factor—will depend directly on the voltage (240 V root mean square (RMS) in the UK) and inversely on the resistance ($I = V/R$), where I = intensity, V = voltage and R = resistance. Thus very much larger currents will flow if the skin is wet, because wetting greatly lowers its resistance; this explains why serious domestic accidents involving electrocution often occur in the bathroom or laundry. Applying Ohm's law the current through a 1000 Ω resistance due to 240 V would be 240 mA which is enough to cause ventricular fibrillation in the heart muscle, and could well be fatal. With dry skin having a resistance of, say, 100 000 Ω the current would be 2.4 mA, causing tingling sensations. Most of the therapeutic currents described in this chapter are applied to wetted, hence low-resistance, skin but are driven by voltages much lower than that of the mains; the maximum output from many faradic-type sources is around 40 or 50 V.

At mains frequency a current density 0.5–1 mA/cm^2 is just detectable and currents around 10 mA cause discomfort or pain. Above this level the current can cause strong painful muscle contractions and at higher levels (50–250 mA) may lead to ventricular fibrillation and hence may be fatal. Currents of still higher intensities tend to provoke complete cardiac arrest and severe heat burns (Ward, 1980). Thus it can be seen why the nature of the electrical contact with the skin is so critical; anything that lowers skin resistance allows larger currents to pass. Voltages higher than that of the mains are proportionally more dangerous because they will cause larger currents; for this reason areas in which high voltages are found, such as transformer substations, are specially protected. It must also be understood that the consequences of electrocution depend on the path the current follows in the body. Thus if the current passes from, say, a hand touching the live wire through the body to earth via the feet standing on the ground, the current then passes through the heart, lungs and abdomen and may well cause cardiac arrest and/or the cessation of respiration and thus prove fatal. Touching both contacts of a lighting socket with one finger would be likely to cause a painful shock and burns to the fingertip.

Immediate treatment of mains current shock

Firstly, the circuit must be disconnected to stop the flow of current through the victim. This may be simply a matter of switching off and unplugging, but it is important to ensure that disconnection has been made before touching the victim otherwise the rescuer may form another path to earth and also receive a shock.

Secondly, the carotid pulse and respiration should be checked. If absent the airway must be cleared, mouth-to-mouth resuscitation and external cardiac massage immediately started and assistance summoned. In all cases the victim should be medically examined as soon as possible—urgently if there has been any loss of consciousness. Musculoskeletal damage can occur as a result of abrupt muscle contraction due to the electric shock as well as cutaneous burns, which are usually evident.

Safety features of electrical apparatus supplied from the mains

The safety of electrical apparatus connected to the mains is ensured in several ways. The metal casing of the apparatus is connected to the large earth terminal of the three-pin plug and socket (see Appendix D). Thus if the live wire were to touch the casing of the machine a large current would flow to earth causing the protective fuse to 'blow' and interrupting the circuit. If an earth wire is not present, or if it is broken, and the casing becomes live, anyone touching the machine may provide a low-resistance pathway to earth.

Small portable pieces of electrical equipment such as radios and hairdriers are often double-insulated and connected to the mains by only two terminals, live and neutral. In these the casing is made of some non-conducting plastic material and the electrical conducting parts are separately insulated. Any exposed metal, such as the cutters of electric razors, is again separately insulated. All mains equipment is protected in one of these ways.

Two further safety measures are of consequence: the use of isolating transformers and core-balance relays.

In the majority of electric shocks involving the mains, current flows from the live to earth through the body tissues. This will occur because the neutral is at earth potential (see Appendix D). It is quite simple to isolate the supply to the apparatus by fitting a transformer (see Appendix C); an even-ratio transformer will give the same mains voltage. This is often referred to as making the current 'earth-free' since it is now necessary to have both terminals touching the skin for the full voltage to be applied. Since most pieces of electrotherapeutic apparatus operating from the mains need a voltage-changing transformer this earth-free condition exists in most of the circuit.

The three-wire fused mains system provides protection if the live connects to the casing but if the current is earthed through some other route which has a relatively high resistance the small currents will not cause the fuse to burn out. To provide protection in this situation a core-balanced relay can be used. The live and neutral wires are passed through a sensing coil; since an equal current in opposite directions is passing in these wires there will be no induced current in the sensing coil. If some of the current flows to earth, perhaps through a person in contact with the live wire, then current flow in the neutral wire is less than that in the live wire, inducing a small current in the sensing coil. This small current is amplified and trips a relay to cut off the mains. These devices can react very rapidly, are relatively cheap, and can be fitted as a separate unit between the power plug and the equipment.

The safety of electromedical equipment is subject to recommendations made by the British Standards Institution (BSI) and the International Electro-technical Commission (IEC). These bodies specify certain safety conditions such as the maximum permissible leakage current both normally and under fault conditions and designate the equipment accordingly. Most of the electrical stimulators referred to in this chapter (designated type BF) would have more stringent protection against delivering an electric shock than equipment to which the patient is not directly connected, electric heating pads for example, but less than the very strict precautions taken for equipment directly connected to the heart such as external cardiac pacemakers (designated type CF). The regulations are covered by BS 5724 and its amendments and supplements (section 2.10, 1988).

Electric shock or damage due to therapeutic nerve and muscle-stimulating currents

As already noted, these do not usually cause damage because the output of the machine will not permit a high-enough current. However, certain situations could lead to pain, alarm and possibly tissue damage.

If current is applied at high intensity very abruptly the sensation and pain caused are likely to frighten the patient. It will be recalled that the sensory nerves are stimulated by lower intensities than the pain nerve endings, so that high currents are more painful. Some pain may well be an appropriate part of treatment (see p. 60), but it should never provoke anxiety or fear. It has already been emphasized that the major resistance to current flow is the skin so that any break in the skin provides a low-resistance pathway and therefore a high local current density, which may be painful. Subjects become accustomed or accommodate to electrical stimulation so that high intensities are easily tolerated if the current is increased gradually over a few minutes. The term 'shock' is often used confusingly; any sudden sensory stimulation may be described as a 'shock' (psychological); this would include electric 'shock' which refers specifically to electrical injury.

There is quite widespread apprehension about contact of the body with electricity. This is doubtless partly a fear of the ill understood. However, it is also culturally engendered in many places to suggest fear (and vitalize monsters!) in old films and new videos. There are even allusions to it in literature; for example, in Shelley's *Epipyschidion*, 'Her touch was as electric poison'. These anxieties may, at first, cause the sensations due to electric currents to be perceived as painful. As current flows so the feelings become familiar and toleration rises. When applying treatment such fears must be taken into account; the patient must be carefully reassured and treatment applied initially at low intensity which can be gradually increased.

As these currents can cause strong muscle contraction it is possible that exceptionally vigorous artificially produced contraction might cause mechanical muscle or joint damage. However, such damage seems unlikely in normal tissues because of the protective mechanism of the Golgi tendon organs, and the fact that electrical muscle stimulation rarely produces a greater contraction than can be produced voluntarily. Further, there seems to be no recorded instance of such injuries happening to normal muscles and joints. With tissues that are already diseased or injured, such as partial muscle rupture, overstrong muscle contraction could be damaging. It is also possible that muscle contraction could dislodge the attachment of a deep vein thrombus, causing an embolus. Prolonged and intensive electrical muscle stimulation can lead to muscle soreness like that due to voluntary activity (Hon Sun Lai *et al.*, 1988).

It is recommended (Wadsworth and Chanmugan, 1980) that infected or inflamed areas should not be treated with low-frequency currents because there is a risk of spreading the infection. This is presumably due to the muscle-pumping effect; there seems no other reason why infection should spread. Certainly, as far as acute inflammation is concerned, any increased activity would be undesirable.

Since these currents provoke nerve impulses it is often recommended that areas in which autonomic nerves might be inappropriately stimulated should be avoided; for example, the region of the carotid sinus (Frampton, 1988). Similarly, treatment close to the pregnant uterus might provoke undesirable uterine movements. While neither circumstance appears to have been reported it would seem proper to be cautious.

If haemorrhage, either on the surface or in the tissues, is occurring or likely to occur then electrical stimulation by causing muscle movement and vasodilation could prevent or disrupt clotting; it should therefore be avoided.

Although there appears to be no evidence for this effect it is usual and reasonable to avoid direct treatment of neoplastic tissue in case metastasis is provoked, or growth encouraged.

Currents applied in the region of an implanted cardiac pacemaker could alter the stimulus leading to cardiac arrhythmia. A separate slight risk is of the electromagnetic field generated by the therapeutic stimulator interfering with demand-type pacemakers; this is a remote possibility with almost any piece of electrical equipment.

A significant danger arises from failure to recognize when the current applied is a direct current, or has a direct current component: with sufficient charge an electrochemical burn can result. Even extremely low current densities, such as that from some TENS machines, can have this effect given sufficient time. In most circumstances the patient's sensation warns of this danger and nothing more than skin irritation occurs. Electrochemical burns seem to develop because the sensations of burning and pain experienced by the patient due to the current are not particularly sharp. There may also be a gradual increase of current, due to falling skin resistance, to which the patient accommodates. It is therefore important that adequate explanation and warning should be given to the patient before treatment and careful checks made during treatment. It is essential that the physiotherapist knows if there is any direct current component in the treatment being applied.

Treatment of insensitive skin or of a particularly tolerant and tough-minded patient could lead to damage (see Chapter 2).

CONTRAINDICATIONS

Contraindications to electrical stimulation may be summarized as circumstances in which:

1 Strong muscle contraction might cause joint or muscle damage; detachment of a thrombus; spread of infection, and haemorrhage.
2 Stimulation of autonomic nerves might cause altered cardiac rhythm or other autonomic effects.
3 Currents might be unduly localized due to open wounds or skin lesions, e.g. eczema.
4 Currents might provoke undesirable metabolic activity in neoplasms or in healed tuberculous infections.
5 Current is not evenly biphasic, leading to possible skin damage or irritation, especially if there is loss of sensation.

REFERENCES

Alon G. (1987). Principles of electrical stimulation. In *Clinical Electrotherapy* (Nelson R. M., Currier D. P., eds) Norwalk, Connecticut USA: Appleton and Lange, pp. 29–80.

Axelgaard J., Brown J. C. (1983). Lateral electrical surface stimulation for the treatment of progressive idiopathic scoliosis. *Spine*, **8**, 242.

Baker L. L. (1987). Clinical uses of neuromuscular electrical stimulation. In *Clinical Electrotherapy* (Nelson R. M., Currier D. P., eds) Norwalk, Connecticut, USA: Appleton and Lange, pp. 115–39.

Baker L. L., Yeh C., Wilson D. *et al.* (1979). Electrical stimulation of wrist and fingers for hemiplegic patients. *Phys. Ther.*, **59**, 1495–9.

Bowsher D. (1988). Modulation of nociceptive input. In *Pain: Management and Control in Physiotherapy* (Wells P. E., Frampton V., Bowsher D., eds) London: Heinemann Medical Books, pp. 30–6.

Currier D. P. (1987). Electrical stimulation for improving muscular strength and blood flow. In *Clinical Electrotherapy* (Nelson R. M., Currier D. P., eds) Norwalk, Connecticut, USA: Appleton and Lange, pp. 141–64.

Currier D. P., Petrilli C. R., Threlkeld A. J. (1986). Effects of medium frequency electrical stimulation on local blood circulation to healthy muscle. *Phys. Ther.*, **66**, 937–43.

De Domenico G. (1982). Pain relief with interferential current. *Aust. J. Physiother.*, **28**, 14–18.

De Domenico G., Strauss G. R. (1986). Maximum torque production in the quadriceps femoris muscle group using a variety of electrical stimulators. *Aust. J. Physiother.*, **32**, 51–6.

Eckerson L. F., Axelgaard J. (1984). Lateral electrical surface stimulation as an alternative to bracing in the treatment of idiopathic scoliosis: treatment protocol and patient acceptance. *Phys. Ther.*, **64**, 483.

Eriksson E., Haggmark T. (1979). Comparison of isometric muscle training and electrical stimulation supplementing isometric muscle training in the recovery after major knee ligament surgery. *Am. J. Sports Med.*, **17**, 169.

Eriksson M., Schuller H. (1978). Hazard from transcutaneous nerve stimulation in patients with pacemakers. *Lancet*, **i**, 1219.

Farragher D. J., Kidd G. L., Tallis R. G. (1987). Eutrophic electrical stimulation for Bell's palsy. *Clin. Rehab.* **1**, 256–71.

Frampton V. (1988). Transcutaneous electrical nerve stimulation and chronic pain. In

Pain: Management and Control in Physiotherapy (Wells P. E., Frampton V., Bowsher D., eds) London: Heinemann Medical Books, pp. 89–112.

Gibson J. N. A., Smith, K., Rennie M. J. (1988). Prevention of disuse muscle atrophy by means of electrical stimulation: maintenance of protein synthesis. *Lancet*, **ii**, 767–9.

Gilles N., Bélanger A. Y. (1987). Rélation entre la force maximale volontaire, force tatanique et douleur lors de l'éléctrostimulation du quadriceps fémoris. *Physiother. Canada*, **39**, 377–82.

Grisogono V. (1989). Physiotherapy treatment for Achilles tendon injuries. *Physiotherapy*, **75**, 562–72.

Hervik J. B. (1989). Rebox II. *Physiotherapy*, **75**, 417.

Health Protection Branch of Health and Welfare Canada (1988). *Physiother. Canada*, **40**, 205–6.

Hon Sun Lai, De Domenico G., Strauss G. R. (1988). The effect of different electromotor stimulation training intensities on strength improvement. *Aust. J. Physiother.*, **34**, 151–64.

Hnik P. (1962). Rate of denervation muscle atrophy. In *The Denervated Muscle* (Gutmann E. ed.) pp. 341–75. Prague: Publishing House of Czechoslovakia.

Johnson D. H., Thurston P., Ashcroft P. J. (1977). The Russian technique of faradism in the treatment of chondromalacia patellae. *Physiother. Canada*, **29**, 266–8.

Kidd G. L., Oldham J. A., Stanley J. K. (1988). Eutrophic electrotherapy and atrophied muscle: a pilot clinical trial. *Clin. Rehab.*, **2**, 219–30.

Kidd G. L., Oldham J. A. (1988a) Motor unit action potential (MUAP) sequence and electrotherapy. *Clin. Rehab.*, **2**, 23–33.

Kidd G. L., Oldham J. A. (1988b). An electrotherapy based on the natural sequence of motor unit action potential; a laboratory trial. *Clin. Rehab.*, **2**, 125–38.

Kidd G. L., Oldham J. A., Stanley J. K. (1989). A comparison of uniform and eutrophic electrotherapies in a procedure of clinical rehabilitation of some hand movements in arthritics. *Clin. Rehab.* **3**, 27–39.

Klein J., Pariser D. (1987). Transcutaneous electrical nerve stimulation. In *Clinical Electrotherapy* (Nelson R. M., Currier P. D., eds.) Norwalk, Connecticut: Appleton and Lange, pp. 209–30.

Kloth L. (1987). Interference current. In *Clinical Electrotherapy* (Nelson R. M., Currier P. D., eds.) Norwalk, Connecticut: Appleton and Lange, pp. 183–207.

Kloth L. C., Feedar J. A. (1988). Acceleration of wound healing with high voltage, monophasic, pulsed current. *Phys. Ther.*, **68**, 503–8.

Lagassé P. P., Roy M. A. (1989). Functional electrical stimulation and the reduction of co-contraction in spastic biceps brachii. *Clin. Rehab.*, **3**, 111–16.

Laycock J., Green R. J. (1988). Interferential therapy in the treatment of incontinence. *Physiotherapy*, **74**, 161–8.

Lloyd T., De Domenico G., Strauss G. R. *et al.* (1986). A review of the use of the electro-motor stimulation in human muscle. *Aust. J. Physiother.*, **32**, 18–30.

McQuire W. A. (1975). Electrotherapy and exercises for stress incontinence and urinary frequency. *Physiotherapy*, **61**, 305–7.

Melzack R., Stillwell R. M., Fox E. J. (1977). Trigger points and acupuncture points for pain: correlations and implications. *Pain*, **3**, 3–23.

Melzack R., Wall P. D. (1965). Pain mechanisms: a new theory. *Science*, **150**, 971.

Meyer G. A., Fields H. L. (1972). Causalgia treated by selective large fiber stimulation of peripheral nerves. *Brain*, **95**, 163–8.

Milner-Brown H. S., Stein B. B. (1975). The relation between the surface electromyogram and muscular force. *J. Physiol.*, **246**, 549.

Montgomery E., Shepherd A. M. (1983). Electrical stimulation and graded pelvic exercise for genuine stress incontinence. *Physiotherapy*, **68**, 112.

Nelson H., Smith M., Bowman B. *et al.* (1980). Electrode effectiveness during transcutaneous motor stimulation. *Arch. Phys. Med. Rehab.*, **61**, 73–7.

Newton R. (1987). High voltage pulsed galvanic stimulation: theoretical bases and clinical applications. In *Clinical Electrotherapy* (Nelson R. M., Currier D. P., eds.) Norwalk, Connecticut: Appleton and Lange, pp. 165–82.

Pärtan J., Schmid J., Warum F. (1953). The treatment of inflammatory and degenerative joint conditions with interferential alternating currents of medium frequency. *Wien. Klin. Wochenschr.*, **31**, 624–8.

Paterson R. P. (1983). Instrumentation for electrotherapy. In *Therapeutic Electricity and Ultra-violet Radiation* (Stillwell K., ed.) Baltimore: Williams & Wilkins, pp. 65–108.

Quirk A. S., Newman R. J., Newman K. J. (1985). An evaluation of interferential therapy, shortwave diathermy and exercise in the treatment of osteoarthrosis of the knee. *Physiotherapy*, **71**, 55–7.

Rennie S. (1988). Diadynamic current therapy. In *Current Physical Therapy* (Peat M., ed.) Toronto: B. C. Decker, pp. 207–11.

Salmons S., Vbrova G. (1969). The influence of activity on some contractile characteristics of mammalian fast and slow muscles. *J. Physiol.*, **210**, 535–49.

Santiesteban A. J. (1981). Application of transcutaneous electrical nerve stimulation for post-operative, cardiopulmonary and obstetric patients. In *Electrotherapy* (Wolf S. L., ed.) London: Churchill Livingstone, pp. 179–97.

Savage B. (1984). *Interferential Therapy*. London: Faber & Faber.

Scott O. M., Vrbova G., Hyde S. A. *et al.* (1985). Effects of chronic low frequency electrical stimulation on normal tibial anterior muscle. *J. Neuro. Psych. Psychiatry*, **48**, 774–81.

Singer K. P. (1986). The influence of unilateral electrical muscle stimulation on motor unit activity patterns in atrophic human quadriceps. *Aust. J. Physiother.*, **32**, 31–7.

Sjölund B. H., Eriksson M. B. E. (1979). The influence of naloxone on analgesia produced by peripheral conditioning stimulation. *Brain Res.*, **173**, 295–301.

Soo C. L., Currier D. P., Threlkeld J. A. (1988). Augmenting voluntary torque of healthy muscles by optimization of electrical stimulation. *Phys. Ther.*, **68**, 3.

Spielholz N. (1987). Electrical stimulation of denervated muscle. In *Clinical Electrotherapy* (Nelson R. M., Currier D. P., eds) Norwalk, Connecticut: Appleton and Lange, pp. 97–113.

Stephens W. G. S. (1965). The use of triangular pulses in electrotherapy. *Physiotherapy*, **51**, 147–50.

Stokes M., Cooper R. (1989). Muscle fatigue as a limiting factor in functional electrical stimulation: a review. *Physiother. Pract.*, **5**, 83–90.

Strauss G. R., De Domenico G. (1986). Torque production in human upper and lower limb muscles with voluntary and electrically stimulated contractions. *Aust. J. Physiother.*, **32**, 38–49.

Sunderland D. S. (1978). *Nerves and Nerve Injuries* 2nd edn. Edinburgh: Churchill Livingstone.

Thorsteinsson G. (1983). Electrical stimulation for analgesia. In *Therapeutic Electricity and Ultra-violet Radiation* (Stillwell K., ed.) Baltimore: Williams & Wilkins, pp. 109–23.

Thorsteinsson G., Stonnington H. H., Stillwell G. K. *et al.* (1977). Transcutaneous electrical stimulation: a double blind trial of its efficacy for pain. *Arch. Phys. Med. Rehab.*, **58**, 8–13.

Tracy J. E., Currier D. P., Threlkeld A. J. (1988). Comparison of selected pulse frequencies from two different electrical stimulators on blood flow in healthy subjects. *Phys. Ther.*, **68**, 1526–32.

Wadsworth H., Chanmugan A. P. P. (1980). *Electrophysical Agents in Physiotherapy* 2nd edn. Marrickville, NSW, Australia: Science Press.

Ward A. (1980). Electricity fields and waves in therapy. Marrickville, NSW, Australia: Science Press.

4.

Evaluation and diagnosis

THE USE OF ELECTRIC CHARGES IN EVALUATION AND DIAGNOSIS

There are two major approaches. Firstly, much information can be gained by measuring the potentials generated by nerve and muscle activity, as noted in Chapter 1. Thus the electrocardiogram (ECG), the electroencephalogram (EEG) and the electromyogram (EMG) are used to study the electrical activity in these tissues. EMG will be considered further. Secondly, information can be gained by stimulating the nerve or muscle with an appropriate electrical pulse and assessing the result. This assessment may be made either by observing the muscle contractions that result or by measuring the electrical response of the muscle or nerve by, for example, the electromyographic record. This latter method allows the time between the stimulus and response to be measured precisely, giving valuable information about the nerve conduction velocity: this method is often called 'evoked action potentials'. They can be divided into motor or sensory conduction velocity tests, electronic reflex tests (such as the H reflex), and centrally evoked responses in which conduction velocities across part of the central nervous system (CNS) are measured. Those tests that involve observation of the muscle contraction have traditionally been the province of the physiotherapist.

Summary

1 Assessment of nerve and muscle potentials: EMG, voluntary and involuntary, used for both diagnosis and re-education.
2 Assessment of results of stimulating nerve and muscle
    a Observing muscle contraction
        i   Establish whether muscle contraction is evident or not.
        ii Establish whether there is nerve continuity or not—nerve excitability.
        iii Establish muscle innervation by strength–duration test—detect innervation changes with time.
    b Evoked potentials
        i   Motor nerve conduction velocity.
        ii Sensory nerve conduction velocity.
        iii Electronic reflex tests.
        iv Evoked responses from CNS.

PATHOLOGICAL CHANGES IN PERIPHERAL NERVES

There are many different ways in which the peripheral nerve may be damaged by injury or disease but conduction in the nerve fibre can only be affected in three ways:

1 It can be slowed, which is usually due to the myelin sheath being affected;
2 It can be stopped over a small section of the nerve fibre—a local block—so that conduction above and below is normal;
3 It can be stopped over the whole distal length of the nerve from the site of injury to skin and muscle.

Temporary mild compression of the nerve will lead to a conduction block, called a *neurapraxia*, due simply to displacement of the myelin sheath and local oedema of the nerve fibre itself. As there is no permanent damage recovery occurs rapidly in a few days or weeks. Since only a section of the nerve fibre is affected conduction beyond the blockage is normal; thus electrical stimulation of motor nerve fibres beyond (distal to) the block will cause muscle contraction. Nerve impulses, however, cannot pass across the block so that electrical stimulation applied proximal to the block does not result in muscle contraction. It must be realized that in an affected mixed peripheral nerve only a proportion of the fibres may be involved; the large-diameter fast-conducting fibres are most susceptible to disruption. Clinically, therefore, a neuropraxia can be a partial block with some conduction across the affected region; the more severe lesions will leave a larger number of nerve fibres affected. Thus the severity of the damage can be quantified, to some extent, by measuring the current intensity (or voltage) needed to provoke a given muscle contraction, as more current is needed to stimulate sufficient of the remaining conducting fibres. This is described below as a nerve excitability test.

If the compression injury is more severe it may cause sufficient damage to the nerve axon so that it is unable to support the metabolic processes of its distal part, resulting in degeneration of the whole length of the nerve fibre, including the myelin sheath, distal to the lesion. This process is called Wallerian degeneration. It takes some days to extend throughout the distal part of the nerve so that for perhaps 3 or 4 days or more the distal section of the nerve remains excitable and can conduct impulses. The fibrous framework of the bundle of nerve fibres remains intact and fills with a chain of Schwann cells so that ultimately nerve fibrils sprouting from the intact proximal part of the nerve are guided in their proper channels to reform the complete nerve processes. This kind of injury is called an *axonotmesis*. The length of time needed for full recovery to occur will depend on the site of the lesion and the length of nerve that has to regrow. The rate of regrowth is somewhat variable, being more rapid at first, up to 5 mm/day, but is usually considered to be on average 1–2 mm/day.

If, instead of compression, the injury is such as to disrupt all tissues of the nerve fibre—such as a cut through the nerve—then the distal segment will degenerate completely, as described already. Since the tissues are totally disrupted the axon filaments will not readily find correct channels down which to regrow so that recovery is at best imperfect. This lesion is called a *neurotmesis*. Such lesions often require surgery to ensure that the two cut ends are sufficiently approximated to allow successful regrowth.

If the nerve cell is damaged by injury or disease all its processes (the peripheral nerve) will suffer and may completely degenerate—an axonotmesis. If the cell dies so will its processes. These points are illustrated in Figure 4.1.

Various toxins, some produced by bacteria or viruses, some due to ingested or inhaled poisons (alcohol or heavy metals) may act systemically to cause damage to a large number of peripheral nerves throughout the body. It is often the myelin sheath that is most affected, reducing the conduction velocities of the large-diameter nerves. This occurs in diseases grouped as the polyneurites, of which the most widely recognized is the Guillain–Barré syndrome.

It can be seen that some nerve lesions may be mixtures, with some fibres being completely interrupted while others suffer only a neurapraxia which leads to different effects on nerve conduction. Electrical tests can elucidate these differences and contribute to making decisions about the prognosis.

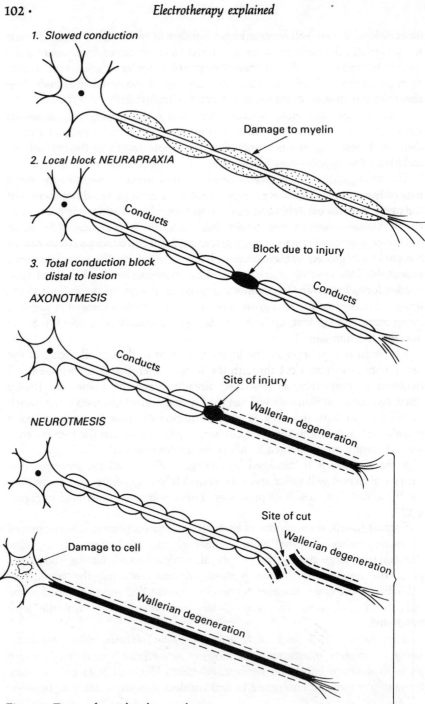

Fig. 4.1 Types of peripheral nerve lesions.

ASSESSMENT OF NERVE AND MUSCLE POTENTIALS

Electromyography

Electromyography involves detecting, amplifying and displaying the electrical changes that occur when a muscle contracts. The signals are tiny, a few microvolts, but are amplified about a thousand times to give millivolt values that can be displayed on an oscilloscope, operate a loudspeaker and be recorded on a chart.

The alpha motor neuron from each anterior horn cell branches at its termination in the muscle to supply a number of individual muscle fibres scattered throughout the muscle. This whole arrangement of neuron and muscle fibres is called a motor unit (Fig. 4.2). The number of muscle fibres served by a single neuron varies; a small number of muscle fibres per nerve are present in those muscles that are concerned with precise control of movement, such as the ocular muscles which may have only five or 10 fibres in each motor unit; large postural muscles on the other hand may have up to 1500 fibres per

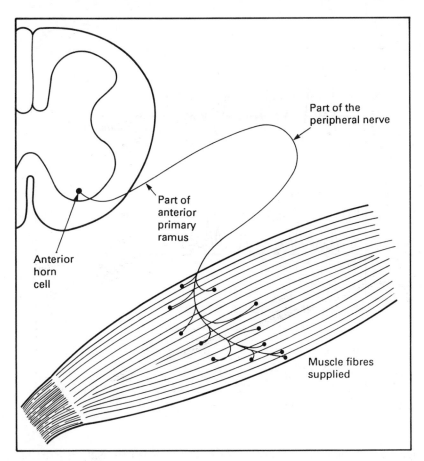

Fig. 4.2 A single motor unit.

motor unit (Williams and Yates, 1973). In normal voluntary activity several motor units are activated asynchronously, resulting in a smooth muscle contraction.

When a normal muscle contracts all the individual muscle fibres of the motor unit depolarize (and then repolarize) at the same time causing a local electrical disturbance in the muscle. This can be detected either by electrodes on the skin or by a needle electrode inserted into the muscle. Surface electrodes are often silver/silver chloride, coated with a suitable conducting gel, and can be taped on to the skin. Needle electrodes consist of fine wires, insulated save at the tip, which are inserted into the chosen muscle by means of a hypodermic needle. In both cases the electrical disturbance recorded is the

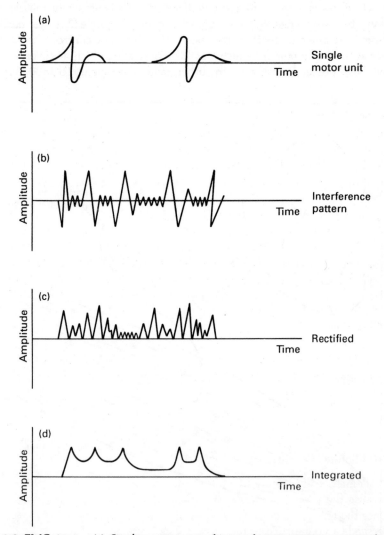

Fig. 4.3 EMG traces. (a) Single motor unit; (b) interference pattern; (c) rectified; (d) integrated.

sum of the potentials due to all the muscle fibres activated. Thus activation of a single motor unit can be recognized because the many muscle fibres contract at nearly the same time producing a single characteristic trace on the recording (Fig. 4.3). The amplitude and duration of this trace vary depending on the number of muscle fibres in the motor unit and how they are oriented in relation to the electrode. Normal motor units give an amplitude of between 0.5 and 3 mV and an average duration of about 4 ms, but may last up to 10 ms. When several motor units are involved the trace will show more complex activity because several motor units give overlapping signals. This is called an interference pattern (Fig. 4.3).

Since skeletal muscles are under voluntary control action potentials can be recorded from muscles during different degrees of contraction. If no muscle contraction is occurring then no electrical activity is detectable. However, in abnormal conditions potentials may be recorded when the muscle is at rest and these can be used in the diagnosis of nerve and muscle pathologies. Denervated muscle membrane becomes hypersensitive to acetylcholine causing spontaneous potentials when the muscle is at rest. These show on the electromyographic record as 1 ms potentials of low amplitude, called fibrillation potentials, the consequence of depolarization of individual muscle fibres. Various other forms of spontaneous activity, such as positive potentials and fasciculation, the spontaneous discharge of whole motor units, also occur in denervated muscle; still other forms are characteristic of muscle disease. Voluntary contraction of disordered muscle may also give a characteristic abnormal EMG record. Thus records taken during reinnervation show large polyphasic potentials. Needle electrodes are generally employed for diagnostic EMG because better localization can be achieved and deeper muscles can be reached.

The normal EMG can be employed by physiotherapists, using surface electrodes, for muscle training—a process called biofeedback (Chapter 5). This is done to train either muscle activity or relaxation. The EMGs are often modified by being rectified and integrated (Wolf, 1987) to produce a stronger average signal which can be displayed to the patient (Fig. 4.3) by a meter, loudspeaker or lights.

ASSESSMENT BY OBSERVING THE RESULTS OF STIMULATING NERVE AND MUSCLE

Muscle contraction

Establishing the integrity of a tendon

Sometimes tendon division is suspected due to injury, but cannot be verified because the patient is unable to produce a voluntary muscle contraction to tense the tendon or cause movement. For example, it may not be possible to persuade a young child to move an injured finger in circumstances where it is important to decide whether primary tendon suture is required. The appropriate muscle can be stimulated at its motor point with a suitable current; faradic-type current is usually used. The muscle pulls on the tendon producing visible movement only if the tendon is intact.

In other circumstances in which the patient may be unable voluntarily to produce muscle contraction, such as hysterical paralysis, muscle-stimulating current may be used to demonstrate normal movement, for either diagnostic or therapeutic reasons.

Establishing the continuity of a nerve

If a peripheral motor nerve is stimulated with a suitable electrical pulse at some point and the muscles that it supplies distally are seen to contract then it can be concluded that the nerve is able to conduct impulses. This is sometimes called a nerve conduction test but should not be confused with a nerve conduction velocity test (see below), which is also sometimes referred to as a nerve conduction test. For example, the ulnar nerve may be stimulated behind the medial epicondyle of the humerus to cause contraction of the hypothenar and intrinsic hand muscles as well as the flexor carpi ulnaris and part of flexor digitorum profundus. Similarly the facial (VII) nerve can be stimulated to cause all the facial muscles to contract. To some extent this can be used as a quantitative test, called a nerve excitability test, since the voltage or current needed to stimulate the normal side can be compared to that needed to give a similar muscle contraction on the affected side. Single 0.1 or 1 ms rectangular pulses with a 1 or 2 s interval between each pulse are used so that the resulting muscle twitch can be assessed. The threshold intensity (or voltage) needed to elicit a minimal muscle contraction is noted for each side. The normal difference in current intensity between the two sides (due to variations in soft tissue thickness, differences in electrode positioning, as well as natural variations in nerve excitability) is considered to lie within 2 mA (Wadsworth and Chanmugan, 1980) and is certainly less than 4 mA (Nash, 1979) for the facial nerve.

The technique used for a facial nerve lesion (Bell's palsy) assessment involves placing a dispersive electrode behind the neck with the patient lying down and applying a small stimulating electrode to the skin below the tragus of the ear just in front of the mastoid process to stimulate the facial nerve as it emerges from the stylomastoid foramen. The current (or voltage) needed to provoke a minimal contraction of the facial muscles is determined first on the normal then on the affected side. This should be repeated a few times to check the consistency of the result; the three trunks of the facial nerve may be assessed separately.

If a neuropraxia is present the difference between the two sides is within the normal variation, i.e. about 2 mA, because stimulation is applied to normally conducting nerve beyond the conduction block. If some axonotmesis is present larger currents, 4–8 mA, will be needed to stimulate sufficient of the remaining conducting fibres to produce a contraction equivalent to that on the normal side. If there is axonotmesis of all the nerve fibres then no muscle contraction will occur unless very high currents, of 10, 20 or more times that of the normal side, are used which would directly stimulate the muscle (Fig. 4.4). Several tests may be done on successive days.

The value of these tests lies in their ability to determine easily the changes in conduction in the early stages of this lesion. Thus a simple neuropraxia will show no conduction loss at any time. The need for a higher current on the affected side indicates conduction loss, hence some degree of axonotmesis, which worsens during the first few days as nerve degeneration occurs. This information would be helpful in deciding whether active decompression measures should be applied (Nash, 1979) and for determining the prognosis of the particular case.

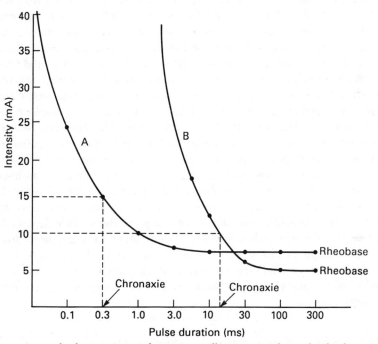

Fig. 4.4 Strength–duration curve for (a) normally innervated muscle; (b) denervated muscle.

Strength–duration (S–D) testing

This is a more sensitive way of determining neuromuscular excitability than the tests just described. The principles have already been considered to some extent in Chapter 3 and Figure 3.13. Although strength–duration tests can be used with both motor and sensory nerves, the former is much better known and more widely used and will be described below. They are known as strength–duration (or intensity–duration) curves, because of the exponential graph that is plotted.

A minimal detectable muscle contraction is used as the standard response and the current or voltage needed to elicit that response at different pulse lengths is plotted on a graph. As already considered in Chapter 3, a certain minimal amount of charge is needed to depolarize the nerve fibre membrane beyond threshold. The magnitude of the charge is a product of current intensity and the time for which it flows. Thus with shorter-duration pulses greater current intensity is needed. However, even if the stimulating pulses were to last a very long time—infinite time—there would still be a minimal amount of energy (charge) necessary to trigger the nerve impulse. Thus, for any given situation (tissue resistance, rate of pulse rise, etc.) there is a minimal current or voltage required and this is known as the *rheobase* (Fig. 4.4).

Long electrical pulses will stimulate excitable tissue, muscle and nerve at the appropriate rheobase current. For muscle tissue pulses of less than, perhaps, 1/20th of a second (50 ms) have insufficient charge at the rheobase current and must be increased to depolarize the muscle membrane; pulses of about 10 ms may need twice as much current and the current needed increases exponentially with shorter and shorter pulses. Nerve tissue, on the other hand, is much more excitable so that pulses as short as 0.1 ms are still an effective stimulus at rheobase currents; shorter pulses, however, need the same exponential current increase as muscle tissue. Therefore if the strength–duration graphs of nerve and muscle are plotted on the same scales they have the same shape but appear on different parts of the abscissa. The graph of current against pulse duration is characteristic but quantitatively different for nerve and muscle tissue. When muscles are made to contract by nerve impulses, as happens when innervated muscle is stimulated, the response will be characteristic of nerve tissue. A typical graph for innervated and denervated muscle is shown in Figure 4.4. It should be noted that such graphs differ slightly depending on whether the electrical pulses are of constant current or constant voltage. In constant-voltage graphs stimuli of somewhat shorter duration can be used before the voltage needs to be increased compared to graphs of constant current, which are said to be more accurate, although in this respect the difference is trivial.

Technique for performing strength–duration tests

The part to be tested needs to be firmly supported and the patient reassured by adequate explanation of what is to happen. Warming and wetting the skin through which current is to pass helps to lower its resistance. One electrode and pad is fixed at one end of the muscle to be tested and the other is moved until a good muscle contraction is obtained using a long duration pulse of 100 or 300 ms. Small electrodes are used to localize the current to the muscle to be tested. A hand-held button electrode with dispersive may be used but fixed electrodes, both suction and adhesive, which free the physiotherapist's hand are recommended. However, this is a matter of preference since there is little evidence for inconsistency within a single test (see below). The muscle contraction is identified visually or by palpation, or both. The pulses are applied at a rate of 1/s, or one every 2 s to allow plenty of time for muscle recovery between contractions. The intensity or voltage is then reduced until the contraction can only just be detected and this value is recorded. A shorter pulse, say 30 ms, is then applied. If the muscle contraction remains the same the strength of the pulse is recorded and a still shorter pulse is applied and so on. If the muscle contraction disappears the current is increased until it returns and is just detectable again. It is usual to take 8 or 10 points from 100 ms to 0.01 ms for constant-voltage machines and from 300 ms to 0.1 ms for constant-current stimulators. It is important to maintain constant position and constant pressure of the electrodes during the test. The current intensities that have been noted (it is often easier to have some other person to note down the readings during the test) are plotted against the appropriate pulse duration on a suitable piece of graph paper. This test does not take very long; perhaps 2–3 min.

Interpretation

The graphs produced will do more than discriminate between innervated and denervated muscle. To some extent they can quantify the state of innervation of a muscle. If only a few fibres are innervated amongst a mass of denervated fibres the first part of the graph will be typical for those denervated fibres, but at higher current intensities with shorter pulses the few innervated fibres are unmasked because the denervated fibres are no longer able to contract. Thus two curves result; one with a low rheobase due to the mass of denervated fibres and a few (masked) innervated fibres, and a second with a high rheobase due to the scattered innervated fibres—the rheobase must be high to provide enough current to reach all the innervated fibres. The typical 'kinked' curves are shown in Figure 4.5. Now the amplitude of the higher rheobase is a function of the number of innervated fibres so that if more fibres become

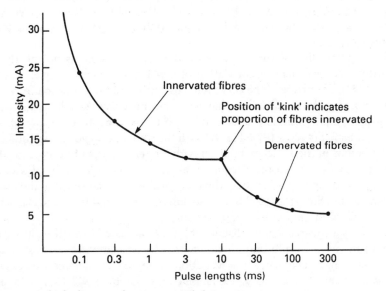

Fig. 4.5 A 'kinked' curve showing partial denervation.

innervated the 'kink' will shift downwards and vice versa. Comparison of a series of S–D curves taken at intervals can indicate progressive denervation or reinnervation.

Chronaxie

The chronaxie is an index of nerve and muscle excitability. It is the pulse duration in milliseconds needed to cause a minimal perceptible muscle contraction with a current (or voltage) of twice the rheobase. It is a very different value, i.e. longer time, for muscle compared to nerve tissue (Fig. 4.4). It is therefore a simple method of discriminating between innervated and denervated muscle. Normal innervated values vary somewhat from one muscle to another (Wadsworth and Chanmugan, 1980) but are well below 1 ms for constant-current and below 0.1 ms for constant-voltage stimulators. Denervated muscle values are around 10 ms or more.

Reliability of strength–duration curves

Since the usefulness of these curves depends on the comparison of one curve with another, it is essential that the variability and what is within normal limits can be recognized. When successive S–D curves are made by different testers on the same subject almost identical figures are obtained. Remarkably high inter-rater reliability has been demonstrated in a careful study (Nelson and Hunt, 1981) which found an average correlation coefficient between testers of 0.945. This quantifies the previously expressed view of one of us (Low, 1979) regarding the impressive consistency of repeated curves made by different testers during training sessions. It has also been shown that two testers making S–D curves for 20 different subjects achieved very similar results (Alexander, 1974). All this evidence indicates that different testers are able to make very much the same S–D curve, contrary to opinions sometimes expressed.

The repeatability of curves made on different occasions is not nearly as consistent. A coefficient of correlation of 0.541 has been found (Nelson and Hunt, 1981). The shape of the curve remains consistent but the absolute values vary. Normal plots will fall within a composite curve based on the 95% confidence limits (Nelson and Hunt, 1981) or the standard deviations (Arsenault and Stevens, 1979; Fig. 4.6). All the sources quoted above note that the variations in rheobase are minimal with longer stimuli but become greater with the higher intensities required at shorter pulse lengths. Different electrode sizes and polarity affect the numerical values and shape of the curve (Arsenault and Stevens, 1979) but these differences are not large and allow the plot to fall within a normal composite curve.

It is easy to increase the reliability of S–D curves and test the 'fit' into a composite curve by plotting all the curves to be compared on a standard rheobase, which eliminates the variations due to the different rheobases (Richardson and Wynn Parry, 1957). Since the rheobase will vary with skin resistance, electrode pressure, the presence of oedema and other factors, this is

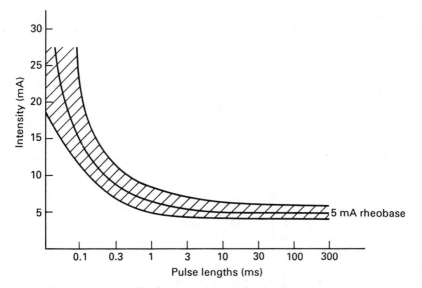

Fig. 4.6 Composite strength–duration curve indicating the area within which all normal curves would lie. Based loosely on 95% confidence limits quoted in Nelson and Hunt (1981) to illustrate the range of normal variation that might be expected about a 5 mA rheobase.

an important correction to make. All that needs to be done is to divide all readings by the rheobase, thus expressing them all as a function of the rheobase, which is unity. The idea is illustrated in Table 4.1, where the results for three graphs with different rheobases are in fact shown to be identical. Making this correction does not, of course, completely remove the variations; as noted earlier, variation is greater at shorter pulse lengths. The mathematical operation of dividing the measured values by the value of the rheobase, although simple to do by hand, is often conveniently done by the machine itself. Thus the figures can be read directly as multiples of the rheobase.

Another way of improving the usefulness of these readings is to plot the graph with the ordinate (i.e., the strength of pulse) as a logarithmic scale. This has the effect of converting the typical exponential curve into two straight lines. The point at which the graph starts to rise is therefore precisely defined. If two curves are evident, as occurs in partial denervation, the three angles— the kinks—and their positions become exactly defined. This is valuable in assessing changes in innervation, as described above (Fig. 4.7).

Comparisons are also more reliable if a constant technique is applied, that is, the electrodes are of the same size and placed in the same position for each test. Constancy is more important than technique employed. With the most careful technique there will be variations in the normal S–D curve from day to day. This is considered to be a normal physiological variation (Nelson and Hunt, 1981) and is hardly surprising when it is realized that nerve conduction velocities have been found to vary quite widely from time to time. Such variations will have little effect on the overall shape of the curve, which is the key parameter in describing nerve excitability.

Table 4.1 The same six pulse durations from three different graphs which are identical when plotted as a function of the rheobase

Pulse duration (ms)	First test		Second test		Third test	
	Reading (mA)	Function of rheobase	Reading (mA)	Function of rheobase	Reading (mA)	Function of rheobase
100	8	1	20	1	12	1
10	8	1	20	1	12	1
3	8	1	20	1	12	1
1	10	1.25	25	1.25	15	1.25
0.3	16	2	40	2	24	2
0.1	40	5	100	5	60	5

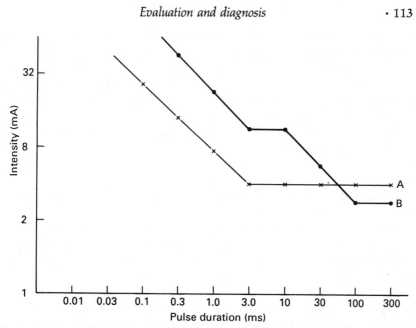

Fig. 4.7 Strength–duration graph plotted on log log scale. A = Normally innervated; B = denervated nerves.

Uses of strength–duration curves

In summary, strength–duration curves can:

1 *Demonstrate the presence of innervated fibres in the muscle being tested.* If all fibres are denervated a typical denervated curve will result. This is then said to show the 'reaction of degeneration' or RD. If a small number of fibres are innervated amongst a mass of denervated fibres a 'kinked' curve may be evident; the position of the kink is a reflection of the number of innervated fibres. If a large number, or all, of the fibres are innervated then a normal curve will result.

2 *Demonstrate changes in innervation by means of successive graphs.* This information is often critically important in the clinical situation where it may be essential to know if reinnervation is occurring. Progressive reinnervation (and denervation) is indicated by changes in the position of the kink. The appearance and movement of a kink towards the normal form in successive plots of the curve can herald reinnervation before any voluntary recovery can be detected.

3 *Indicate the value of the rheobase, chronaxie and utilization time.* As already discussed, the rheobase varies with a number of factors, such as skin resistance, position and size of stimulating electrodes, skin temperature, presence of oedema or skin atrophy and other factors. The rheobase, therefore, has limited value as an indicator of nerve excitability except when the two sides can be directly compared, as in the nerve excitability tests considered above. It should be noted that the rheobase for denervated

muscle is lower than that of innervated muscle (Stephens, 1973). The chronaxie has already been described as the pulse duration at which a current of twice the rheobase is required to elicit a twitch (Stephens, 1973); it can simply be read off the graph. It provides a single number to indicate the state of innervation. The utilization time is the duration of the shortest pulse that causes a muscle contraction with the rheobase current. If therapeutic stimulation of the muscle is to be performed it is the appropriate pulse length to use.

Strength–duration testing using accommodation or triangular pulses

The property of accommodation of nerve and muscle membranes has already been considered (Chapter 3; Fig. 3.14). If the electrical stimulus is made to rise relatively slowly the membrane threshold rises so that greater current intensities are needed to trigger the nerve impulse or muscle contraction. So far S–D curves using square wave pulses have been considered; these are described as rising almost instantaneously. If the pulse takes about 10 ms to rise, the rheobase is little changed from that due to square wave pulses for nerve membrane. However, if the current rises at such a rate that it takes 0.3 s (33 ms) to reach the square wave rheobase, then it will need twice the current to trigger the nerve impulse. If the rate of rise is just a little less the nerve threshold is not reached unless very large currents are applied. Thus there is a certain minimum rate of rise which must be exceeded if the electric pulse is to initiate the nerve impulse. The same applies to the muscle fibre membrane, except that the rate of rise must be very much slower (taking about 100 ms to reach the square wave rheobase) before the membrane can accommodate and the threshold keep up with the rising current. Thus if triangular pulses instead of rectangular pulses are used to plot an S–D curve, a somewhat different graph (U-shaped if plotted on logarithmic scales) to that of the square wave plot is seen. There is very clear discrimination between the innervated nerves with a minimum of between 1 and 10 ms and the denervated nerves with a minimum around 100–200 ms and a very much lower (5–10 times) threshold (Stephens, 1973). Such plots are very effective in discriminating between nerve and muscle (Fig. 4.8).

EVOKED POTENTIALS

In these tests the peripheral nerve is electrically stimulated and the resulting nerve impulse or muscle potential is measured. These tests can provide a measurement of the velocity of the nerve impulse and information about its amplitude and nature.

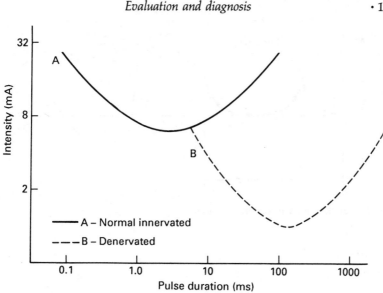

Fig. 4.8 Strength–duration curves using accommodation pulses. A = normally inner-vated; B = denervated nerves.

Nerve conduction velocity studies

Nerve conduction velocity studies are performed on peripheral nerves only, as opposed to reflex testing or centrally recorded evoked responses which involve the central nervous system. Both motor and sensory conduction velocities can be recorded. The stimulus is applied to the nerve by two small electrodes fixed on the skin about 2 or 3 cm apart. The pulse duration used can be varied from 0.05 to 2 ms; the frequency is also variable but 1 or 2 Hz is often used. The recording is made from a different set of electrodes—often silver/silver chloride of about 1 cm diameter—which are placed over the stimulated muscle or sensory nerve. Both the stimulating and response signals are displayed on an oscilloscope; some method of making a permanent record, whether photographic or pen and chart, is included. From this permanent trace conduction velocity and other measurements can be made. More sophisticated equipment is able to display such measures automatically and almost instantly.

To determine motor conduction velocity the nerve is stimulated with single pulses which will initiate impulses in many axons to activate the motor end-plates of many thousands of muscle fibres, causing a brisk muscle contraction. This can be displayed with the stimulus to show the conduction time between stimulus and the start of muscle contraction, which is called latency (Fig. 4.9). This includes the time it takes the impulse to cross the motor end-plate and provoke muscle contraction. To measure the time that is due to nerve conduction only, stimulation is given at two points along the course of a nerve. The linear distance between these two points is measured on the body surface. The latency is then found from each of the two points so that the time difference between them can be divided into the distance. This will give a

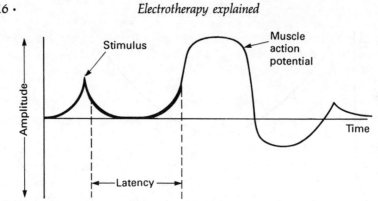

Fig. 4.9 Evoked muscle action potential.

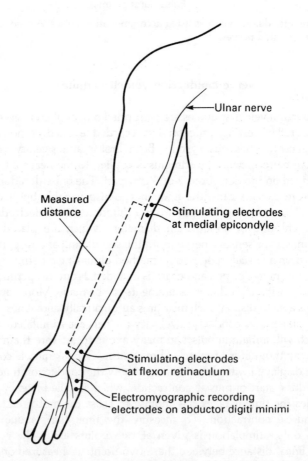

Fig. 4.10 Nerve conduction velocity calculation.

reasonably accurate conduction velocity (Fig. 4.10). For example, if stimulation of two sites 20 cm apart were to give latencies of 7 ms from the proximal and 3 ms from the distal site then the velocity would be found by: 20 cm/7–3 ms = 5 cm/ms = 50 m/s.

Conduction velocities of the two sides can be compared with published normal values. Conduction velocities are often reduced in compression lesions, such as carpal tunnel syndrome, and may indicate the diagnosis.

Sensory nerve conduction tests are performed in a similar way except that the recording is made from the nerve itself, i.e. the nerve impulses. This can be done either by stimulating at the periphery and recording from the proximal nerve trunk—the orthodromic direction—or it can be done antidromically. The nerve impulse is, of course, a much smaller electrical disturbance than the action potential of many muscle fibres acting together but with modern equipment it can easily be recorded and gives a direct measure of the conduction velocity.

Not only are the latency and velocity of nerve impulses measured but also the shape and amplitude of the impulses which may vary in some disease processes.

Electrical reflex testing

The H reflex

The H reflex refers to testing a stretch reflex, such as the ankle jerk, by electrically stimulating the afferent (Ia) fibres from the muscle spindles. A tap on the tendon causes stretch of the muscle and hence muscle spindles, which send impulses through a monosynaptic reflex in the spinal cord to cause a muscle twitch. If the nerve proximal to the muscle, e.g. the posterior tibial nerve for the tendocalcaneous reflex, is stimulated with a low-intensity short (say 0.1 ms) pulse the Ia afferent nerves can be selectively stimulated. The current must be kept below the threshold for the alpha motor neuron fibres, otherwise these will directly initiate a muscle twitch and the reflex will be lost. Thus the afferent side of the stretch reflex is stimulated beyond the spindles, leading to a muscle twitch which is recorded electromyographically and appears after a delay of approximately 30 ms (Nelson, 1987).

The reflex is most evident in those muscles that have many muscle spindles. It can be used to assess conduction rates. This is useful if nerve compression in the intervertebral foramen is suspected since peripheral nerve conduction velocity through this region cannot otherwise be assessed. The H of this reflex refers to Hoffman who first suggested the test; it should not be confused with the Hoffman reflex. The blink reflex has also been examined by electrical stimulation in a somewhat similar way.

The F wave

The F wave is not strictly a reflex. If motor nerves are strongly stimulated

Electrotherapy explained

electrically and the resulting muscle membrane potentials are carefully recorded electromyographically a small inconsistent potential is seen to follow some 30 ms after the main muscle contraction. This is thought to be due to the antidromic impulses set up in the motor nerves provoking a further orthodromic response when they reach and stimulate the anterior horn cells (Echternach, 1981).

Evoked potentials in the CNS

Electrical potentials can be recorded with the use of modern sensitive electronic equipment from sites over the spinal cord, brainstem and cortex. The impulses passing in nerve tracts produce an electrical disturbance which can be measured at the body surface. The amplitude of this measured signal is due to the sum of all the action potentials occurring at that time. It has been calculated that changes of around 100 mV in a nerve fibre would result in a change of a few microvolts on the nearest body surface (Lehmkuhl, 1981).

A stimulus is applied outside the CNS, either by electrical stimulation of a peripheral nerve or by direct stimulation of a sense organ, and this stimulus is exactly timed and repeated. The consequent responses of a series of such stimuli are added together electronically so that the random noise signals cancel one another out but any response repeated at exactly the same time after the stimulus is enhanced and becomes clearly evident.

In general, diseases involving demyelination are characterized by lower conduction velocities, hence longer latencies, whereas those involving loss of neurons are associated with a lower signal amplitude.

Spinal-evoked potentials

Recording electrodes are placed on the skin over the spinous processes at appropriate levels and a peripheral nerve is stimulated. For instance, the tibial nerve may be stimulated in the popliteal space and recordings made from electrodes over the lower thoracic spinous processes. Similarly, mechanical stimulation of sensory receptors may be used as the exciting stimulus.

Evoked potentials recorded from the sensory cortex

Recording electrodes are fixed to the scalp over the region of the sensory cortex and a peripheral nerve on the opposite side of the body is stimulated. The major response recorded from, say, the median nerve may occur some 15–20 ms after the stimulus more generalized responses also occur.

Visual-evoked potentials

Recordings are made from electrodes placed over the occipital region and provoked either by flashes of light or by pattern reversals. The eyes can be tested separately and compared. Demyelinating diseases such as multiple sclerosis can lead to increased latency.

REFERENCES

Alexander J. (1974). Reproducibility of strength–duration curves. *Arch. Phys. Med. Rehab.*, **55**, 56–60.

Arsenault A. B., Stevens J. (1979). A study of the variability of the strength–duration curve parameters. *Physiother. Canada*, **31**, 125–30.

Basmajian J. V. (1974). *Muscles Alive: Their Functions Revealed by Electromyography*, Baltimore: Williams and Wilkins.

Echternach J. L. (1981). The use of conduction velocity measurements as an evaluative tool. In *Electrotherapy* (Wolf S., ed.) London: Churchill Livingstone, pp. 73–97.

Lehmkuhl L. D. (1981). Evoked spinal, brainstem and cerebral potentials. In *Electrotherapy* (Wolf S. L., ed.) London: Churchill Livingstone, pp. 123–54.

Low J. (1979). A review of the uses and reliability of strength–duration curves. *N.Z. J. Physiother.*, **13**, 16–20.

Nash J. D. (1979). Prognostic nerve conduction test. *Physiotherapy*, **65**, 82.

Nelson R. M. (1987). Electrophysiologic evaluation: an overview. In *Clinical Electrotherapy* (Nelson R. M., Currier D. P., eds.) Norwalk, Connecticut: Appleton and Lange, pp. 243–57.

Nelson R. M., Hunt G. C. (1981). Strength–duration curve; intrarater and interrater reliability. *Phys. Ther.*, **61**, 894–7.

Richardson A. T., Wynn-Parry C. B. (1957). The theory and practice of electrodiagnosis. *Am. Phys. Med.* **4**, 3–16.

Stephens W. G. S. (1973). The assessment of muscle denervation by electrical stimulation. *Physiotherapy*, **59**, 292–4.

Wadsworth H., Chanmugan A. P. P. (1980). Electrophysical agents in physiotherapy. Marrickville, NSW, Australia: Science Press.

Williams N. E., Yates D. A. H. (1973). Electrodiagnosis and electromyography. *Physiotherapy*, **59**, 288–91.

Wolf D. (1987). Electromyographic biofeedback: an overview. In *Clinical Electrotherapy* (Nelson R. M., Currier D. P. eds.) Norwalk, Conn.: Appleton and Lange, pp. 259–78.

5.   *Biofeedback*

Uses of biofeedback
   Biofeedback for the control of muscle activity and movement
      Uses of EMG biofeedback for motor control
      Application of EMG biofeedback
      Other forms of biofeedback for control of activity
   Biofeedback for the treatment of stress-related conditions
      Essential hypertension
      Cardiac arrhythmias
      Raynaud's disease
      Migraine
      Tension headache
      Epilepsy
   Technique of application of temperature biofeedback
Effectiveness of biofeedback
Evaluation of EMG biofeedback for muscle control

The word 'feedback' has been defined (Wiener, 1948) as 'a method of controlling the system by re-inserting into it the results of its past perform-ance'. This concept has already been considered in Chapter 3 as 'negative feedback' in which a deviation of the system in one direction leads to a correction of this deviation. Biofeedback refers to the application of this idea, originally reported in engineering, to biological systems and specifically to the conscious control of some of those systems which are usually considered to be autonomically (automatically) regulated.

As an example, the temperature of the skin of the fingers is under sympathetic regulation which is largely dependent on the local and general environmental temperature, as described in Chapter 7. If a sensitive skin thermometer is applied to the skin of the finger most people are able to make a small alteration of the skin temperature at will (Fig. 5.1). This may take a little time and some practice but can be done providing the subject can see the thermometer reading and thus has immediate information of any change in skin temperature; this is the 'feedback'.

Many physiological changes of which people are normally unaware can be made visible or audible with suitable electronic instruments. This has enabled biofeedback control to be practised for a whole range of activities such as the control of blood pressure, heart rate, skin temperature but principally for the contraction and relaxation of voluntary muscle electromyographically.

The concept can be expressed in principle by the feedback loop shown in Table 5.1. The physiological change is detected or measured by some device, e.g. the skin temperature alters the resistance of the thermistor. The output of this measurement is displayed on a digital indicator, the subject perceives this information about the temperature and he or she now makes conscious

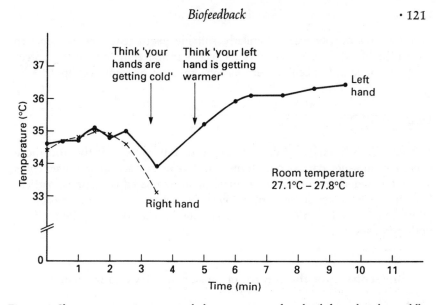

Fig. 5.1 Skin temperature as recorded over 10 min for the left and right middle fingers of a 58-year-old normal subject. Room temperature was 27.1–27.8°C.

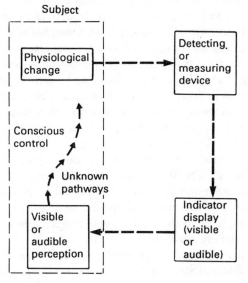

Table 5.1 Feedback loop

attempts to alter it, i.e. to warm or cool the finger (Fig. 5.1). Exactly which neuronal pathways are involved in this last part of the loop is not understood but the fact that it is possible to exert some control, albeit to a limited extent, indicates that such pathways exist.

This is not different in principle from the re-education given by physiotherapists in providing feedback for the correction of posture or the initiation of a muscle contraction. The development of relatively cheap electronic circuitry allows electromyography with surface electrodes to record motor unit action potentials reasonably easily. Similarly suitable instruments are available to record the blood pressure, heart rate (electrocardiograph) and electric potentials developed in the central nervous system (electroencephalograph).

USES OF BIOFEEDBACK

Biofeedback is used for two separate broad purposes: firstly, for those conditions in which control over some defective muscle action or movement is attempted and secondly, for the control of stress-related conditions, particularly those in which some control over the autonomic nervous system is attempted. There is some overlap in that muscle relaxation may be used for both purposes.

Biofeedback for the control of muscle activity and movement

The method used in this context is electromyographic biofeedback. It will be recalled from Chapter 4 that diagnostic use can be made of the electrical signals generated when a motor unit fires. (A motor unit comprises the axon of an anterior horn cell and its several branches to individual muscle fibres; Fig. 4.2.) When one of these fires, the muscle fibres it supplies all contract together causing an electrical disturbance called the motor unit action potential. When a muscle contracts normally many hundreds of these motor units fire asynchronously, producing electrical potentials which can be detected either by needle electrodes in the muscle tissue or from surface electrodes. These signals can be displayed on an oscilloscope screen or recorded on a strip of paper (chart recorder) as well as being fed to a loudspeaker to generate a series of audible clicks, as explained in Chapter 4 (see also Fig. 4.3). The electromyographic display bears an approximate relationship to the magnitude of the muscle contraction causing it. The relationship is quite complicated because the muscle unit action potentials that occur will not all be equally detected and recorded. However for biofeedback purposes the overall effect of stronger contractions leading to more and louder clicks, merging into a roar, and a large display on the screen are adequate.

Electromyographic machines specifically built for biofeedback usually provide both audible and visual outputs, the latter often as a moving meter needle rather than an oscilloscope trace. The smooth movement of the needle is achieved by rectifying and averaging the motor unit electrical activity from the muscles, thus producing an output which varies smoothly with the average muscle activity (Fig. 4.3). Surface electrodes are usually used so that localization of the electromyogram (EMG) signal is not exact. It is also only applicable for reasonably superficial muscles.

Uses of EMG biofeedback for motor control

The majority of published accounts of the use of EMG biofeedback have been for the *treatment of hemiplegic patients*; most commonly as attempts to re-educate controlled dorsiflexion of the foot and thus improve the gait. This can involve two approaches: encouraging activity in the tibialis anterior and other dorsiflexors and/or discouraging the unwanted spasticity of the plantarflexors. Biofeedback can be applied to any superficial muscle of the hemiplegic patient; the deltoid has been treated in order to improve shoulder control, for example. Most studies have found biofeedback to be a successful method of treatment; some found it more successful than conventional treatment (e.g. Basmajian *et al.*, 1975). However, not all patients appear able to improve with biofeedback and it is difficult to separate any specific gain from that due to the enthusiasm engendered by any new treatment. One striking point that emerged from several studies was the extent to which improvement occurred with any treatment in patients who had been selected on the assumption that further improvement was unlikely (Marcer, 1986).

Attempts have been made to *reduce and control spasticity* from causes other than cerebrovascular accidents, e.g. head injury, multiple sclerosis or cerebral palsy. In the case of cerebral palsied children teaching the technique of biofeedback may be difficult and any improvement may be particularly hard to distinguish from that due to growth and maturation. It should be noted that in all neurological disorders treated by biofeedback it is assumed that there are some intact neuronal pathways available to suppress the spasticity. If this is known not to be the case—in a complete transection of the spinal cord, for example—biofeedback would be pointless.

Dystonic conditions in which the patient suffers uncontrollable movements or postures have also been treated by EMG biofeedback (Moon, 1980). Spasmodic torticollis is the most widely known of these conditions and has been treated by biofeedback to the sternocleidomastoid muscles. This has enabled patients voluntarily to inhibit the forceful inappropriate neck movements and proved to be a successful treatment given the intractable nature of the condition.

Writer's cramp and blepharospasm are other dystonias which have been treated with biofeedback (Marcer, 1986).

As might be expected, biofeedback has been used in the treatment of *recovering peripheral nerve injuries*. Once motor unit activity has been detected on the electromyograph voluntary repetition can be encouraged. This use nicely illustrates the point that the principle of biofeedback is used in physiotherapy without its being described as such. Once a trivial muscle contraction or a flicker can be detected manually the physiotherapist encourages the patient to further effort, thus providing the feedback by recognizing the muscle contraction and informing the patient. What EMG biofeedback provides is a means of extending the recognition to the least possible motor activity (single motor unit) and of quantifying it to some extent. In cases of nerve transplant biofeedback can be used to help the patient learn the new muscle action. Notice that this contrasts with and complements the use of muscle-stimulating currents (see Chapter 3) to provoke artificial muscle contraction of the newly innervated muscle which the patient attempts to copy. Biofeedback informs the patient when he or she is making the correct response.

Training specific muscle activity: after trauma to a muscle or its attachments or after a tendon or muscle transplant it may not be possible for the patient to perform a particular voluntary movement. Similarly some voluntary movements which are therapeutically useful, such as abduction of the great toe, are not easy for some patients to perform at will. In all these circumstances biofeedback can be used provided the muscle is sufficiently superficial to give a reasonably isolated output. In all cases the patient is able to detect from the EMG output when the voluntary effort is producing a contraction in the appropriate muscle.

Posture control: for this, monitors are worn which signal tilt away from the vertical. The inclination monitor is worn on the trunk and the head-position trainer is worn as a helmet.

Biofeedback has also been utilized in the treatment of patients with functional breathing disorders such as hyperventilation or shallow breathing (Moon, 1981). A medical gas analyser (mass spectrometer) was used to measure the partial pressure of carbon dioxide in the expired air. The patient was shown how varying the respiration rate altered the amount of expired carbon dioxide and was encouraged to slow the rate in order to increase the carbon dioxide to bring it nearer to the normal level of 40 mmHg. Others have used biofeedback in the teaching of diaphragmatic breathing (Johnston and Kyu-ha Lee, 1976).

It is sometimes considered that biofeedback works by making the patient aware of his or her own sensations when the dysfunction occurs, e.g. the spasticity, and then consciously preventing it from occurring. Thus once learned, control can be maintained. In many patients, however, control is gradually lost when the immediate feedback is stopped. It has been suggested by Colgan (1980) that EMG biofeedback works by operant (behavioural) conditioning because it has been found that the motor response can be conditioned without awareness on the part of the patient. In order to maintain control the feedback must be withdrawn from some of the trials so that the patient gradually learns the response with progressively fewer feedback reinforcements; this is called generalization training.

It is also considered that feedback should be proportional to the response. Thus a strong muscle contraction should produce a strong signal. Further, visual signals such as a digital meter are better than auditory feedback because direct comparisons can be made from one trial to another. Colgan (1980) also pointed out that direct sensory information from the muscle is needed for control and without it, it seems unlikely that significant therapeutic benefits can occur. This conforms with the successful effects of muscle practice and artificial stimulation considered below.

Application of EMG biofeedback

Instruments for providing EMG biofeedback vary in complexity. The simplest give only averaged motor unit responses on a meter. The more complex machines allow changes in sensitivity from showing a single motor unit response to those coupled to computing facilities and chart recorders which provide a permanent record of each training session and printouts of measures such as the average EMG activity during each minute of the session. The action potentials are only a few microvolts so essentially the EMG instrument is simply a very powerful amplifier. This means that any extraneous electrical signals will also be amplified and tend to interfere with the output. It is therefore important that good electrical contact be maintained with the skin and that other sources of electric fields be kept away. In the physiotherapy department pulsed shortwave is a likely source of interference, but any electrical field can have an effect. Several types of electrodes are available to make the good electrical contact with the skin surface that is essential for biofeedback. Silver/silver chloride electrodes are electrically the most suitable (Hurrell, 1980) but others, e.g. steel, are quite satisfactory. To make good electrical contact the skin must be cleaned with an alcohol wipe (gentle rubbing with a pumice stone is recommended) and saline gel (or saline) smeared between the electrode and the skin. It is important that the electrode be fixed firmly in place with sticky tape because movement over the skin will lead to interference. De Weerdt and Harrison (1986) recommend taping the signal wires to the patient to reduce movement.

The position and support of the patient must be carefully chosen for this treatment. If relaxation is to be attempted then the whole body must be fully supported lying or half-lying so that all postural muscles will be relaxed. If a movement is to be attempted then it is essential to position the patient so that this particular movement can occur unhindered and be visible to the patient; further, the need for fixator or synergistic activity in other muscles should be diminished. For example, if the deltoid is to be re-educated the upper limb should be supported in about 60° abduction and slight flexion at the shoulder. Most importantly the patient must be able to see the biofeedback meter or other signal. A full explanation of the purpose of the treatment and what is expected of the patient is given and the electrodes are fixed in place as described above. The positioning of the electrodes depends on the muscles involved and requires a knowledge of muscle anatomy. Generally the strongest signals will be had from electrodes placed close to the belly of the muscle and where it is most superficial. It may be helpful for the initial treatment if the working of the EMG biofeedback machine is shown to the patient and trials made by taking signals from a muscle which can easily be controlled by the patient.

The need to remain still to prevent unwanted potentials from other muscles interfering is explained to the patient. The sensitivity of the instrument can be altered by adjusting a dial to give an appropriate signal. Some muscles will generate strong outputs because many motor units are active and are close to the surface. In other circumstances, such as recovering nerve lesions, only a few isolated spike potentials may be present and the sensitivity must be increased to recognize them.

The training session consists of a series of attempts by the patient to increase the signal, or decrease it if relaxation is the objective. The physiotherapist encourages the patient verbally and suggests attempting activities which may lead to the desired muscle contraction, such as trying the activity on the opposing normal limb. Other ways of facilitating muscle contraction such as passive stretching may be used providing they do not create unwanted EMG signals. As voluntary control of a muscle contraction improves, the sensitivity of the device can be deliberately reduced to provide the patient with a new goal. If relaxation is the aim then the sensitivity would be increased as the patient improves. In the treatment of spasticity it is suggested that once the motor unit activity in the muscle at rest is under control, the physiotherapist stretches the muscle and the patient attempts to reduce the electrical activity in the muscle during various degrees and rates of stretch (Currier, 1988). Since the patient has to concentrate hard during all biofeedback treatments it is important to judge the length of time for which the patient can make the best effort. Overlong treatments may be unsuccessful and thus unrewarding and frustrating.

Other forms of biofeedback for control of activity

The pressure of balloon-like devices in the rectum can be measured and used for biofeedback treatment for the control of incontinence. As far as urinary incontinence is concerned the method was no more successful than simple bladder training (Marcer, 1986) or, probably, electrical stimulation of the perineal muscles. Vaginismus has also been successfully treated with biofeedback.

Muscle-strengthening and endurance-training devices have electronic displays which indicate the strength or power developed which can, in a sense, act as biofeedback devices as the subject can exercise at a predetermined rate, for example at 50% of maximum, thus learning to maintain a particular training schedule.

The amount of weight taken through one foot can be monitored with a pressure-sensitive pad in the shoe. This is connected to a circuit and battery carried in a small box (some are about 40 by 80 mm) which is attached either to the leg or at the waist. The circuit generates an audible signal when a pre-set pressure is reached. This can be used to encourage weight-bearing with, for example, hemiplegic patients (Triptree and Harrison, 1980) or in training patients in partial weight-bearing. In the former case the sound occurs when the patient takes sufficient weight and the sensitivity of the device can be decreased as he or she improves. In the latter the signal is set to sound when too much weight is taken on the leg. In both cases the patient is receiving feedback to show how to modify the activity, in this case walking. The pad can also be used to re-educate sitting or kneeling posture or the proportion of weight taken through the heel compared to that through the forefoot.

Recently attempts have been made to use the EMG output from intact muscles to control artificial limbs. This has been called the myoelectric artificial limb.

Biofeedback for the treatment of stress-related conditions

In these conditions some form of relaxation is found to be beneficial and biofeedback may well provide the means and motivation for the continued practice of relaxation.

Essential hypertension

The blood pressure is monitored and displayed to the patient who ultimately learns some voluntary control. Harvey (1978) reports that subjects can learn to reduce blood pressure by anything up to 35 mmHg.

Cardiac arrhythmias

The heart rate is monitored and displayed to the patient who can learn to gain some control mainly by slowing the heart rate. Schwartz (1977) suggests that it can be more helpful to train patients to reduce heart rate and blood pressure simultaneously.

Raynaud's disease

Biofeedback is appropriate for idiopathic Raynaud's disease, not the disorder due to arterial disease or vibration trauma. The temperature of the fingers is monitored using a suitable skin thermometer and the patient attempts voluntarily to increase the temperature, as described later.

Migraine

Hand-warming has also been used for the treatment of migraine with some success but with much less obvious connection (Marcer, 1986).

Tension headache

Relaxation of the occipitofrontalis muscle and posterior neck muscles is taught with biofeedback displaying the EMGs of these muscles. This has been a widely used treatment based on the hypothesis that tension in these muscles is the cause of the headaches. Chronic pain associated with muscle tension at other sites, notably chronic back pain, has also been treated with biofeedback.

Epilepsy

Sterman *et al.* (1974) discovered it was possible for patients to reduce the frequency of epileptic fits by producing a special rhythm in the electroencephalogram—the sensorimotor rhythm.

Many of these conditions have been found to benefit from relaxation training; indeed several exponents have combined biofeedback and relaxation training and found this to be the most successful treatment. In several studies of the effectiveness of biofeedback a small number of patients have demonstrated quite dramatic and continued improvement while most patients have achieved some benefit. It is arguable that biofeedback acts in the same way in all these conditions by encouraging and rewarding relaxation (see Marcer, 1986 for discussion).

Technique of application of temperature biofeedback

Although the instruments monitoring blood pressure or heart rate will differ from the thermometer measuring skin temperature the principles of application are the same. The physiotherapist first explains the rationale of the biofeedback treatment emphasizing its harmless and painless nature. It should also be stressed that it may take some time, perhaps several sessions, to achieve control. The patient is supported in a comfortable sitting or half-lying position in a room which remains at a comfortable constant temperature and where interruptions will not occur. The thermistor is attached to the skin of any fingertip (the middle finger of the dominant hand is recommended) with sticky tape. After a few seconds the reading on the thermometer is taken and recorded as the baseline. The patient is then asked to close the eyes, relax, and imagine circumstances in which his or her hands and fingers are being warmed. Various situations can be suggested to the patient, such as holding the hands in front of a warm fire or washing them in warm water. It is often helpful to ask the patient to repeat phrases such as: 'I feel relaxed and my hands are getting warmer'. The thermometer reading should be recorded every 30 s and the attention of the patient drawn to any slight temperature increase (Fig. 5.1).

Once the patient is accustomed to the treatment he or she is encouraged to watch the thermometer. The physiotherapist must ensure that relaxation is maintained with the patient's eyes open. The kind of imagery that is used will clearly depend on social, geographical and cultural factors. Some suggestions (from Currier, 1988) are given below:

'Imagine you are jogging on a hot day'.
'Imagine rubbing your hands over a warm fire'.
'Think about lying on a hot beach'.
'Imagine cutting grass on a hot August day'.

Other examples will readily come to mind and those appropriate to the patient's experience should be chosen. It may be helpful to warm the opposite hand with hot water or an infrared lamp to provide the patient with a warm sensation to aim for, but it must be remembered that this will lead to some reflex heating of the treated hand which may be mistaken for voluntary control.

Treatment sessions may last anything from 10 to 30 minutes. In the early stages if relaxation is impossible and no success in hand-warming is being achieved it may be wise to use short treatment sessions. It may take several sessions before the patient is able to control the hand-warming; once control is gained, longer sessions are more useful.

When some control has been gained there is no need for temperature recording to be made every 30 s: a record of the initial and final temperature of each treatment is all that is needed. While the patient is learning, the 30 s or 1 min record can show the small amounts of successful warming as they occur. The patient is encouraged to practise the hand-warming at home, especially in situations where digital vasospasm may be provoked, such as going out into the cold.

Gradually the treatment sessions are reduced in frequency as the patient becomes able to control finger temperature at will. Some patients with Raynaud's disease (and some migraine sufferers) have marked and dramatic reduction in the number and severity of their attacks as a result of biofeedback training but others have less immediate beneficial results or less long-lasting relief. However, in view of the fact that biofeedback is a simple non-invasive painless treatment with no deleterious side-effects it would seem worthy of trial for most patients.

To summarize the uses of biofeedback:

1 *For control of muscle activity and movement*
   a To re-educate activity or weight-bearing with pressure sensor.
   b For the myoelectric artificial limb.

   } Control of movement by pressure measurement
   Control of artificial limb by EMG activity

   c To re-educate movement loss in cerebrovascular accident patients.
   d For the control of spasticity from any cause.
   e For dystonic disorders: control of movement.
   f For recovering peripheral nerve lesions.
   g To re-educate specific muscle activity.

   Control of motor unit activity with EMG

2 *For stress-related conditions*
   a For muscle relaxation for pain relief, headache or other pain.
   b For blood pressure control for hypertension.
   c For heart rate control for cardiac arrhythmias.
   d For vasodilation of hands for Raynaud's disease and migraine.

   } Control of autonomic system

EFFECTIVENESS OF BIOFEEDBACK

The division of biofeedback strategies into those associated with control of the autonomic system and those concerned with control of movement has been deliberately followed in the belief that the mechanisms and pathways of the central nervous system involved in control are different. It must be recognized, however, that there is no evident difference in success between these two groups.

In all studies the successful outcomes occur in some, but not all, patients treated and the success that does occur is often modest. This happens in most therapeutic situations and is quite appropriate. It only needs to be noted to counter previously made claims that biofeedback was a new, universally successful, powerful panacea for all problems. What is, perhaps, different and important about biofeedback is that it sets out to teach patients control of their own body, be it movement control or autonomic, thus giving long-term benefits in both psychological and economic terms.

EVALUATION OF EMG BIOFEEDBACK FOR MUSCLE CONTROL

Using EMG, subjects can be taught to contract a single motor unit and to control the rate of firing of that unit at will (Basmajian, 1963). The subject is only consciously aware of this contraction through the feedback of the oscilloscope and loudspeaker. Single motor units can be identified because each causes a single spike potential. Almost all normal subjects are able to control a single motor unit and many can control two or more (Basmajian, 1974). With practice some especially able subjects can apparently follow complex rhythms with the firing of a single motor unit and even, amazingly, continue to control the unit from memory, with no visual or audible feedback. On being asked how they can do this they are only able to say that they thought about a motor unit they had previously learned to control.

Superficially EMG biofeedback would seem appropriate as a means of training skilled muscle action since activity in the desired muscle can be quantified. Two points must be recognized in this connection: firstly, it is not easy to be certain that the EMG signals are arising entirely in the muscle intended unless intramuscular electrodes are used. Secondly, training in skilled repetitive movements involves inhibition of unwanted activity in antagonistic muscles (Basmajian, 1975), thus it is more a matter of decreasing unwanted muscular contractions than increasing the activity. It is reasonable to suppose that what applied to training in normal healthy neuromuscular systems would also apply to re-education of the damaged systems.

Control of abduction of the great toe was used to compare the effectiveness of EMG biofeedback with other methods of training normal subjects (Middaugh, 1978). In this study the range of abduction of the hallux was measured by placing the bare foot on paper and tracing along the medial border; voluntary abduction was then attempted and a second outline drawn. The angular change was measured with a protractor. Four different treatments were then applied to four groups of 10 subjects: EMG feedback; manually applied sensory stimulation and practised muscle contractions; unassisted, practised muscle contractions, and no activity. A second measurement of toe abduction was then carried out in the same way. All treatments led to an increased range of voluntary abduction, including the control group in which nothing but attempted movement for the measurement had occurred. The average initial range of movement at the pretest was 7° with considerable differences between subjects (1–14°). This conforms with data collected by one of us (JL), using the same method of measurement in 102 normal young adult subjects. Immediately after the pretest of these subjects the abductor hallucis was stimulated with faradic-type current and voluntary abduction attempted. One week later, without further training, the post-test was conducted in the same way (Table 5.2).

Table 5.2 Range of motion of abduction before and after electrical stimulation and practice ($n = 102$)

	Pretest		Post-test	
	Left toe	*Right toe*	*Left toe*	*Right toe*
Mean	8.67°	8.98°	10.35°	11.05°
Range	0–20°	0–17°	0–22°	0–24°
Standard deviation		3.98°		4.12°

As shown, gains were made and retained. On average the right great toes increased in range of abduction by 2° (about 22%) and this difference is statistically (*t*-test) highly significant ($p > 0.001$; *t*-test). It is, however, largely accounted for by those subjects who had the least movement initially, which again conforms with the results of Middaugh (1978). This is hardly surprising since training would not be expected to increase an already large range of movement.

Thus it seems that movement control can be developed by voluntary practice, sensory stimulation, electrical muscle stimulation and biofeedback, all of which provide conscious proprioceptive feedback (feeling the toe move) and visual feedback (seeing it move), but the biofeedback adds further information of muscle contraction.

As well as evaluating the range of movement Middaugh also measured the EMG activity in the muscle and was thus able to monitor changes in total muscle activity. From this, it was concluded that EMG biofeedback was very effective in increasing the electrical response (muscle activity) in subjects who had little ability to use the abductor hallucis initially, i.e. those who had a poor range of movement on the pretest. However as training for a relatively brief contraction, such as that needed to measure the range of movement, EMG biofeedback was no better than unassisted practice of the contraction. In those subjects who had considerable control already, i.e. those with a good range of movement on the pretest, unassisted practice was most effective; in fact it was suggested that EMG biofeedback may interfere with training in this group.

It is suggested that EMG biofeedback is likely to be most effective when feedback from other sources is at a minimum, which would accord with these results. If there was little or no movement to start with there will be little feedback either from the joint or from seeing the toe move so any additional feedback helps. A sustained muscle contraction leads to less sensory feedback than brief (phasic) movement so that EMG biofeedback is an effective teaching method for a sustained contraction. On the other hand, when good movement already exists feedback can add little, so voluntary practice works better.

The therapeutic implications of this would seem to be that EMG biofeedback is a valuable additional method of movement training for those situations in which other feedback is lacking—in many neurological conditions, some hemiplegic patients and recovering nerve lesions. If normal sources of feedback are present EMG seems to have no advantage.

REFERENCES

Basmajian J. V. (1963). Control and training of individual motor units. *Science*, **141**, 440–1.

Basmajian J. V., Kukulka C. G., Narayan M. G., Takebe K. (1975). Biofeedback treatment of foot-drop after stroke compared with standard rehabilitation technique effects on voluntary control and strength. *Arch. Phys. Med. Rehab.*, **56**, 231–6.

Colgan M. (1980). Biofeedback treatment of neuro-muscular dysfunction. *N.Z. J. Physiother.*, **8**, 12–15.

Currier D. P. (1988). Nerve and muscle stimulating currents—biofeedback. In *Physical Agents for Physical Therapists* (Griffin J. E., Karselis T. C., eds) pp. 132–166. Springfield, Illinois: Charles C. Thomas.

De Weerdt W., Harrison M. A. (1986). Electromyographic feedback for stroke patients: some practical considerations. *Physiotherapy*, **72**, 106–8.

Harvey P. G. (1978). Biofeedback—trick or treatment? *Physiotherapy*, **64**, 333–5.

Hurrell M. (1980). Electromyographic feedback in rehabilitation. *Physiotherapy*, **66**, 293–8.

Johnston R., Kyu-ha Lee (1976). Myofeedback: a new method of teaching breathing exercises in emphysematous patients. *Phys. Ther.*, **56**, 826–9.

Marcer D. (1986). *Biofeedback and Related Therapies in Clinical Practice*. London: Croom Helm.

Middaugh S. J. (1978). EMG feedback as a muscle re-education technique. *Phys. Ther.*, **58**, 15–22.

Moon M. H. (1980). The therapist and EMG: biofeedback training for spasmodic torticollis. *N.Z. J. Physiother.*, **8**, 21–4.

Moon M. H. (1981). Biofeedback using a respiratory parameter in the treatment of behavioural breathing disorders. *N.Z. J. Physiother.*, **9**, 19–20.

Schwartz G. E. (1977). Biofeedback and the self-management of disregulation disorders. In *Behavioural Self-management* (Stuart R. B., ed.) New York: Brunner/Mazel.

Sterman M. B., MacDonald L. R., Stone R. K. (1974). Biofeedback training of the sensorimotor electroencephalogram rhythm in man: effects on epilepsy. *Epilepsia*, **15**, 393–416.

Triptree V. J., Harrison M. A. (1980). The use of sensor pads in the treatment of adult hemiplegia. *Physiotherapy*, **66**, 299.

Wiener N. (1948). *Cybernetics or Control and Communication in the Animal and the Machine*. New York: Wiley.

6.

Therapeutic ultrasound

Spread of infection
Vascular problems
Radiotherapy
The nervous system
Specialized tissue
Implants
Anaesthetic areas

Ultrasound refers to mechanical vibrations which are essentially the same as sound waves but of a higher frequency. Such waves are beyond the range of human hearing and can therefore also be called ultrasonic. Vibration merges with sound at frequencies around 20 Hz; vibration below this frequency is often called infrasound or infrasonic. The upper limit of frequency for human hearing, and hence the range of frequencies defined as sound, varies considerably. It is higher in children and lower in old age; it is about 16–20 kHz. Most of the frequencies involved in speech and music lie in the range of 30 to 4000 Hz. Ultrasonic energy or ultrasound describes any vibration at a frequency above the sound range but it is frequencies of a few megahertz that are typically used in physiotherapy: several different frequencies are employed in the range from 0.5 to 5 MHz (Table 6.1). The terms 'sonic' and 'sound' are often used interchangeably, a course followed here, but strictly sound refers to audible frequencies.

Table 6.1 Frequency and wavelength of ultrasound at 1500 m/s

Frequency (MHz)	Wavelength (mm)	Period (μs)
0.5	3.0	2
0.75	2.0	1.33
0.87	1.724	1.15
1.0	1.5	1
1.5	1.0	0.66
2.0	0.75	0.5
3.0	0.5	0.33
5.0	0.3	0.2

THE NATURE OF SONIC WAVES

Sonic waves are a series of mechanical compressions and rarefactions in the direction of travel of the wave, hence they are called longitudinal waves (Fig. 6.1). They can occur in solids, liquids and gases and are due to regular compression and separation of molecules. (In solids, but not fluids, transverse waves can also occur; ter Haar, 1987.) The passage of these waves of compression through matter is, of course, invisible but the effect can be seen in a Slinky spring, a very flexible spring which is sold as a toy. If the spring is held up and a few coils are gathered together and then released the

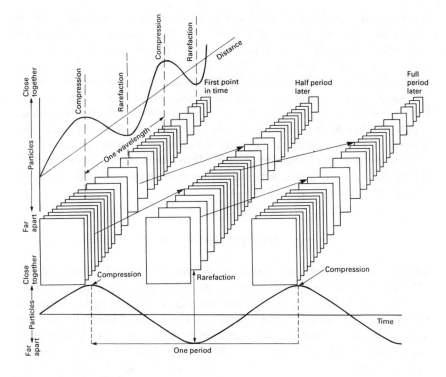

Fig. 6.1 Longitudinal wave.

compression will pass down the length of the spring and, if the spring is supported below can be seen to bounce back up the spring. A series of such compression waves simulates what happens when sonic waves pass in a material (Fig. 6.1). It is important to understand that it is energy that travels as the wave, not matter: this is true of any waves, not just sonic waves. Thus each coil of the spring oscillates about a fixed point when given wave energy (in the same way water or air molecules vibrate about their average position as a result of the sonic wave).

As sound waves pass through any material their energy is dissipated or attenuated. Sometimes all the energy is absorbed at once; sometimes the sound wave passes with almost no loss. The molecules of all matter are in constant random motion; the amount of molecular agitation is what is measured as heat—the greater the molecular movement, the greater the heat (see Chapter 7). This molecular motion is oscillatory but in several different ways and at many different frequencies. For instance, the whole molecule may move to and fro, or it may rotate to and fro, or the molecule may change shape in an oscillatory way. As the molecules jostle one another energy will be transferred from one to another so that some will oscillate at higher frequencies and with greater amplitude because they have gained energy while others will be at lower frequencies and amplitudes because their energy has been transferred by collision. When sonic vibration is applied to the material it is superimposed on the existing motions and will add to them where the sonic vibration matches the natural frequency of some of the molecular movements. The ultimate result is that the regular sonic wave energy tends to become randomized as the energy it gives to particular molecular motions becomes spread out in collisions with other molecules. In this way the sonic energy is steadily converted to heat energy. It can be seen that the sonic energy will be attenuated as it passes through the material which becomes heated; further, the rate at which this exchange occurs will depend on both the nature of the material, i.e. the way the molecules oscillate, and the frequency of the sonic wave. Thus the ratio of transmission to absorption of sonic waves differs in different materials and varies with the frequency of the sonic energy.

Description of waves

In order to characterize any wave several features must be described. The frequency, that is the number of complete cycles in a second, given in hertz (Hz), has already been noted. The time taken for a complete cycle is known as the period. This describes the relation of the wave motion to time. The distance through which the wave motion repeats itself—the distance from, say, one wave peak to the next—is called the wavelength and is often denoted by λ (lambda). In the case of longitudinal waves passing in a medium it is the distance from, say, the central point of one compression of molecules to the next. This describes the motion in relation to distance (Fig. 6.1).

It is obvious that the velocity at which the wave passes through the material will depend on the frequency and wavelength: either a higher frequency or a greater wavelength, or both, will lead to a greater velocity. For any given velocity the wave could travel with either a high frequency and small wavelength or a low frequency and long wavelength. The fundamental equation for wave motion is thus expressed as:

$$\text{Velocity} = \text{frequency} \times \text{wavelength}$$

$$V = f\lambda$$

The amplitude is the magnitude of the wave. It can be described as the distance from the mean position that a particle is made to move by the wave.

Sound waves will pass more rapidly through material in which the molecules are close together, thus their velocity is higher in solids and liquids than in gases. Sound waves in air, for example, have a velocity of 343 m/s. The velocity of sound waves in salt water is approximately 1500 m/s and is almost the same in most soft tissues. From what has been noted above it is simple to deduce the wavelengths of those frequencies employed in physiotherapy (Table 6.1).

At other frequencies ultrasound is used for various purposes. In industry low-frequency ultrasound is used for many cleaning and mixing processes since efficient vibration of very small particles is achieved. It can also be used for cutting and engraving as well as detecting cracks in metal such as welding defects.

The other major medical use of ultrasound is in body imaging and dental drills/descalers. These latter usually operate at between 20 and 60 kHz (Williams, 1987).

PRODUCTION OF THERAPEUTIC ULTRASOUND

There is no difficulty in producing low-frequency ultrasound by means of mechanical vibration, an extension of the familiar ways in which sound is produced, such as vibrating reeds or whistles. With somewhat higher frequencies it is not possible to make the mechanical part, or column of air, change its direction sufficiently quickly.

Piezoelectric transducers are used to achieve the high-frequency ultrasound energy needed for surgery, imaging and therapy. These are suitably cut crystals which change shape under the influence of an electric charge. The piezoelectric effect was first described by Pierre and Paul-Jacques Curie in 1880. They showed that certain crystals generated a small voltage when subject to pressure. The reverse of this effect, first used in 1910 by Langevin, is used to produce high-frequency oscillation of the crystal by applying a high-frequency alternating charge to it. This effect is due to the molecular configuration of the crystal being altered by the electric charge.

Many types of crystal can be used but the most favoured are quartz, which occurs naturally, and some synthetic ceramic materials such as barium titanate and lead zirconate titanate (PZT). The crystal must be cut to suitable dimensions—the most important being thickness—so that it will resonate at the chosen frequency and so achieve maximum vibration. In order to apply the electric charges, metal electrodes must be fixed to the crystal. If a suitable metal plate is fixed to one surface of the crystal while the opposite surface is in air, then almost all the vibrational energy is transmitted from the crystal to the plate and thence to any solid or liquid to which it is applied. This is the treatment head which is used to transmit sonic energy to the tissues.

The other essential part of a therapeutic ultrasound generator is a circuit to produce oscillating voltages to drive the transducer. It is also necessary to provide a controlling circuit, based on an astable multivibrator (see Chapter 3) which can turn the oscillator on and off to give pulses of ultrasound output. The power supply from the mains needs to be rectified and modified to be suitable for the oscillator and control circuits. Switches to turn the whole system on and off and to change from continuous to pulsed output are also needed. Most importantly a means of controlling the output or intensity of ultrasound and a meter to measure this are provided.

A basic oscillator circuit consists of an inductance and a capacitor. If the charged capacitor is allowed to discharge through the inductance a magnetic field will be set up. As the charge on the capacitor falls this magnetic field collapses inducing a current in the coil which recharges the capacitor with the opposite polarity. The capacitor now discharges through the coil in the other direction, and the process is repeated over and over again. There is, therefore, a regular change from electrical energy in the form of a charge on the capacitor to magnetic energy in the form of the magnetic field. This is a typical oscillating system in that there is a regular energy change—potential to kinetic energy and back again—like a pendulum swinging to and fro.

For any given system the time taken for each cycle of events is constant and depends on the size of the system, in the same way that the frequency of a pendulum is inversely proportional to its length. The time taken for the electrical cycle and hence its frequency depends on the size of the capacitor (in farads) and the inductance of the coil (in henries). Electrical circuits can be made to oscillate at any chosen frequency by using the appropriate values for capacitance and inductance. The smaller these values are, the shorter each oscillation and the higher the frequency. The frequency is thus inversely proportional to the product of inductance and capacitance. The frequency of this circuit is expressed as:

$$f = \frac{1}{2\pi\sqrt{LC}}$$

where f = frequency, L = inductance and C = capacitance.

It will also be evident that some energy is bound to be lost at each oscillation due to 'friction' in the system. Energy is lost from the capacitor and from the wires, appearing as heat in the circuit, and also from the magnetic field around the inductance. Thus the oscillations are damped. Note that it is the amplitude, i.e. the amount of energy, that diminishes whereas the frequency remains constant; also note that the energy loss is approximately exponential due to the fact that proportionally less energy is lost as the current becomes less.

In order to maintain a constant amplitude energy must be added to the circuit to replace that which is removed for driving the piezoelectric crystal. This is achieved with a transistor to switch additional current through the oscillator coil at appropriate moments—see Chapter 10 p. 226 and Fig. 10.1.

Thus it can be seen how a suitable circuit can maintain a constantly oscillating electric charge to cause the piezoelectric crystal to change shape at the same frequency and so drive the metal plate backwards and forwards also at the same high frequency, producing a train of sonic compression waves in any medium with which it is in contact.

A suitable resistance circuit is provided to control the amplitude of the electrical oscillations which in turn control the magnitude of the mechanical vibration of the crystal and hence the amplitude of the sonic wave. This amplitude is referred to as the intensity and measured in watt per square centimetre.

Current supplied to the oscillator circuit can be switched on and off by the astable multivibrator (see Chapter 3) in order to produce a pulsed output. This can be varied to give different pulse ratios: 1:1 and 1:4 are in common use.

A meter is often included which measures the electrical oscillations applied to the crystal but not the vibration of the crystal. (This means, of course, that if the crystal has failed the lack of output is not evident from the meter.) Some meters indicate average current (see below) so that the indicated output is less with pulsed ultrasound.

TRANSMISSION OF SONIC WAVES

The metal plate of the treatment head moves backwards and forwards to generate a stream of compression waves that forms the sonic beam. Due to the fact that the wavelength of these waves is much smaller than the transducer face, the sonic beam is roughly cylindrical and of the same diameter as the transducer (Williams, 1987). Even the smallest therapeutic transducers are 2 or 3 cm across and, as can be seen from Table 6.1, wavelengths are only a few millimetres. (For audible sound with wavelengths much larger than the source producing them—about 1.34 m for middle C—the sound waves spread out in all directions so that sound can be heard equally well at all places equidistant from the source.)

This beam of ultrasound emitted from the transducer is by no means uniform even in a homogeneous medium. Waves emitted from the different places on the face of the transducer will travel to the same point in space in front of the transducer face by different paths and hence arrive out of phase. Some waves cancel out, others reinforce so that the net result is a very irregular pattern of sonic waves in the region close to the transducer face, called the near field or Fresnel zone. In the region beyond this, the far field or Fraunhofer zone, the sonic field spreads out somewhat and becomes much more regular because the differing path lengths from points on the transducer become insignificant at greater distances. The length of the near field will depend on the square of the radius (r) of the transducer face and inversely on the wavelength:

$$\text{Length of Fresnel zone} = r^2/\lambda$$

Therefore, a 30 mm diameter transducer at 1 MHz in water, or soft tissues, would have a near field of 150 mm from the treatment head (15 mm = r; 15^2 = 225; λ = 1.5 mm (see Table 6.1); 225/1.5 = 150 mm).

At higher frequencies the near zone would be longer still. For all practical purposes therapeutic ultrasound utilizes the near field and hence is irregular. This is one reason why the treatment head must be moved continuously during treatment to 'iron out' some of the irregularities.

Boundaries between media

As has already been explained, a wave is a transfer of energy. Sonic waves involve vibratory motion of molecules so that there is a characteristic velocity of wave progression for each particular medium. It depends on the density and elasticity of the medium and together these specify what is known as the acoustic impedance of the medium. This acoustic impedance describes the nature of the material, i.e. how easily the molecules move in relation to one another, so it is not surprising that it is linked to the velocity of sonic waves in that particular material. The acoustic impedance can be found by multiplying the density of a medium by the velocity of sonic waves through it. When sonic waves travelling at a velocity characteristic for the particular medium come to the boundary they cross it to continue at the same frequency. However, they do not continue at the same velocity so the wavelength and amplitude must change.

Some of the energy is reflected back. The amount of energy reflected is proportional to the difference in acoustic impedance between the two media. Thus water and glass have rather different acoustic impedances so that over 63% of the original sonic energy is reflected at this interface. Water and soft tissue, on the other hand, have very similar impedance so that only 0.2% is reflected (Williams, 1987). This applies to waves that strike boundaries at right angles.

If the wave front strikes the boundary at some other angle the reflected wave will travel away from the boundary at the same angle; that is, the angle of incidence of a beam equals the angle of reflection and is in the same plane (see Fig. 11.2). Refraction also occurs with sonic waves due to the difference in acoustic impedance. The beam of sonic energy that passes through the second medium does not continue in a straight line but changes direction at the boundary because of the different velocities in the two media. If the boundary between air and water is considered, a sonic wave travelling in air at 343 m/s striking the water surface at an angle of incidence of about 10° would be refracted in water through an angle of about 50° (Fig. 11.2). If the acoustic impedances are closely matched little refraction will occur.

The turning back of a wave in the same medium has a further consequence. Two waves, the original and the reflected, are travelling in opposite directions so that at some points they will be combined, adding to each other; at other points they will cancel one another out. This tends to produce a stationary wave pattern, logically called a standing wave. Such waves are certainly generated in the tissues by therapeutic ultrasound and may have significant consequences.

It can be seen that the transmission of ultrasound through differing media, like the tissues, with many boundaries, or interfaces as they are often called, can alter the direction and intensity of the beam by reflection, refraction and the formation of standing waves. For a particularly clear and detailed description of these concepts see Ward (1986).

Absorption of sonic waves in a parallel beam

It has been seen already that ultrasound will increase the motion of molecules causing more molecular vibration and molecular collisions, resulting in heat. Thus kinetic energy is converted to heat energy as it passes through the material. The energy will decrease exponentially with distance from the source because a fixed proportion of it is absorbed at each unit distance so that the remaining amount will become a smaller and smaller percentage of the initial energy (see Fig. 11.4). There is an inverse relationship between the amount of energy that penetrates a material and the amount that is absorbed. Thus if a beam of ultrasound is passed through the tissues it will be steadily reduced in intensity in the manner shown in Figure 11.4. This can be expressed as the absorption coefficient. There is no point at which all the energy has been absorbed so it is usual to specify a half-value depth, that is, the depth or distance at which half the initial energy has been absorbed. The half-value depth can be used to describe the exponential curve of energy transmitted against distance penetrated, and is analogous to the half-life of radioactive material. (Cf. penetration depth, Chapter 11.)

Since the conversion of sonic energy to heat is due to increased molecular motion it follows that the amount converted will depend on the nature of those molecules and on the frequency/wavelength of the ultrasound. Thus the half-value depth will be different in different tissues for any given ultrasound frequency (Table 6.2).

Table 6.2 Half-value depth of penetration (given in mm)

f (MHz)	Skin	Fat	Muscle	Tendon	Cartilage	Bone	Source
1	11.1	50	9 (24.6*)	6.2	6	2.1	Hoogland (1986)
3	4	16.5	3 (8*)	2	2		
1		48	9				McDiarmid and Burns (1987)
3		16	3				
1	40						ter Haar (1978)
3	25						
1		153	28			0.4	Ward (1986)
3		26.4	7.7			0.04	
				Average value			
1				65			Wadsworth and Chanmugan (1980)
3				30			

f = Frequency.

*In line of muscle fibres (not the usual direction of clinical application).

Attenuation of ultrasound in the tissues

From what has been said already it is evident that the attenuation of ultrasound in the human tissues is complex.

Firstly, energy from the ultrasound beam is not only absorbed by the various tissues through which it passes, but it is also scattered out of the beam by multiple reflections and refractions. Of course, the scattered energy may also be absorbed but not in the region to which the ultrasound beam is applied.

Secondly, the tissues through which the beam passes are far from homogeneous so that the half-value depths can only be a rough guide. Furthermore differences in acoustic impedance between soft tissue and bone are quite large which leads to reflection of the sonic energy as explained earlier. There can also be the formation of shear waves (Williams, 1987) which transmit energy along the periosteal surface at right angles to the ultrasound beam. Due to the fact that this reflection is quite large (25%; Ward, 1986) and that sonic energy is absorbed almost immediately in bone, there is marked heating at the bone surface (Fig. 6.2). This mechanism is considered to account for the periosteal pain that can arise with excessive doses of therapeutic ultrasound. Differences of acoustic impedance between other soft tissues are much smaller.

The attenuation increases with the amount of structural protein in the tissue and with decreasing water content. Thus tissues can be listed in order of increasing absorption of ultrasound energy (Frizzel and Dunn, 1982).

Increasing protein content

Blood–fat–nerve–muscle–skin–tendon–cartilage–bone

Low ————————————————————————————→High

Absorption of ultrasound

It may be seen that this conforms with Table 6.2.

Calculations of the relative rate of heating for a fat–muscle–bone system have been made (Ward, 1986) and these are shown in Figure 6.2. The important factor is the rate of tissue-heating which is influenced both by the blood flow, which constantly carries heat away, and by heat conduction. Both of these will reduce the peaks and troughs of the heating rate predicted on absorption and reflection characteristics. In highly vascular tissues such as muscle it is likely that heat would be rapidly dissipated preventing any large temperature rise; on the other hand, less vascular tissue, such as dense connective tissue in the form of tendon or ligament, may experience a relatively greater temperature rise.

Thirdly, it was noted earlier that moving the transducer head during treatment was important to smooth out the irregularities of the near field. It will also reduce some of the irregularities of absorption that might occur due to reflection at interfaces, standing waves, refraction, differences in tissue thermal conduction or blood flow. Thus the resulting heating pattern is likely to be much more evenly distributed than that indicated in Figure 6.2.

The calculation of temperature rise in the tissues as a result of ultrasound absorption can be done from typical tissue measurements, the density, the specific heat per unit mass and the absorption coefficient for a given intensity. From such calculations it is estimated that for an output of $1 \, W/cm^2$ there is a temperature rise of $0.8°C/min$ if vascular cooling effects are ignored (ter Haar, 1987).

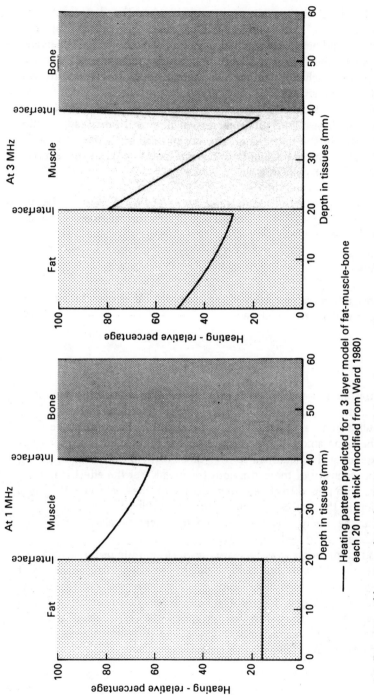

—— Heating pattern predicted for a 3 layer model of fat-muscle-bone
each 20 mm thick (modified from Ward 1980)

Fig. 6.2 Proportional heating of 1 and 3 MHz ultrasound through tissues. Continuous line = heating pattern predicted for a three-layer model of fat–muscle–bone, each 20 mm thick. Modified from Ward (1986).

Pulsed ultrasound

A circuit in the ultrasonic generator is arranged to turn the ultrasound on in short bursts or pulses; 2 ms pulses are often used. This reduces the time average intensity and hence the amount of energy available to heat the tissues while ensuring that the energy available in each pulse (pulse average intensity) is high enough for mechanical rather than thermal effects to predominate (see also discussion, Chapter 10).

Most therapeutic ultrasound generators produce 2 ms pulses and vary the intervals between pulses. This can be expressed either as the mark:space ratio, which is the ratio of the pulse length to the interval, or as the duty cycle, which is the ratio of the pulse length to the total length of pulse plus interval, expressed as a percentage. Thus:

Pulse	Interval	Mark:space ratio	Ratio of pulse to total period	Duty cycle
2 ms and 2 ms gives		1:1	1 in 2	50%
2 ms and 8 ms gives		1:4	1 in 5	20%

Many other ratios are possible and pulse lengths other than 2 ms may be available more widely in the future.

Effects of pulsing

If pulsed ultrasound is applied at a mark:space ratio of 1:4 the amount of introduced energy is one-fifth of that which would be introduced by continuous ultrasound applied for the same length of time and at the same intensity. The same amount of energy could be introduced into the tissues either by extending the treatment for five times the length of time or giving five times the intensity of the continuous treatment. Yet the effect is not the same because with pulsed treatment there is time for the heat to be dissipated by conduction in the tissues and in the circulating blood. Therefore, higher intensities can be safely used in a pulsed treatment because the average heating produced is reduced.

Ultrasound application can increase rates of ion diffusion across cell membranes (Dyson, 1985); this could be due to increased particle movement on either side of the membrane and possibly, increased motion of the phospholipids and proteins that form the membrane. It is possible that mild mechanical agitation of the tissues has certain effects which remain the same no matter how long the agitation is continued but that short bursts of more vigorous agitation have different, more significant effects.

Therapeutic mechanisms

There have been two schools of thought which have developed historically concerning the therapeutic mechanisms of ultrasound. One considers heating to be the only effect. This view is found in much of the American writing on the subject. High doses are recommended and little value is seen in low-intensity and pulsed treatments. The term 'ultrasonic diathermy' is often used and emphasizes the heating effect. The other school of thought, largely European, is more concerned with low-intensity treatments causing mechanical or biological effects and with pulsed treatments. These different views and their historical development are well described by Fyfe and Bullock (1985).

It is evident that many uncertainties remain concerning ultrasound. The part played by heat versus the mechanical effects, ignorance of the distribution of ultrasonic energy in the tissues and inaccurate calibration of ultrasound machines are all areas in which little is known. A lack of clinical research also contributes (Partridge, 1987).

PHYSIOLOGICAL EFFECTS

The result of absorption of ultrasound in the tissues, as has already been discussed, is the oscillation of particles about their mean position. This oscillation, or sonic energy, is converted into heat energy which is proportional to the intensity of the ultrasound. If all this heat is not dissipated by the normal physiological means a local rise in temperature will occur and thermal effects will result. If heat dissipation equals heat generation there is no net rise in temperature and any effects are said to be non-thermal. Non-thermal effects are achieved by using low intensities or pulsing the output.

Thermal effects

If local temperature is raised to between 40 and 45°C hyperaemia will result (Lehmann and Guy, 1972). Temperatures above 45°C are destructive. To achieve a useful therapeutic effect the tissue temperature has to be maintained between these values for at least 5 min (Lehmann and deLateur, 1982). Heating fibrous tissue structures such as joint capsules, ligaments, tendons and scar tissue can cause a temporary increase in their extensibility, and hence a decrease in joint stiffness. The advantage of using ultrasound to achieve this heating is due to the preferential heating of collagen tissue and to the effective penetration of this energy to deeply placed structures. However, ultrasound-absorbing structures can prevent the treatment reaching deeply placed target tissues if they intervene in the path of the sonic beam (Dyson, 1987). Mild heating can also have the effect of reducing pain and muscle spasm and promoting healing processes.

Non-thermal effects

Cavitation

Cavitation is the formation of tiny gas bubbles in the tissues as a result of ultrasound vibration. These bubbles, generally of a micron (10^{-6} m) or so in diameter (ter Haar, 1987), although they can grow much larger under some circumstances, are of two kinds—stable or transient cavitation.

Stable cavitation occurs when the bubbles oscillate to and fro within the ultrasound pressure waves but remain intact.

Transient (or collapse) cavitation occurs when the volume of the bubble changes rapidly and then collapses (implodes) causing high pressure and temperature changes and resulting in gross damage to tissues.

The former kind, associated with acoustic streaming, is considered to have therapeutic value (see below) but the latter, which is only likely to occur at high intensities, can be damaging. Cavitation can be easily demonstrated experimentally and it has now been established that it occurs in the tissues as a result of ultrasound therapy (ter Haar and Daniels, 1981). Pulsing reduces the risk of damage due to cavitation.

Acoustic streaming

This is a steady circulatory flow due to radiation torque. Additionally, as a result of either type of cavitation there is a localized, unidirectional fluid movement around the vibrating bubble. These very small fluid movements around cells are called microstreaming and are believed to play a significant role in the therapeutic effect of ultrasound (Dyson, 1987). Such streaming is said to affect the permeability of cell membranes where it is particularly marked. Its effect is to alter the rate of diffusion of ions across the membrane, for example, calcium which, as a second messenger, may result in the stimulation of repair processes and sodium which possibly alters electrical activity in nerves and could, therefore, be involved in pain relief.

Standing waves

Standing waves have already been described as being due to reflected waves being superimposed on the incident waves. The result is a set of standing or stationary waves with peaks of high pressure (antinodes), half a wavelength apart, between which are zones of no pressure (nodes). This pressure pattern has been shown to cause stasis of cells in blood vessels at the pressure nodes (Dyson and Pond, 1973). The endothelium of the blood vessels exposed to standing waves can also be damaged leading to thrombus formation (Dyson *et al.*, 1974). It must be realized that if the transducer is moved during treatment standing waves are unlikely to form.

Micromassage

The waves of compression and rarefaction may produce a form of micro-massage which could reduce oedema (Summer and Patrick, 1964).

Effects of ultrasound on inflammation and repair processes

Acute stage

Ultrasound releases histamine and presumably other growth factors from the mast cells. This may follow the increased calcium ion diffusion across the cell membrane causing degranulation. In this way ultrasound can accelerate normal resolution of inflammation providing that the inflammatory stimulus is removed (Dyson, 1987). This acceleration could also be due to the gentle agitation of the tissue fluid which may increase the rate of phagocytosis and the movement of particles and cells (Evans, 1980). It should be noted that ultrasound has a pro-inflammatory action, not an anti-inflammatory one; there is evidence that it accelerates the inflammatory phase of repair (Young, 1988).

Granulation stage

This begins approximately 3 days after injury and is the stage at which the connective tissue framework is laid down by fibroblasts for the new blood vessels. During repair, fibroblasts may be stimulated to produce more collagen; it has been shown that ultrasound can promote collagen synthesis (Harvey *et al.*, 1975). This is thought to be due to increased cell membrane permeability, caused by ultrasound, allowing the entry of calcium ions which control cellular activity (Dyson, 1987). Not only is more collagen formed but it is also of greater tensile strength after ultrasound treatment.

Ultrasound is also believed to encourage the growth of new capillaries in chronic ischaemic tissue and the same could happen during repair of soft tissues after injury (Dyson, 1987). The enhanced release of growth factors from macrophages following exposure to therapeutic ultrasound has also been observed (Young, 1988).

Remodelling stage

This stage can last months or years until the new tissue is as near in structure as possible to the original tissue. Ultrasound is considered to improve the extensibility of mature collagen such as is found in scar tissue (Lehmann and deLateur, 1982). This is believed to occur by promoting the reorientation of the fibres (remodelling) which leads to greater elasticity without loss of strength.

THERAPEUTIC USES

Therapeutic ultrasound has been applied to an enormous range of conditions with claims of successful outcomes. At any stage a placebo effect may also occur. For a recent review of the clinical applications of ultrasound see McDiarmid and Burns (1987).

Acute and subacute traumatic and inflammatory conditions

This is, perhaps, the area in which successful treatment has been most clearly demonstrated. For the following conditions the reader is referred directly to the references cited.

1 Soft tissue, sports injuries: Patrick (1978).
2 Occupational injuries: Middlemast and Chatterjee (1978).
3 Postpartum: McLaren (1984) and Creates (1987).
4 Surgical wounds, episiotomies: Ferguson (1981).
5 Dental extractions: El Hag *et al.* (1985) and Hashish *et al.* (1986).
6 Painful shoulders: Munting (1978) and Downing and Weinstein (1986), who found little benefit.
7 Subacromial bursitis: Bearzy (1953).

Chronic rheumatoid and arthritic conditions

1 Rheumatic conditions: De Preux (1952).
2 Osteoarthritis: Griffin *et al.* (1970).
3 Rheumatoid nodules: Clarke and Stenner (1976).

Venous ulcers and pressure sores

1 Venous ulcers: Dyson and Suckling (1978), Roche and West (1984) and Callam *et al.* (1987).
2 Pressure sores: McDiarmid *et al.* (1985).

Scar tissue and excessive fibrous tissue

1 Scar tissue: Bierman (1954) and Patrick (1978).
2 Dupuytren's contracture: Markham and Wood (1980).
3 Painful, indurated episiotomy scars: Fieldhouse (1979).
4 Contractures: Lehmann (1965).
5 Plantar fasciitis: Clarke and Stenner (1976).

Pain relief

1 Herpes zoster: Garrett and Garrett (1982), Jones (1984) and Payne (1984).
2 Phantom limb pain: Rubin and Kuitert (1955).
3 Low back pain: Patrick (1978).

Phonophoresis

Phonophoresis is the movement of drugs through skin into the subcutaneous tissues under the influence of ultrasound. Many drugs are absorbed through the skin only very slowly; high-frequency sonic vibration will accelerate this process. Such treatment has been in use since the early 1950s but not by many physiotherapists. It is also known as sonophoresis or ultrasonophoresis.

In Chapter 2 it was explained how iontophoresis achieved this same effect, that of driving drugs through the skin, by means of electrical forces. Phonophoresis relies on pertubation of the tissues causing more rapid particle movement and thus encouraging absorption of the drug. The effects of phonophoresis are those of the particular drug employed, combined with the effects of ultrasound. In studies on various musculoskeletal lesions it is difficult to separate these effects, but one study (Griffin et al., 1967) compared the clinical effects of ultrasonically driven hydrocortisone with ultrasound alone in over 100 patients. Some two-thirds of these, mainly osteoarthritis patients, benefited significantly from ultrasonically driven hydrocortisone, while just over a quarter had similar benefit from ultrasound alone.

Penetration of phonophoretically driven drugs

The depth to which drugs can be made to penetrate is a matter of particular uncertainty. As occurs with iontophoresis (see Chapter 2), once the drug has passed through the epidermis it is likely to be dispersed in the circulation to an extent which depends on the vascularity of the tissues concerned and the ease with which molecules of the drug can enter blood vessels. In any case dispersion will occur in the tissues. However, several studies quoted by Skauen and Zentner (1984) showed that cortisol could be driven into pig muscle and nerve by phonophoresis; further the therapeutic effects reported by several studies, e.g. Kleinkort and Wood (1975), could only result if significant quantities of anti-inflammatory drug had penetrated to the affected tissue. In some of these studies ultrasonic frequencies rather lower than those customarily employed, 0.33 or 0.25 MHz, were found to be more effective. In fact, it has been concluded that lower frequencies lead to greater penetration (Skauen and Zentner, 1984).

It must be realized that deeper penetration does not necessarily infer greater effectiveness. If the therapeutic effects occur in the dermis and epidermis, such as the cutaneous anaesthetic effect of lignocaine, then it might be expected that higher frequencies would be a more effective delivery system since the ultrasound energy is largely absorbed in the superficial tissues. This has been shown to occur in that 1.5 and 3 MHz ultrasound appeared to be more effective in achieving absorption of local anaesthetic than 0.75 MHz (Benson et al., 1988). Interestingly, this same study showed that pulsed was rather more effective than continuous ultrasound in achieving transfer of this particular cream. Not only did the 1:1 pulsing used give half the energy of the continuous, but the pulsed intensity used was lower than that given with

Electrotherapy explained

continuous ultrasound. The fact that pulsing can lead to better penetration is good evidence for a specific effect due to pulsation of ultrasound.

Drugs used in phonophoresis

The anti-inflammatory drug hydrocortisone has been widely used and reported on; it seems that high concentrations of the drug are effectively driven through the skin with high-dosage ultrasound and the amount is proportional to the time and intensity of treatment. However, low concentrations and low-intensity ultrasound seem to be less effective or ineffective (Skauen and Zentner, 1984). Kleinkort and Wood (1975) found 10% hydrocortisone ointment to be more effective than 1%. Many inflammatory skin conditions have been treated with hydrocortisone.

Numerous other steroid-type drugs can be applied by phonophoresis as well as many non-steroidal anti-inflammatory drugs, mainly salicylates.

Phonophoresis of hydrocortisone has been used in the treatment of many skin conditions including psoriasis, scleroderma and pruritis. It would seem to be a simple, sensible and logical way to increase the rate of absorption of the drug into the dermis. A lotion containing zinc oxide, tannic acid, urea and menthol has been applied by phonophoresis to treat herpes simplex virus type II in both oral and genital infections with good results (Fahim, 1980). Antibiotics such as penicillin have been given by phonophoresis for the treatment of skin infections.

Some suggested products appear not to be transmitted; e.g. Difflam Cream (benzydamine hydrochloride). This was tested in a double-blind controlled study (Benson *et al.*, 1989) in which the drug in a gel was recovered from the skin surface and measured; no significant difference was found between treatments with the ultrasound on and those with it off. As suggested above, if the base, cream or ointment in which the drug is dissolved is not a good ultrasonic transmitter then it seems unlikely that treatment would work effectively.

Application

The drug to be driven into the tissues is combined in a suitable gel or cream which forms the couplant. It is smeared on to the part, using a spatula so that it is not applied to the physiotherapist's fingers, and some may be smeared on to the treatment head. The treatment head is moved over the skin in the usual manner. Relatively high intensities of 1 and 1.5 W/cm^2 have been used. The depth of the target tissue determines the frequency used. The time of treatment depends on the area over which phonophoresis is to be applied; 1 min treatment for every 10 cm^2 area is reasonable, although Griffin *et al.* (1967) suggest 5 min for each 25 in^2, i.e. about 1 min for 30 cm^2. Most reported applications of phonophoresis have used continuous ultrasonic energy but Benson *et al.* (1988) used both continuous and pulsed energy to produce skin anaesthesia with Emla cream; the pulsed mode appeared to be more effective in these circumstances, as noted above.

When treatment is completed the remaining couplant, containing the drug, should be removed from both the patient's skin and the ultrasound transducer. It is essential to ensure complete removal from the treatment head since any drug remaining may be inadvertently and inappropriately applied to the next patient treated.

Since the cream or gel containing the drug is being used as the couplant it is important that it transmits ultrasound adequately. This has been considered by Benson and McElnay (1988) who investigated the transmission characteristics of 38 different products and found wide variations. In general they found that gels were better than creams and that many were extremely poor transmitters of ultrasound. Some examples from this study are given in Table 6.3, but for fuller information the original article should be consulted.

Table 6.3 Transmission characteristics of various compounds

Product	Active ingredients	Transmission relative to water (%)		
		0.75 MHz	1.5 MHz	3 MHz
Steroids				
Cobadex cream	Hydrocortisone, dimethicone	55	67	75
Locoid lipocream	Hydrocortisone butyrate	38	61	71
Anti-inflammatory drugs				
Intralgin gel	Benzocaine salicylamide	87	11	120 sic
Movelat cream	Corticosteroids, heparinoid, salicylic acid	33	48	69
Local anaesthetics				
Emla cream	Lignocaine, prilocaine	83	90	95
Xylocaine ointment	Lignocaine hydrochloride	2	2	0

From Benson and McElnay (1988).

Contraindications

The same considerations apply when giving phonophoresis as apply when giving ultrasound for its intrinsic effect (see p. 158). The effect of the drug must also be considered; for example, anti-inflammatory drugs may suppress necessary inflammatory reactions, such as local skin infections, allowing them to become more serious. If local skin-anaesthetizing drugs are being driven in by ultrasound it must be remembered that skin sensation under the treatment head will gradually be lost so that the patient may no longer detect excessive heat; high intensities should not therefore be used for these drugs.

PRINCIPLES OF APPLICATION

Adequate transmission of ultrasonic energy to the tissues depends on having a couplant that provides a good match of acoustic impedance between the metal of the transducer head and the skin. There is virtually no transmission of ultrasound from the transducer to air; the energy being reflected causes heating of, and possibly damage to, the transducer itself. Water is a good couplant (see below) but has to be held in place between the treatment head and the tissues in some way. It is therefore made into a gel, held in a plastic or rubber bag or the whole body part is immersed in water with the treatment head (Fig. 6.3). All three methods are in use but the first, called the direct contact method, is most commonly found. With all methods it is important to move the treatment head continuously relative to the tissues for the following reasons:

1 The ultrasound beam is very irregular in the near zone.
2 The pattern of energy absorption in the tissues is very irregular due to reflection and refraction.
3 Standing waves can be formed that might lead to temporary stasis of circulating blood cells and to endothelial damage.
4 At high intensities unstable cavitation or excess heating could occur causing tissue damage.

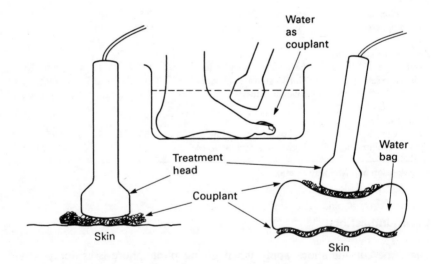

Fig. 6.3 Direct contact, immersion and water bag applications.

Steady movement of the treatment head will even out the dose delivered to the target tissues and will eliminate the risks of damage due to local high-intensity 'hot spots'.

Direct contact application

Thixotropic substances are gels that become fluid on vibration and thus make ideal couplants for ultrasound. Various agents of high molecular weight may be added to water to form a suitable gel provided they are non-irritant to the tissues and not corrosive to the metal of the treatment head. While tests have shown differences in the ability of different gels to transmit ultrasound (Docker and Patrick, 1982), most of the commercial gels are acceptable. KY gel has the advantage of very high viscosity and is available in sterile form. Creams, which are emulsions of light oils in water, are also widely used. The requirements for the couplant are an acoustic impedance similar to the tissues, high transmissivity and viscosity, low susceptibility to bubbles and a hygienic dispenser.

Transmission of ultrasound is sometimes expressed as a percentage of that of water, which is taken to be 100%. Tap water has been shown to be a satisfactory couplant for ultrasound, being significantly better than mineral oil or glycerin (Griffin, 1980). Although all studies do not agree on the superiority of water (Reid and Cummings, 1977) the differences are small and the safety, cheapness and convenience of water outweigh any possible loss of transmission.

The couplant also serves the important purpose of acting as a lubricant to allow the treatment head to move smoothly over the skin.

Technique

Prior to any treatment it is sensible to check that there is an output from the machine. This can be done by placing the treatment head just below the water surface in a suitable container and observing the disturbance which appears in the water. This, and similar methods, only indicates the presence of an output but to quantify it a radiation balance is needed.

The skin surface to be treated should be inspected; inflammatory skin conditions should be avoided, and the nature of the treatment explained to the patient. Oakley (1978) recommends that 'all patients should be tested for sensitivity before treatment'.

The couplant should be applied to the skin surface and/or the treatment head, which is placed on the skin before the machine is turned on. This is to avoid damage to the transducer which can occur if the energy is reflected back into the transducer at its interface with air. The treatment head is moved continuously over the surface while even pressure is maintained. The emitting surface must be kept parallel to the skin surface to reduce reflection and pressed sufficiently firmly to exclude any air. The rate of movement must be slow enough to allow the tissues to deform and thus remain in complete contact with the rigid treatment head but fast enough to prevent 'hot spots' developing when using a higher-intensity, continuous-mode treatment. Patrick (1978) states that with pulsed ultrasound used at minimal dosage the movement of the transducer should be so slow as to be almost imperceptible.

The pattern of movement can be a series of overlapping parallel strokes, circles or figures-of-eight. It is helpful if the position of the patient can be arranged so that the treatment head is applied downwards and moved horizontally as the weight of the treatment head contributes to the pressure, making it easier for the physiotherapist to control it. Furthermore, the couplant is more easily kept in place as it does not tend to move downwards away from the area. The physiotherapist should be comfortably seated with arm supported as skill is needed to apply efficient ultrasound, ensuring close contact, appropriate movement and correct angle of the transducer at all times.

Water bath application

As the part to be treated is immersed in water this can only reasonably be applied to the hand, forearm, foot and ankle. Testing the output of the machine and inspection of the part to be treated precede treatment, as above. The patient is seated and the part is put in water of a comfortable temperature, in such a position that it is suitably supported. The treatment head is placed in the water and moved parallel to the surface of the part which is being treated and about 2 cm or less away from the skin. The treatment head and skin will need to be wiped periodically to remove air bubbles which will reflect much ultrasound. If degassed water is used no bubbles can form but procuring fully degassed water for each patient is expensive and time-consuming so that it is simpler to remove the bubbles by hand when they are seen.

Ultrasound is easily transmitted through water so that little energy is lost. Treatment by this method is valuable because very irregular surfaces and tender areas can be comfortably treated as the treatment head does not exert pressure on the skin.

Water bag application

Another method of applying ultrasound to irregular surfaces which cannot conveniently be placed in a water bath is to use a plastic or rubber bag filled with water, forming a water cushion between the treatment head and the skin (Fig. 6.3). The water bag can be an ordinary rubber balloon but condoms are more satisfactory because the rubber is thinner and of better quality. Special devices which perform the same function are made. The bag should be filled with warm water, degassed if possible. All visible air bubbles should be squeezed out before knotting the neck of the bag to seal it. Couplant is smeared on to the surface of the bag, skin and treatment head. The bag is then held in place over the irregular surface to be treated; this takes a separate pair of hands, which can be the patient's in some circumstances. The treatment head is then pressed firmly on to the bag so that a layer of water about 1 cm thick separates it from the surface. Inevitably some bubbles will form and it is important to ensure that these are in the sides of the bag and not in the region transmitting the ultrasound. The treatment head is then moved mainly by deforming the bag although it can also be moved over the surface of the bag. It is likely that there will be increased energy losses at the many interfaces but as there seems to be no information on their magnitude it is suggested that the output intensity should be increased by perhaps 50% over what would be appropriate for a direct contact treatment.

Solid sterile gel as couplant

Ultrasound treatment cannot conveniently be given over open wounds or injured skin because there is a risk of transmitting infection and the moving treatment head may cause further damage. To solve these problems a polyacrylamide agar gel in a 3.3 mm sheet can be used as a couplant. In a hydrated form this material is sold in sterile packs as Geliperm and it is used for wound dressings and over skin grafts. It is 96% water but impermeable to bacteria, and is conveniently transparent.

The flexible sheet, cut to an appropriate size, is placed over the open wound with a little sterile saline to ensure that there are no air bubbles between the gel sheet and the raw surface. The slightly wetted outside surface of the gel sheet will allow the treatment head to move smoothly over it. The gel has been found to transmit 95% of the applied ultrasound energy (Brueton and Campbell, 1987).

DOSAGE

Having determined the condition, position and depth of the target tissue, the various parameters of ultrasound must be decided on. These include mode, frequency, intensity and time. As there is no certain way of knowing how much energy is absorbed in any particular tissue, decisions about dosage become a matter of judgement to some extent. This judgement must be based on the known factors governing ultrasound absorption.

Mode—continuous or pulsed output

As noted earlier, ultrasound treatments may be given as continuous or pulsed output. Continuous produces some heat in the tissues but pulsed ultrasound allows higher instantaneous intensities but much lower time-averaged intensity (see below), hence negligible heating.

Frequency

As attenuation increases with rising frequency effectively the lower frequencies penetrate further (Table 6.2). Thus much of the energy carried in 3 MHz ultrasound is absorbed in the superficial tissues whereas 0.75 MHz ultrasound will penetrate deeply through the tissue; that is, it has a large half-value depth. While it makes sense to use higher-frequency ultrasound, such as 3 MHz, to treat superficial tissue it must be remembered that significant amounts of energy from lower-frequency therapeutic ultrasound are also absorbed by the superficial layers.

Intensity

Power, that is the total energy per second supplied by the machine, is measured in watts. Since this is spread over the whole face of the transducer, and transducers are of different sizes, it is more useful to give the intensity in W/cm^2. Most therapeutic sources emit up to a spatial average maximum of $3 W/cm^2$. It has already been explained that the ultrasound beam is very irregular so a useful measure is the average intensity of the peaks and troughs of the sonic field over a specific area, usually the transducer face; this is the space-averaged intensity.

Time-averaged intensity is an important value in pulsed treatments. The intensity shown on the meter is usually the space-averaged time-averaged (SATA) intensity. During pulsed treatments the SATA intensity is obviously much lower; this may be indicated by the meter, although on some machines the meter may continue to indicate the average intensity during the pulse—called pulse-averaged intensity (ter Haar, 1987). It is reasonable to increase the intensity to compensate for losses due to absorption and scattering when treating more deeply placed targets. By estimating the depth of the target tissue from the surface and knowing the half-value depth, an appropriate intensity can be selected. For example, if an intensity of $0.25 W/cm^2$ is required for a lesion 40 mm deep, using a 1 MHz frequency, the surface intensity would have to be $0.5 W/cm^2$, assuming a half value depth of 40 mm.

When treating 'thin' areas, such as the hand, it may be necessary to reduce the surface intensity to allow for possible reflection of the ultrasound beam from the further skin–air interface.

Dyson (1987) states that intensities towards the upper end of the range available on most ultrasound machines are potentially damaging. The lowest intensity and highest frequency required to produce the desired therapeutic effect should therefore be used. Low, but still therapeutically effective, temporal average intensities can be achieved by using a pulse-averaged intensity of $0.5 W/cm^2$ (2 ms on, 8 ms off) to give a temporal average intensity of $0.1 W/cm^2$.

Time

The amount of energy applied to the tissues and hence the effects will depend not only on the intensity but also on the length of time for which it has been applied. Quite short treatment times of a few minutes are usually considered to be sufficient. As the treatment head is moved continuously over the treated area the size of this area must be the most important determinant of the treatment time. There are differing opinions but a convenient guide is to give 1–2 min of treatment for every 10 cm² of surface covered (many transducer heads have an area of 5 cm² and the palm of a small hand is about 50 cm²). Minimum treatment times are considered to be 1–2 min, maximum 10–15 min and an average would be in the region of 5 min.

Table 6.4 summarizes some of these points. The dosage chosen is often a compromise, taking account of several different factors. In general, the smallest effective dose should be used.

Table 6.4 Summary of choice of dose

Heating of the tissues	Mode	
Desirable	Continuous	
Not required	Pulsed	

Depth of lesion	Frequency	Assumed half value depth
Superficial	3 MHz	25 mm
Medium	1 MHz	40 mm
Very deep	0.75 MHz	100 mm

Nature of condition	Intensity
Acute	Low (see text)
Chronic	Higher (see text)
Surface intensity adjustment to take account of	
Depth of lesion	
Frequency of wave form	

Depth in mm	Intensity at various depths (W/cm²) (1 W/cm² at surface)		
	3 MHz	1 MHz	0.75 MHz
20	0.5		
40	0.25	0.5	
60			
80	0.125	0.25	
100	0.06		0.5

	Time
Surface area of lesion	1–2 min/10 cm²

Progress	Action
No change	Increase dose
Better	Same dose
Worse	Decrease dose

Progression and timing

Recent injuries and acute conditions should be treated as soon as possible after the occurrence and thereafter once or twice daily. Chronic conditions may be treated on alternate days.

Progression is based on the outcome of previous treatment. If there is subjective and objective improvement the treatment should be continued at the same dose. If the symptoms are unpredictably worse the treatment should be reduced or discontinued. If there is no change when one would be expected the dose should be increased one parameter at a time until some change is apparent or until a number of applications have been tried without result, in which case the ultrasound should be discontinued.

POSSIBLE DANGERS

There seems to be no reported evidence of damage due directly to therapeutic ultrasound but it is reasonable to suppose that injury could occur under some conditions.

1 Burns could occur if the heat generated exceeded the physiological ability to dissipate it.
2 Tissue destruction would result from transient cavitation.
3 Blood cell stasis and endothelial damage may occur if there is standing wave formation.

These dangers would be more likely with high-intensity continuous-output with a stationary head or over bony prominences. If the patient feels any pain, aching or prickling during the application the intensity should be reduced or the treatment terminated.

CONTRAINDICATIONS

Rapidly dividing tissue

Since ultrasound has been shown to affect tissue repair it is possible that it could affect abnormal tissue activity so that it might encourage neoplastic growth and provoke metastases. Therefore, treatment over tumours or over tissue in precancerous states should be avoided.

Similarly, any risk to the rapidly dividing and differentiating cells of the embryo and fetus should be avoided by not applying treatment over the pregnant uterus. Diagnostic ultrasound is entirely safe and it is probable that low doses of therapeutic ultrasound would have no ill effects.

It may be wise to avoid the epiphyseal plates.

Spread of infection

It has been suggested that bacterial or viral infection could be spread by ultrasound, presumably by facilitating micro-organism movement across membranes and through the tissues. In spite of the lack of evidence this seems a reasonable supposition so infected areas should not be treated with ultrasound.

Due to the possible risk of reactivating encapsulated lesions tuberculous regions should also not be treated.

Vascular problems

Circumstances in which haemorrhage might be provoked should not be treated—for example, where bleeding is still occurring or has only recently been controlled, such as an enlarging haemarthrosis or haematoma or uncontrollable haemophilia.

Severely ischaemic tissues should be avoided because of the poor heat transfer and possible greater risk of arterial thrombosis due to stasis and endothelial damage.

Treatment over recent venous thrombosis might extend the thrombus or disrupt its attachment to the vein wall forming an embolus. Areas of atherosclerosis are best avoided for the same reason.

Radiotherapy

Areas that have received radiotherapy in the last 6 months should not be treated.

The nervous system

Normal doses of ultrasound have been applied for many years to the tissues around the spinal cord without any ill effects. In fact treatment of the spinal nerve roots and over the apophyseal joints is particularly common. Since the central nervous system is deeply buried beneath thick muscle and, more importantly, bone tissue it seems reasonable to suppose that only trivial amounts of energy could reach it. Where nerve tissue is exposed, e.g. over a spina bifida or after a laminectomy, ultrasound should be avoided. Statements are sometimes made to the effect that treatment over the cervical ganglia or vagus nerve might be dangerous in cardiac disease (Forster and Palastanga, 1985).

Specialized tissue

The fluid-filled eye offers exceptionally good ultrasound transmission and retinal damage could occur.

Treatment over the gonads is not recommended.

Implants

Although metal implants in the tissues would reflect the ultrasound at their interfaces and thus lead to more energy absorption in these areas, this does not lead to a large temperature rise in the region because the metal conducts the heat very easily to other cooler areas. Experiments with implanted metal in pigs showed no ill effects when ultrasound was applied (Lehmann and deLateur, 1982). The effects might, however, be different with smaller and more superficial implants, like metal bone-fixing pins subcutaneously placed; as a precaution, low doses should be used in these circumstances.

Plastics used in replacement surgery, such as high-density polyethylene and acrylic, should also be avoided since their effect on ultrasound absorption is unknown (Lehmann and deLateur, 1982).

Treatment over implanted cardiac pacemakers should not be given because the sonic vibration may interfere with the pacemaker's stimulating frequency.

Anaesthetic areas

There are some circumstances in which caution should be exercised. High doses should not be given over anaesthetic areas. It must be realized that the most common pain produced by high-intensity ultrasound is deep periosteal pain, probably due to the large amount of energy absorbed at the bone–tissue interface where there is not only reflection but shear waves may also occur, as explained earlier. Thus the cutaneous thermal sensation is of no consequence as regards protection, except where heating is occurring in or on the skin.

REFERENCES

Bearzy H. J. (1953). Clinical applications of ultrasonic energy in treatment of acute and chronic subacromial bursitis. *Arch. Phys. Med. Rehab.*, **34**, 228–31.

Benson H. A. E., McElnay J. C. (1988). Transmission of ultrasound energy through pharmaceutical products. *Physiotherapy*, **74**, 587–9.

Benson H. A. E., McElnay J. C., Harland R. (1988). Phonophoresis of lignocaine and prilocaine from Emla cream. *Int. J. Pharm.*, **44**, 65–9.

Benson H. A. E., McElnay J. C., Harland D. R. (1989). Use of ultrasound to enhance percutaneous absorption of benzydamine. *Phys. Ther.*, **69**, 113–18.

Brueton R. N., Campbell B. (1987). The use of Geliperm as a sterile coupling agent for therapeutic ultrasound. *Physiotherapy*, **73**, 653–4.

Bierman W. (1954). Ultrasound in the treatment of scars. *Arch. Phys. Med. Rehab.*, **35**, 209–13.

Callam M. J., Harper D. R., Dale J. J. *et al.* (1987). A controlled trial of weekly ultrasound therapy in chronic leg ulceration. *Lancet*, **ii**, 204–6.

Clarke G. R., Stenner L. (1976). Use of therapeutic ultrasound. *Physiotherapy*, **62**, 185–90.

Creates V. (1987). A study of ultrasound treatment to the painful perineum after childbirth. *Physiotherapy*, **73**, 162–5.

De Preux T. (1952). Ultrasonic wave therapy in osteo-arthritis of the hip joint. *Br. J. Phys. Med.*, **15**, 14–19.

Docker M. F., Patrick M. K. (1982). Ultrasound couplants for physiotherapy. *Physiotherapy*, **68**, 124–5.

Downing D. S., Weinstein A. (1986). Ultrasound therapy of subacromial bursitis: a double-blind trial. *Phys. Ther.*, **66**, 194–9.

Dyson M. (1985). Therapeutic applications of ultrasound. In *Biological Effects of Ultrasound* (Nyborg W. L., Ziskin M. C., eds.) London: Churchill Livingstone.

Dyson M. (1987). Mechanisms involved in therapeutic ultrasound. *Physiotherapy*, **73**, 116–20.

Dyson M., Pond J. B. (1970). The effect of pulsed ultrasound on tissue regeneration. *Physiotherapy*, **56**, 136–42.

Dyson M., Pond J. B. (1973). The effects of ultrasound on circulation. *Physiotherapy*, **59**, 284–7.

Dyson M., Pond J., Woodward B. *et al.* (1974). The production of blood cell stasis and endothelial cell damage in the blood vessels of chick embryos treated with ultrasound in a stationary wavefield. *Ultrasound Med. Biol.*, **1**, 133–48.

Dyson M., Suckling J. (1978). Stimulation of tissue repair by ultrasound: a survey of the mechanisms involved. *Physiotherapy*, **64**, 105–8.

El Hag M., Coghlan K., Christmas P. *et al.* (1985). The anti-inflammatory effects of dexamethasone and therapeutic ultrasound in oral surgery. *Br. J. Oral Maxillo. Surg.*, **23**, 17–23.

Evans P. (1980). The healing process at cellular level: a review. *Physiotherapy*, **66**, 256–9.

Fahim M. (1980). New treatment for herpes simplex virus type 2. (Ultrasound and zinc, urea and tannic acid ointment.) Part II. Female patients. *J. Med.*, **11**, 143–67.

Ferguson H. N. (1981). Ultrasound in the treatment of surgical wounds. *Physiotherapy*, **67**, 12.

Fieldhouse C. (1979). Ultrasound for relief of painful episiotomy scars. *Physiotherapy*, **65**, 217.

Forster A., Palastanga N. (1985). *Clayton's Electrotherapy: Theory and Practice*. London: Baillière Tindall.

Frizzel L. A., Dunn F. (1982). Biophysics of ultrasound. In *Therapeutic Heat and Cold* (Lehmann J. F., ed.) Baltimore: Williams & Wilkins.

Fyfe M. C., Bullock M. I. (1985). Therapeutic ultrasound: some historical background and development in knowledge of its effects on healing. *Aust. J. Physiother.*, **31**, 220–4.

Garrett A. S., Garrett M. (1982). Ultrasound for herpes zoster pain. *J.R. Coll. Gen. Pract.*, **32**, 709, 711.

Griffin J. E. (1980). Transmissiveness of ultrasound through tap water, glycerin and mineral oil. *Phys. Ther.*, **60**, 1010–16.

Griffin J. E., Echternach J. L., Price R. E. *et al.* (1967). Patients treated with ultrasonic driven hydrocortisone and with ultrasound alone. *Phys. Ther.*, **74**, 594–601.

Griffin J. E., Echternach J. L., Bowmaker K. L. (1970). Results of frequency differences in ultrasonic therapy. *Phys. Ther.*, **50**, 481–6.

Harvey W., Dyson M., Pond J. B., Grahame R. (1975). The 'in vitro' stimulation of protein synthesis in human fibroblasts by therapeutic levels of ultrasound. *Proceedings of 2nd European Congress on Ultrasonics in Medicine*, pp. 10–21.

Hashish I., Harvey W., Harris M. (1986). Anti-inflammatory effects of ultrasound therapy: evidence for a major placebo effect. *Br. J. Rheumatol.*, **25**, 77–88.

Hoogland R. (1986). *Ultrasound Therapy.* Delft: Enraf Nonius.

Jones R. J. (1984). Treatment of acute herpes zoster using ultrasonic therapy. *Physiotherapy,* **70,** 94–6.

Kleinkort J. R., Wood F. (1975). Phonophoresis with 1 per cent versus 10 per cent hydrocortisone. *Phys. Ther.,* **55,** 1320–4.

Lehmann J. F. (1965). Ultrasound therapy. In *Therapeutic Heat and Cold* (Licht S. ed.) pp. 321–86. Baltimore: Elizabeth Licht Publisher, Waverly Press Incorporated.

Lehmann J. F., deLateur B. J. (1982). Therapeutic heat. In *Therapeutic Heat and Cold* 3rd edn (Lehmann J. F., ed.) Baltimore: Williams & Wilkins.

Lehmann J. F., Guy A. W. (1972). Ultrasonic therapy in interaction of ultrasound and biological tissues. *Workshop Proceedings* (Reid J. M., Sikov M. R., eds). US Dept of Health Education and Welfare publication (FDA) 73,73-8008, pp. 141–52.

Markham D. E., Wood M. R. (1980). Ultrasound for Dupuytren's contracture. *Physiotherapy,* **66,** 55–8.

McDiarmid T., Burns P. N. (1987). Clinical applications of therapeutic ultrasound. *Physiotherapy,* **73,** 155–62.

McDiarmid T., Burns P. N., Lewith G. T. *et al.* (1985). Ultrasound and the treatment of pressure sores. *Physiotherapy,* **71,** 66–70.

McLaren J. (1984). Randomised controlled trial of ultrasound therapy for the damaged perineum. *Clin. Phys. Physiol. Measure.,* **5,** 40.

Middlemast S. J., Chatterjee D. S. (1978). Comparison of ultrasound and thermography for soft tissue injuries. *Physiotherapy,* **64,** 331–2.

Munting E. (1978). Ultrasound therapy for painful shoulders. *Physiotherapy,* **64,** 180–1.

Oakley E. M. (1978). Application of continuous beam ultrasound at therapeutic levels. *Physiotherapy,* **64,** 103–4.

Partridge C. J. (1987). Evaluation of the efficacy of ultrasound. *Physiotherapy,* **73,** 166–8.

Patrick M. K. (1978). Applications of therapeutic pulsed ultrasound. *Physiotherapy,* **64,** 103–4.

Payne C. (1984). Ultrasound for post-herpetic neuralgia. *Physiotherapy,* **70,** 96–7.

Reid D. C., Cummings G. E. (1977). Efficiency of ultrasound coupling agents. *Physiotherapy,* **63,** 255–7.

Roche C., West J. (1984). A controlled trial investigating the effect of ultrasound on venous ulcers referred from general practitioners. *Physiotherapy,* **70,** 475–7.

Rubin D., Kuitert J. H. (1955). Use of ultrasonic vibration in the treatment of pain arising from phantom limbs, scars and neuromas: a preliminary report. *Arch. Phys. Med. Rehab.,* **36,** 445.

Skauen D. M., Zentner G. M. (1984). Phonophoresis. *Int. J. Pharm.,* **20,** 235–45.

Summer W., Patrick M. K. (1964). *Ultrasonic Therapy. A Textbook for Physiotherapists.* London: Elsevier.

ter Haar G. (1978). Basic physics of therapeutic ultrasound. *Physiotherapy,* **64,** 100–3.

ter Haar G. R. (1987). Basic physics of therapeutic ultrasound. *Physiotherapy,* **73,** 110–13.

ter Haar G. R., Daniels S. (1981). Evidence for ultrasonically induced cavitation in vivo. *Physics Med. Biol.,* **26,** 1145–9.

Wadsworth H., Chanmugan A. P. P. (1980). *Electrophysical Agents in Physiotherapy.* Marrickville, NSW, Australia: Science Press.

Ward A. R. (1986). *Electricity Fields and Waves in Therapy.* Marrickville, NSW, Australia: Science Press.

Williams R. (1987). Production and transmission of ultrasound. *Physiotherapy,* **73,** 113–16.

Young S. R. (1988). The effect of therapeutic ultrasound on the biological mechanisms involved in dermal regeneration. PhD Thesis, University of London.

7.   *Heat and cold*

GENERAL PRINCIPLES

Despite the fact that heat and cold are very familiar ideas, the fundamental nature of heat is often not well understood.

To understand what happens when matter becomes hot it is necessary to consider the microstructure of matter.

Solids are formed of collections of atoms or molecules closely packed together in a regular pattern, so that each can only move a short distance. Under normal circumstances the average interatomic force is zero. If the atoms move closer together, e.g. when the solid is compressed, repulsion forces push them apart again and as they separate the force of attraction between them becomes greater and draws them together. Thus the atoms or molecules vibrate about their equilibrium positions and it is these movements—kinetic energy—which are recognized as heat. If more heat energy is added the amount of motion increases and usually (but not in all circumstances) the matter becomes hotter, i.e. the temperature increases.

163

Electrotherapy explained

In *liquids* the atoms or molecules have a rather greater amplitude of vibration and can partly overcome the interatomic forces of their immediate neighbours. The atoms have greater speeds because of their increased temperature and move randomly.

In *gases* the atoms are widely spaced and move randomly over much larger distances. Again adding heat causes more motion so that the average positions of the atoms becomes further apart so the matter has expanded. This is very evident in gases because of the large interatomic distances but less obvious in liquids and still less in solids. This property of expansion is utilized in engines to convert heat energy to mechanical energy and in the measurement of temperature.

The idea that heat is a form of energy and is conserved is asserted by the first law of thermodynamics.

Temperature

Temperature is a measure of the level of heat. Humans assess this level through special temperature receptors in the skin. The judgement made by the central nervous system is not absolute; rather it is a comparison of skin temperatures. If the right hand is immersed in hot and the left in cold water and both hands are then placed in tepid water it feels cold to the right hand and hot to the left. This illustrates a general feature of perception in the nervous system which tends to recognize contrasts.

Most simple thermometers utilize expansion to measure temperature, mercury in glass being the familiar form. Mercury expands much more than glass on being heated and if it is only allowed to expand along a very narrow tube quite a small temperature change will cause a large movement of mercury along the tube. To measure temperature two fixed points, the melting point of ice and the boiling point of water are found, and the region between them divided into 100 parts, called degrees. Such a scale was first described by Andreas Celsius, a Swedish astronomer of the early 18th century, and is known as the Celsius scale, abbreviated to C. (In English-speaking countries it was formerly known as the centigrade scale but Celsius has now been universally adopted by international agreement.) Gabriel Fahrenheit invented the mercury-in-glass thermometer about 1714 but used the freezing point of brine as his zero and the body temperature of a healthy human as his other fixed point; he divided the interval into 96 degrees. This led to the freezing point of water being 32°F, its boiling point at 212°F and, subsequently corrected, body temperature to 98.4°F. While the Fahrenheit scale has long been discarded for scientific purposes it is still found describing room and water temperatures, in the hydrotherapy pool for example, and in other situations. It is important, therefore, to understand the relationship between these two scales.

It will be realized that if temperature is due to the kinetic energy of atoms and molecules there is no upper limit, since more heat leads to more motion. There is, however, a definite lower limit as less heat gives less motion until

ultimately there is no motion at all. This point is called absolute zero, and is
− 273.2°C. For much scientific work the more logical kelvin scale is used; this
is the SI unit of temperature. This treats absolute zero as 0°K and uses the same
degrees as the Celsius scale so that the freezing point of water becomes 273K
and its boiling point 373K. It is called after Lord Kelvin, formerly William
Thomson, who deduced the effect.

Quantity of heat

If a kettleful of boiling water is poured into a bath of tepid water the bath
water may become perceptibly warmer but not nearly as hot as the water in
the kettle. Clearly when a small quantity of water is added it carries a small
quantity of heat which when spread throughout the larger volumes leads to
little rise in temperature. To describe the quantity of heat a unit called the
calorie was formerly used. This is the amount of heat needed to raise the
temperature of 1 g of water 1°C; but since it is an energy measurement the
appropriate SI units are now used, i.e. 4.18 kJ/kg/°C for water. In dietetics the
kilocalorie is still widely used and is confusingly called the Calorie (with a
capital C); this is therefore equal to 4.18 kJ. This amount of heat energy
applied to unit mass of a material to raise the temperature 1°C is known as the
specific heat of the material. Water has a much greater specific heat than other
common materials (Table 7.1) so that it takes a great deal of heat energy to
raise the temperature of water and conversely hot water stores much heat per
unit mass. The amount of heat needed to raise the temperature of a material
per unit volume is known as the heat capacity and is found by multiplying the
specific heat by the density of the material.

The specific heat of the human body is close to 3.5 kJ/kg/°C (Sekins and
Emery, 1982) which is not surprising since it is 70% water. To raise the

Table 7.1 Specific heat

	Specific heat (kJ/kg/1°C)
Water	4.185
Air	1.01
Aluminium	0.904
Copper	0.402
Mercury	0.14
Glass	0.77
Paraffin wax	about 2.7
Rubber	2.01
Whole human body	3.56
Skin	3.77
Fat	2.3
Muscle	3.75
Bone	1.59
Whole blood	3.64

Data from Sekins and Emery (1982).

temperature of a 50 kg woman 2°C it takes 350 kJ of energy (50 × 3.5 × 2). Notice that this would be additional to the energy continuously being generated in the body. In fact, even at rest the basal metabolic rate leads to the emission of heat.

The conversion of any form of energy—electrical, chemical, magnetic etc.—to any other form leads to the general law of conservation of energy, which briefly can be expressed as follows: energy can neither be created nor destroyed. Similarly, there is a law of conservation of mass stating that it is impossible to create or destroy matter. However, it was recognized that mass and energy are two forms of the same thing; this was postulated by Albert Einstein's special theory of relativity in 1905. This is quantified by the expression $E = mc^2$, where E is energy, m is mass and c the velocity of electromagnetic radiation, i.e. $3 × 10^8$ m/s. Thus huge amounts of energy in the form of heat and radiation are released by a nuclear explosion at the expense of a very small amount of matter. The continuous production of heat and light by the sun, the source of all energy on earth, is due to the continuous conversion of matter into radiation. In fact, matter can be considered as concentrated energy. (It has been calculated that 1 kg of mass contains enough energy to operate a million 100 W light bulbs for 30 years.)

The addition of heat

When heat is added to matter it can cause expansion (an increase in volume or, if the volume is restricted, an increase in pressure) or it may change the physical state of the material, by melting or vaporizing it or it may cause a temperature rise in the material, or any combination of these. Temperature rise combined with expansion is perhaps the most familiar. Causing gas to expand and do useful mechanical work is the basis of many familiar engines, the internal combustion engine of cars or the steam turbines of power stations for example. Much ingenuity goes into designing engines that convert as much heat energy into expansion with as little temperature increase as possible but this can never be 100% efficient (see below). When water boils a change of state occurs in which the liquid is changed into a gas. The heat energy is used in separating the molecules, disrupting the bonding forces and changing the state from liquid to gas, rather than increasing the kinetic energy; therefore there is no rise of temperature during the process. Exactly the same thing happens when the solid form, i.e. ice, is melted to water and when any other substance is vaporized or melted. As the energy used to make these physical changes does not appear as temperature rises the energy is stored in the microstructure of the material and can be returned as heat if the process is reversed. It is therefore known as latent heat. The quantity of heat per unit mass is characteristic for any material. For water it takes approximately 540 Cal (2260 J) to change each gram into water vapour and about 80 Cal/g for the change from ice to water. Other substances have different latent heats; for example, the vaporization of liquid ammonia needs 340 Cal/g. Some material can pass from a solid directly to a gaseous state; this process is called sublimation.

In solids atoms are more strictly confined by neighbouring atoms so that the addition of heat leads to each atom oscillating more vigorously, increasing the average separation from other atoms, and hence expanding the whole material. When heat energy is added it not only goes to increasing the kinetic motion of the molecules, thus raising the temperature, but also to increasing the intramolecular and intra-atomic energies.

Liquids have rather more space between molecules than solids but much less than in gases. Almost all liquid states are therefore less dense than the solid states. Water is exceptional in that the molecules are more closely packed together at around 4°C than when the crystalline solid, ice, is formed; thus ice will float on water. The same thing happens when molten bismuth solidifies.

Energy conversions

Having described heat as the energy of the microstructure of matter it is important to understand how it is related to other energy forms. There is no difficulty in converting other forms of energy, such as mechanical or electrical energy, to heat energy in their entirety, with 100% efficiency; but it is not possible to do the reverse, turning all the heat energy in the microstructure of matter to some other energy form. Similarly, if one form of energy is converted to another, say chemical to mechanical, there is always some part converted to heat in the material so that such conversions can never be 100% efficient. Some of these concepts are expressed in Figure 7.1, which also shows some familiar energy conversions.

Since all energy ultimately ends as heat in the structure of matter it is sometimes described as the basic form of energy, but it is simply the tendency to randomization. Thus ordered molecular motion, such as the movement of a pendulum or the pendular motion of a swinging arm, are all the molecules moving in the same direction at the same time. Molecular motion is steadily converted to heat by friction in the air and at the moving joints. So, the regular ordered motion is changed to disordered (random) motion of the molecules of the material, that is heat energy. This idea is expressed in various ways as the second law of thermodynamics; if a system is free to change itself it will end in a state of higher probability, i.e. the energy will be randomized. If a metal spoon is put into a cup of hot coffee the motion of the water molecules striking the spoon transfer energy by making the metal atoms move about more (see below) so that the heat energy is averaged out between the spoon, which becomes hotter, and the coffee, which is cooled. It is said that heat has passed from the hotter to the cooler material. For a clear, authoritative and more extensive explanation of these phenomena see Swartz and Goldfarb (1974).

Heat transfer

1 One method of transferring heat from place to place has been noted above; that is, by the kinetic motion of atoms and molecules being passed from one

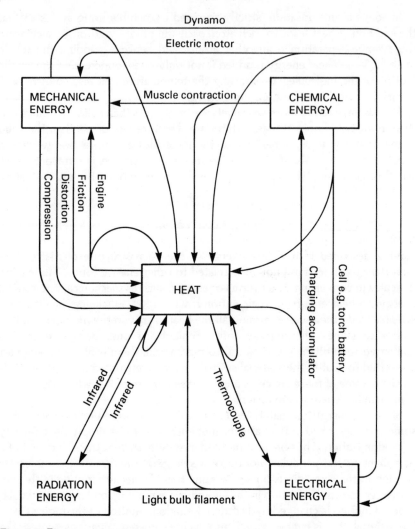

Fig. 7.1 Energy conversions.

to the next, dramatically described as 'atoms jostling one another'. This is called *conduction* and is easily demonstrated, especially in metals; if one end of a metal bar is heated the other end becomes hotter in time. (This concept is familiar to most of us as a consequence of leaving metal spoons and forks in the cooking pot!) Conduction is an inevitable consequence of molecular and atomic motion in the microstructure of any material and it would be expected that 'jostling' would be more effective in transmitting energy if the molecules are closer together, as happens in solids, and this is broadly the case. Metals make good heat conductors while liquids and gases are much less effective. Notice that if two different materials are in contact heat can be transferred from one to the other in the same way, the molecules of the hotter material knocking into and so giving kinetic energy to those of the cooler. Heat flow through matter varies with the nature of the material and is called thermal conductivity. It is expressed in Cal/s/cm/°C. It can also be expressed in W/m/°C (1 W = 1 J/s). Very roughly, the thermal conductivity of liquids is about 100 times that of gases and that of solids is about 100 times that of liquids. This explains why gas, e.g. air, makes such an effective thermal insulator.

2 A second way of transferring heat energy is by bulk movement of the moving molecules themselves. When hotter atoms or molecules move from one place to another, as can easily occur with liquids and gases, the heat energy is said to be moved by *convection*. The fluid movement can be due to being pumped—the distribution of heat around the body is due to the heart circulating the warm blood—or it can be due to the fact that the heated liquid or gas, being less dense, tends to float upwards on the cooler fluid. This latter is called thermal convection and is familiar in many situations, from making marmalade to meteorology.

3 The third way in which heat energy can be transferred is by *radiation*. This is really the conversion of heat energy to an electromagnetic radiation. The most familiar radiations are infrared radiations which can be produced by heating and lead to heating when they are absorbed; both visible and microwave radiations can also lead to heating when they are absorbed. When sufficient energy is added to matter to alter rotational and vibrational levels within the molecule, some of the energy can be emitted as microwave and infrared radiations. Similarly, disturbing the electron configuration of atoms leads to the production of visible radiations. All objects are emitting radiation all the time but they are also absorbing it. In many everyday circumstances objects are radiating infrared and absorbing the same amount radiated from other objects, thus maintaining a balance.

The amount of radiation depends on the temperature of the object; it is proportional to the fourth power of the kelvin temperature. The wavelength is also dependent on temperature so that emissions of shorter and shorter wavelength are given off with higher temperatures. (These relationships are defined in Stephen's law and Wien's laws respectively.) This conforms with common experience in that the radiation given off at low temperatures is not detectable and at higher temperatures the infrared can be sensed; at even higher temperatures objects become red-hot with both infrared and visible radiations being given off; at still higher temperatures heated objects give off yellow light and eventually become white-hot.

Radiations can travel through space. In this way heat can be transferred without any intervening matter. This is of considerable consequence since all energy on earth is ultimately derived from the radiation energy given out continuously by the sun. (The sun generates energy by converting matter into energy in a sort of ongoing nuclear fission emitting enormous amounts of radiation due to its high temperature of around 6000°K.)

Although heat transmission is customarily described in terms of conduction, mainly in solids, convection in fluids and radiation it must be recognized that in many real-life situations all three operate as complex chains of heat

Electrotherapy explained

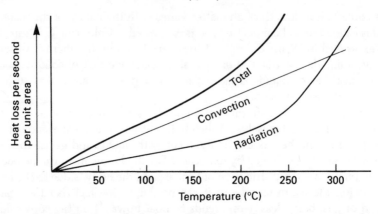

Fig. 7.2 Graph of heat transfer from an object kept at the same temperature above the surroundings showing the different contributions of convection and radiation.

exchanges. For example, central heating radiators are warmed by hot water pumped through them (forced convection) and they warm air in contact with their surfaces (conduction) which rises (thermal convection) to warm the room. The radiator also emits infrared radiations which are absorbed by other objects and people in the room, which causes further heating. Obviously the contribution from both radiation and convection will increase with increasing temperature but whereas convection increases approximately linearly, radiation increases exponentially; thus at low temperatures energy is transferred predominantly by convection (Fig. 7.2).

Summary

Adding energy to matter increases the kinetic energy of its microstructure. This can result in:

1 A rise in temperature—heating.
2 Expansion of the material.
3 A change of physical state—melting or vaporization.

The amount of heat energy needed to produce a given temperature rise depends on the specific heat of the material. Similarly there is a characteristic value for the amount of expansion for different materials—the coefficient of linear or volume expansion. The change of state will occur at characteristic temperatures for different substances. At these temperatures all the energy goes into overcoming the binding forces so that there is no temperature rise during this period.

Heat may be transferred by:

1 Conduction.
2 Convection.
3 Radiation.

In conduction the molecular or atomic agitation travels directly through the material at a rate which depends on the nature of the material and is described as the thermal conductivity.

Convection is the bulk transport of fluids, and hence of the heat of their microstructure. Although easy to visualize, thermal convection currents are difficult to quantify. Forced convection refers to the liquid or gas being pumped from one place to another.

Radiation involves heat being converted to electromagnetic radiation, largely infrared radiation, which will pass through space and when absorbed by matter cause heating. Other radiations, like microwave and visible light, will also cause heating when they are absorbed, in the same way as infrared. Ionizing radiation such as ultraviolet and X-rays also does this to a small extent but it is overshadowed by the dramatic chemical and other effects they produce (Chapter 15).

The idea of cold is due to human perception and skin temperature and is simply the absence of heat.

Thermometers

A thermometer is an instrument that measures temperature. It may utilize any physical change that correlates with heating and cooling. By far the most familiar is the mercury-in-glass thermometer used clinically to measure body temperature and also in laboratories. This device depends on the expansion of mercury which is much greater than that of glass when both are heated. The mercury-filled bulb is heated and the expansion is made visible because a thin line of mercury is forced along a narrow glass capillary tube. A typical clinical thermometer with a range of 30–45°C has a constriction in the capillary tube which breaks the mercury thread, preventing its return to the bulb as cooling occurs. This allows an accurate reading of the maximum temperature reached. The glass cylinder acts as a lens to enlarge the mercury thread. These thermometers can be extremely accurate: when new the vast majority are accurate to within 0.1°C (Cetas, 1982). The disadvantages are the dangers when breakages occur and the fact that these thermometers cannot easily be coupled into electronic systems for continuous patient monitoring. Alcohol-in-glass thermometers work in the same way, are usually larger and can be made easier to read by colouring the alcohol. They are often used for checking room or waterbath temperatures.

Another widely used thermometer depends on the difference in expansion of two metals when they are heated. Strips of brass and invar are firmly fixed together so that the whole bimetallic strip will bend on heating because the brass expands more than the invar. The bimetallic strip can be wound into a spiral with one end fixed and the other end moving a pointer over a temperature scale. Such thermometers are sturdy but often inaccurate. The bimetallic strip is in widespread use as a thermostat, that is a device to open or close a switch at a pre-set temperature. The switch may be closed, say to turn on current for water heating; as the water temperature rises it affects the

Electrotherapy explained

bimetallic strip causing it to bend away from the electrical contact, thus opening the switch and turning off the heater current. This kind of system is found in many situations controlling the temperature of domestic water heaters, room temperature, electric blankets, electric heater pads and the paraffin wax baths used in physiotherapy departments, as well as many other situations.

This idea is a good example of a common and important mechanism, known as a negative feedback system or a servo mechanism. Numerous physiological mechanisms which maintain body constancy are of this kind, for example, the appropriate level of a particular hormone in the blood, or the body temperature itself. The general features are:

1 Continuously monitoring some factor—water temperature, hormone level etc.
2 Responding to any change in a way that opposes or negates that change, e.g. shutting off heater current if water temperature rises.

Many other examples of such systems will come to mind, from rocking chairs to autopilots. All of them have a tendency to oscillate about the mean position because there is inevitably some delay between the change and the response.

The opposite system is a positive feedback mechanism in which a change causes a response to increase (reinforce) the initial change. This leads to a rapid acceleration to the limits of the system; for example, the opening of the sodium gates across the nerve fibre membrane during the development of a nerve impulse (see Chapter 1).

Other thermometers use different effects. When metals are heated the ohmic resistance rises with temperature. Platinum resistance thermometers are used to achieve great accuracy in laboratory work.

In the thermistor, a semiconductor, the electrical resistance decreases exponentially with rise in temperature. At low temperatures the electrons in a semiconductor are bound to the atoms but as the temperature rises more and more electrons are freed to wander from atom to atom—as they do in metal conductors—so the resistance falls. They can be manufactured to be very small—a tiny bead or disc on the end of two fine wires—and are relatively accurate. For these reasons they are used as thermal probes in hypodermic needles for testing temperature deep in the tissues. They are also found in the little discs of epoxy resin of some digital readout skin thermometers.

The thermocouple is a device that utilizes the electromotive force which develops between two different metals if their junction at one end is at a different temperature to the opposite end. They have been largely superseded by thermistors for clinical work.

Thermography

Thermography is the term used for the process of sensing the temperature of quite large areas of the body by photographing the surface using an infrared sensitive film. The film can be made to give a colour response to different temperatures, thus giving a colourful map of the temperature of the surface being investigated. This technique is used in the detection of underlying areas of inflammation or hot spots and for other purposes.

Certain liquid crystals will change colour on being heated and can therefore be used as temperature sensors.

A pyrometer, which is simply another word for thermometer, usually refers to measurement of heat from the emitted radiation, usually for high temperatures.

Numerous other types of thermometers have been developed for special purposes. For clinical and general use electronic thermometers are no more accurate, and sometimes less reliable, than the mercury-in-glass type originally developed over 300 years ago (Cetas, 1982; Table 7.2).

Table 7.2   Thermometers and their mode of action

Type	Change due to heat
Mercury-in-glass	Expansion
Alcohol-in-glass	Expansion
Bimetallic strip	Expansion
Platinum resistance	Electrical resistance increases
Thermistor	Electrical resistance decreases
Thermocouple	Electric potential difference between dissimilar metals
Thermography	Infrared radiation emitted
Liquid crystal display	Reflection of visible light

THE PHYSIOLOGICAL EFFECTS OF HEAT AND COLD

Body temperature

It is well understood that humans are homeothermic in respect of their core temperature, that is, the temperature of the deeply placed structures and organs. Skin and subcutaneous tissue temperatures are much more variable. Normally there is a circadian variation in the core temperature of about 1°C, being lower in the early morning and higher in the afternoon (Hardy, 1982). Most people have core temperatures around 36.8°C but individuals vary and children tend to have slightly higher temperatures. Oral and rectal temperatures, which are conveniently measured, approximate to the real core temperature but are more variable. Vigorous exercise will temporarily raise the core temperature above these limits. It is largely through the skin that heat exchange with the environment takes place so skin temperature is much more variable.

Maintenance of homeothermy

The core temperature is dependent on a balance between heat loss and gain. The main features are identified in Table 7.3.

Although all the effects noted in Table 7.3 occur, the major heat gain is from metabolism, which is vastly increased during vigorous exercise: some 75% of the energy applied to muscle contraction appears as heat. At moderate environmental temperatures radiation accounts for some 60% of heat loss (Hubbard and Mechan, 1987). As the outside temperature rises, approximating the body surface temperature, the effectiveness of radiation and conduction becomes less and less. If the outside temperature is above body temperature the body gains further heat by radiation from the surroundings. In these circumstances heat loss is entirely due to the evaporation of sweat from the skin. This is a very efficient method of heat loss as the evaporation of each gram of sweat at body temperature takes some 2.5 kJ of heat energy; under suitable conditions a man can lose 1 kg of sweat per hour, thus achieving a cooling rate of nearly 700 W (2500 J × 1000 g/3600 s = 694.4 W; Holwill and Silvester, 1973).

Table 7.3 Causes of heat gain and loss

Causes of heat gain	*Causes of heat loss*
Basal metabolism	Radiation to the environment
Metabolism of muscle contraction	Conduction to cooler objects
Metabolism of other tissues beyond basal, e.g. digestion	Conduction to air, continually removed by convection
Absorption of radiation from the environment	Evaporation of water from skin— 'insensible perspiration'—vapour carried away by convection
Conduction from hotter objects	Evaporation of sweat—water vapour carried away by convection
	Exhaled warm air—forced convection
	Excretion of urine, faeces and other fluids

The difference between the core temperature and the normally lower body surface temperature is critical in controlling the heat loss from the body because the rate at which heat can be lost from the body surface depends on the temperature difference between that surface and the environment. A large temperature difference can be maintained between the core and the outer shell of the body because of the low thermal conductivity of tissue, especially fat tissue. The flow of heat from the deep tissue to the skin is largely due to the blood flow—forced convection. Heat is thus transmitted through the thermal barrier provided by the subcutaneous fat. This concept of a temperature gradient between the core and periphery can be expressed schematically by the isothermal lines shown in Figure 7.3. Additionally there is a progressive fall in temperature towards the periphery so that at toe-level skin temperature can be at room temperature.

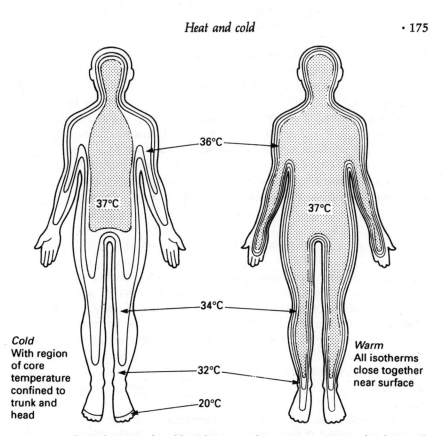

36°C

37°C   37°C

34°C

Cold
With region
of core
temperature
confined to
trunk and
head

Warm
All isotherms
close together
near surface

32°C

20°C

Fig. 7.3 Body isotherms. Left: cold, with region of core temperature confined to trunk and head. Right: warm, with all isotherms close together near surface.

When the body is exposed to cold the loss of heat can be much reduced by vasoconstriction which greatly reduces the blood flow to the extremities and skin of the trunk so allowing skin and subcutaneous tissue temperature to fall. Conversely if the body retains too much heat vasodilation of skin vessels vastly increases the blood flow and hence the skin temperature. The isothermic lines are close to the surface, showing that there is now less difference between the surface and the core temperature (Fig. 7.3). The thicker layer of subcutaneous fat in women gives them better thermal control than men. At low environmental temperatures their skin is colder but becomes warmer in hotter environments (Hardy, 1982).

Counter-current heat exchange

Counter-current heat exchange is another aspect of thermal regulation in the body. Heat can be exchanged between the warm arterial blood moving from the body core to the periphery and the cooler venous blood returning from the extremities. If arteries and veins lie close together, as in the limbs, where the venae comitantes are situated on each side of a medium artery, heat can pass from the warmer artery to the cooler vein. Since arterial blood loses heat as it passes to the periphery and venous blood gains heat as it moves centrally, the heat gradient between them remains much the same, thus heat exchange continues throughout the length of the vessels. The value of this arrangement is that body core heat in the arterial blood is conserved in the central parts by being used to heat the incoming venous blood instead of the extremities which are maintained at a lower temperature than the core.

While this counter-current mechanism is of great importance in some animals its effectiveness in humans is in question. Estimates of the heat savings vary from a negligible 5% to a significant 50% (Hardy, 1982).

Cutaneous thermoreceptors

Receptors in the skin signal temperature changes; some are heat receptors but many more (about eight times as many) are cold receptors. At one time it was considered that heat receptors could be identified anatomically as Ruffini end-organs and cold receptors as Krause's bulb end-organs, but now free nerve endings in the region of the basal layer of the epidermis are considered to be important. Many of those are identical to pain nerve endings (C fibres; group IV unmyelinated) and thermal perception seems to involve interpretation of the impulses from cold, warm and pain receptors by the central nervous system.

Cutaneous thermoreceptors have two separate roles. They signal temperature sensation, which is the conscious perception of whether the skin is being warmed or cooled. Secondly they contribute to the control of body temperature, which is unconscious. For the former it is the temperature change that needs to be measured and for the latter it is the absolute skin temperature that is needed. The perception of thermal sensations is also affected by the size of the area stimulated and, importantly, the rate of change of the stimulation; that is, both the temperature difference and the time it takes to change.

Pain nerve endings discharge at the extremes of the temperature range— where the temperature stimulus becomes merged with pain—at approximately 45°C for heating and 15°C for cooling. The numerous cold receptors discharge over a wide range, many with peak excitation around 25–35°C. Different neurons have different ranges and different peak discharges. The warm receptors, which also vary, tend to have peak discharges around 38°C (Fig. 7.4). Note that cold receptors also have discharge peaks at the extremes of both hot and cold where pain is perceived.

The continuous discharge of receptors shown in Figure 7.4 depends on the absolute skin temperature as shown but if the skin is suddenly heated there is an abrupt decrease in cold receptor activity and a corresponding increased frequency of warm receptor discharge. Both frequencies slowly return to the frequency appropriate for the new absolute skin temperature. Thus information from these receptors is used to perceive skin temperature and temperature changes as well as contribute to subconscious temperature regulation (Fischer and Solomon, 1965). The perception of temperature change on the skin is

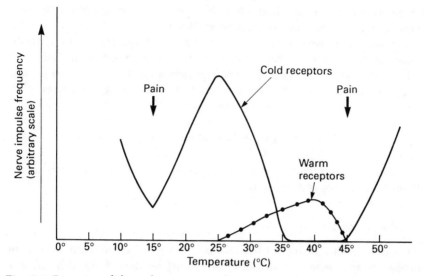

Fig. 7.4 Response of thermal receptors in skin.

extraordinarily sensitive. At skin temperatures around 30°C changes of as little as 1°C can be recognized under some conditions. At colder or hotter skin temperatures, and if the change is slow, larger changes of 5 or 10°C are needed before temperature change is recognized.

The usual method of testing thermal sensitivity by applying warm and cold water-filled test tubes to the skin, being about 10°C above and below skin

Table 7.4 Temperature ranges

Temperature (°C)	Body and environmental temperatures		Subjective feeling associated with surface temperatures
60		Behavioural regulation	
55			
50			
45			Tissue damage, burning pain
40			Very hot
35	Normal range of resting temperature of body 36.3–37.3°C	Approximate region of physiological temperature regulation	Hot
30			Warm
			Neutral
25	Region of thermal environmental comfort		Cool
20			Cold
15			
10			Very cold
5		Behavioural regulation	Very cold + pain →tissue damage
0			

temperature respectively, should thus allow easy recognition of the temperatures unless there is a significant sensory deficit.

The sensations associated with different surface temperatures are shown in Table 7.4 but it must be realized that this is a very subjective matter.

For humans there are two facets of heat regulation: *physiological*, controlled by the hypothalamus and *behavioural*, controlled in the higher centres.

Physiological control

The major ways in which physiological control is effected are metabolic and vasomotor control and sweating.

Metabolic control

When much heat is being lost from the body some restoration can be made by increasing the metabolic activity. The most evident form this takes is shivering, in which irregular muscle contractions are provoked by stimulation of the sympathetic nervous system. Over short periods shivering can produce quite good heating but for several hours of cold exposure it can only double the resting metabolism on average (Hardy, 1982). Brown adipose tissue is fatty tissue with more than the usual vascularity, hence making it look brown. It is found in a number of sites in the trunk close to the heart and kidney and between the scapulae. Fat metabolism can occur locally in this tissue in a way that releases energy entirely as heat. While important in newborn infants the value of this mechanism to adults is uncertain. It is stimulated by adrenaline release.

At rest most body heat (about 70%) is produced in the viscera of the trunk and in the brain. On activity most of the heat (about 90%) is produced by the muscles and skin which move the sites of major heat production nearer to the surface and to the extremities (Hardy, 1982). Of course, the increased blood flow needed to maintain oxygenation and nutrition to sustain continuous muscle contraction serves to dissipate heat from the working muscles to the rest of the body.

Vasomotor control

The blood flow in the skin not only serves the usual nutritional role but also acts as a heat transfer system. Arterioles feed capillary loops in the dermis forming papillae which drain via venules to a network of small veins. Slightly more deeply placed are rather larger venous plexuses: blood moving through these transfers heat to the overlying skin. Over most of the skin surface the blood flow is regulated by the lumen of the arteriole which is under the control of the sympathetic nervous system. In the skin of the hands, feet, ears, lips and some mucous membrane surfaces arteriovenous anastomoses are present between the arteriole and the large venous plexuses. These are regulated by vasoconstrictor impulses from the sympathetic nervous system so that when closed, in cold conditions, the flow of blood in the veins is reduced to almost nothing but the nutritive blood flow through the papillae is maintained. On dilation they allow a large flow of venous blood through plexuses causing a marked rise in skin temperature and thus loss of heat from the surface. At rest the skin contains some 20 times as much blood as is needed for nutrition alone. Under cold conditions the blood flow to each 100 g of skin can be reduced to as little as 1 ml/min whereas in hot conditions this can rise to 150 ml/min (Hubbard and Mechan, 1987).

Sweating

As noted earlier, water evaporation from the skin surface is a very efficient way of losing heat; in fact it is the only way when the environmental temperature is the same as or even greater than the skin temperature. It is not difficult to see why so much energy (2.5 kJ/g) is used since the energy leads to increased movement of the water molecules, giving them a range of kinetic energies. The ones with the highest kinetic energy will be 'thrown off' the water surface to form vapour which moves away from the skin surface by convection. At all times under all circumstances the body is losing heat by evaporation (about 500 g/day for a 1.5 m² surface area, e.g. the 50 kg woman considered previously). About half of this is the water vapour of expired air while the remainder is due to the steady transpiration of water through the skin, the so-called insensible perspiration. This is more or less constant at environmental temperatures below about 30°C but at higher temperatures, or when metabolic heat is produced by vigorous exercise, active sweating occurs and the amount of sweat vaporized increases with temperature.

There are about 2 500 000 eccrine sweat glands in the skin of an average man; these glands are under the control of the sympathetic nervous system by cholinergic nerves (those of the palms and soles may have additionally adrenergic fibres). Quite large amounts of sweat can be produced if needed. The glands themselves consist of little coiled tubes in the dermis which pass straight up through the epidermis to open on to the surface. They are numerous on the palms and soles and tend to be larger in areas that sweat most extensively, like the axillae. Sweat is 99% water with some sodium chloride and traces of compounds such as urea and lactic acid. It must be remembered that when visible sweat occurs on the skin and drips off or is wiped off it is not being vaporized and hence is not taking much heat from the body. Vaporization depends not only on the temperature but also on the humidity of the air. In dry air conditions body cooling is therefore much more efficient.

Behavioural control

These are familiar responses which depend on sensations of heat and cold being interpreted as discomfort (Table 7.4). In temperate and cold climates the main method of behavioural regulation is wearing clothes, which provide thermal insulation by trapping a layer of air close to the skin surface. In other words, clothes prevent heat loss due to thermal and forced convection of air warmed by the skin. The effectiveness of air as an insulator is noticed when clothes become wet and immediately feel much colder. Similarly, restricting the movement of cold air close to the body by maintaining a draught-free environment or wrapping the body in blankets acts in the same way. Using a material that reflects infrared radiations (survival sleeping bags) cuts down the heat loss further by blocking radiation emission from the body. Vigorous voluntary muscular activity is also used to increase metabolic heat.

Opposite behaviours encourage heat loss in a hot environment. Thus air-trapping by thick clothing is reduced; light loose-fitting clothing reduces absorption of radiation while allowing air convection currents close to the skin. Applying a steady draught of air by a fan or other means assists cooling. Avoiding radiation by remaining in the shade and limiting activity in hot environments also helps to control body temperature.

Temperature regulation

The temperature-regulating centre is largely in the hypothalamus. It is effectively a thermostat responding to lowered blood temperatures by initiating heat-generating and conserving mechanisms and in the opposite way to raised blood temperatures. Reflex responses to cold are apparently controlled from the posterior hypothalamus (Wadsworth and Chanmugan, 1980) and adrenaline release is an important endocrine response to cooling. From what has been noted above there is also involvement of the higher centres.

Bacterial or viral infections of sufficient virulence lead to the release of substances which in some ill–understood way re-set the thermostat of the temperature-regulating centre. Thus the patient shivers and feels cold and the heat-conserving mechanisms come into play; cutaneous vasoconstriction makes the patient look pale. Consequently the core temperature rises to a new, higher level for a time. When the infection has been overcome, aided by the higher metabolic rate and consequent increased activity of the immune system, the patient feels hot and cutaneous vasodilation occurs with sweating to bring the body temperature down as the thermostat is re-set back to the normal level.

Body temperature regulation is helped by the high specific heat (3.5 kJ/kg/°C) which means that it takes a large quantity of heat to raise, or heat loss to lower, the body temperature. (For the 50 kg woman cited previously it would take 175 kJ to raise her temperature by 1°C.) Furthermore small temporary changes of core temperature, such as occur with exercise, are physiologically normal.

Since the principal source of heat is metabolism, which depends on tissue mass, and the principal source of heat loss is from the whole of the skin, which depends on the surface area, it is evident that body size will have an important effect. Babies have a large surface area for their mass but as growth occurs the amount of tissue increases proportionally more than the surface area. (If this is not immediately obvious consider the reverse; if an apple is cut in half each piece has half the original amount of matter but much more than half the surface area due to the new cut surface.) It would be expected that babies would be at more risk from excessive heat loss than from becoming overheated, but they appear to compensate by maintaining a higher metabolic rate and perhaps by means of the brown adipose tissue referred to above. Large mammals often have specialized physiology or behaviour to prevent them overheating, e.g. large-surface-area ears in elephants or wallowing by hippopotamus. Camels living in hot arid climates can store heat by allowing their body temperature to rise during the day and losing heat at night.

Even in healthy subjects the heat-regulating mechanisms can become overwhelmed by extremes of heat or cold. Feeling faint due to lowered cerebral blood pressure following prolonged standing or abrupt postural changes in the heat is familiar to most people. It can be called heat syncope and is caused by venous pooling; recovery is rapid once the subject lies down. A much more dangerous syndrome is heat stroke, when heat regulation fails, the person stops sweating and body temperature starts to rise. Urgent treatment to cool the patient and maintain body fluids is life-saving.

During hard work at high outside temperatures, body temperature is controlled by sweating and if water and salt are not replaced muscle cramps and fatigue result. Under extremely cold conditions the core temperature starts to fall, unconsciousness follows and unless rewarming can be effected thermal regulation is completely lost; this condition is fatal.

Stress due to extremes of temperature is a far more serious problem for those who have some deficiency in their normal response, either due to disease or old age. It has been noted that mortality rates go up during heatwaves or very cold spells, particularly amongst the elderly and those with chronic cardiovascular disease. As might be anticipated hypothermia is much the more significant problem in the UK, particularly among elderly people living alone. They may be unable to maintain their home at a suitable temperature so that body temperature falls leading to confusion and inertia, exacerbating the problem. It has been found (Fox *et al.*, 1973) that many of these elderly people have some failure of their temperature-regulating system—falling body temperatures do not provoke the normal shivering and vasoconstriction responses as quickly as usual.

There are a number of conditions in which exposure to extremes of heat or cold may lead to particular difficulties. For example, cystic fibrosis is associated with inefficient production of sweat and hence inadequate control in extreme heat.

For those who are otherwise fit, acclimatization and adaptation can occur to some degree in extremes of temperature. Working in hot situations for several hours at a time over a period of a few weeks can lead to more rapid cutaneous vasodilation and increased sweating capacity. Mechanisms of cold adaptation seem less well understood and may be largely a matter of tolerating low skin temperatures.

THE PHYSIOLOGICAL EFFECTS OF TEMPERATURE CHANGE ON THE BODY TISSUES

A complicated set of physiological changes will ensue from any temperature change and these interact to produce still more complex responses. The basic changes and some of their consequences are considered below.

Metabolic activity

The rate of any chemical action that can be affected is increased by a temperature rise (Van't Hoff's law). Metabolism, being a series of chemical reactions, will increase with a rise and decrease with a fall of temperature. The actual change is about one-eighth (13%) for each 1°C so increasing the tissue temperature by, say, 4°C would increase the metabolic rate by some 60%. However, it is not as simple as this in the living organism because increasing temperature tends to denature proteins and thus interfere with the enzyme (protein)-controlled metabolic processes. Thus after some increased activity an optimum temperature is reached at which metabolic activity is maximally stimulated by the heat and yet not sufficiently hot to destroy the necessary enzymes. This temperature point will differ for different reactions. At temperatures above 45°C so much protein damage occurs that there is destruction of cells and tissues. At low temperatures metabolism is progressively reduced and tissue destruction occurs if the intra- or extracellular fluid becomes frozen. From a therapeutic point of view the local temperature changes that can, or should, be achieved are limited in the deeper tissues to about 5 or 6°C above or below core temperature; for skin and subcutaneous tissue much lower temperatures are in use.

Viscosity

Viscosity is temperature-dependent. In liquids (but not gases) raising the temperature lowers the viscosity. Although the effect appears to be quite small, it affects all the tissue fluids and notably blood flow in the narrow capillaries.

Nerve stimulation

Plainly heat and cold stimulate the sensory receptors of the skin since these sensations can be recognized (see p. 176). Furthermore these receptors pass information to the heat-regulating centres, contributing to the control of body temperature. Afferent nerves stimulated by heat may have an analgesic effect by acting on the gate control mechanism in the same way as the mechanoreceptors (see Chapter 3); in the past, this effect was called a counter-irritant mechanism (Gammon and Starr, 1941). There is some evidence that stimulating heat receptors inhibits nociceptive impulses in rats (Kanui, 1985). This could account for the analgesic effects of local heating.

Superficial heat is widely used for the relief of pain. Several surveys of patients with persistent pain have found that some form of heat ranks highly, after analgesia, amongst the measures used by the patient to control pain. For example, Barbour *et al.* (1986) found that heat was the most effective non-analgesic method of pain control being used in 68% of the cancer outpatients in their sample.

It has been suggested that heating the secondary afferent muscle spindle nerve endings and Golgi tendon endings could be the way in which muscle spasm is reduced by heating (Lehmann and de Lateur, 1982).

Cooling has marked effects on peripheral nerves. Initially cold receptors are stimulated, adding to the overall sensory input, but at lower temperatures conduction rates are depressed. This occurs at first in the small myelinated fibres and later in large myelinated fibres. With sufficient cooling some nerve conduction is abolished so that numbness occurs. The therapeutic implications are considered in Chapter 9.

Blood vessel changes

Heat and cold applied to the skin have obvious effects. With heating the skin surface reddens, i.e. an erythema is produced, and with cooling it becomes pale due to vasoconstriction, although subsequent vasodilation due to cold may occur (see Chapter 9). The striking cutaneous hyperaemia due to heat leads to the idea that similar effects occur in other tissues but this is not the case. As noted already, the skin is specially adapted for heat regulation and what is being seen is a heat-blocking response. The vasodilation occurs not only to distribute the additional heat around the body, allowing compensatory heat loss from other regions, but also to protect the heated skin. This is important because the skin surface is naturally heated from the outside and heat conduction is not effective through the subcutaneous fat; in fact the two mechanisms may be somewhat separate in that it has been found that directly heating the skin causes capillary dilation but the arteriovenous anastomoses are opened by reduced sympathetic tone for total body temperature regulation. The vasodilation due to heat is caused by several mechanisms. There is thought to be a direct effect on capillaries, arterioles and venules, causing them all to dilate (Lehmann and de Lateur, 1982). The increased metabolism will lead to increased release of carbon dioxide, lactate and greater acidity of the heated tissues, tending to provoke dilation. As heating can damage proteins this may cause an inflammatory reaction due to the release of histamine-like substances and bradykinin which leads to the vasodilation (Lehmann and de Lateur, 1982). The axon reflex has also been invoked to account for dilation (Wadsworth and Chanmugan, 1980). It must also be recognized that the reduced viscosity of blood would contribute to the increase of blood flow. The foregoing accounts for the area being heated; other skin areas may well show cutaneous vasodilation to lose heat in response to impulses from the heat-regulating centre.

Cold cutaneous vasodilation is somewhat different and the mechanisms are discussed in Chapter 9.

Increased blood flow in tissues other than skin has been shown to occur as a consequence of heating (Millard, 1961) but is much less marked and in some cases uncertain.

Collagenous tissue changes

The extensibility of collagenous tissue has been shown to increase with heating (Lehmann *et al.*, 1970). This only occurs if the tissue is simultaneously stretched and requires temperatures near the therapeutic limit, but it is an important therapeutic effect. Joint stiffness has been found to be reduced by heating (Wright and Johns, 1961): on cooling joint stiffness is increased.

Blood

Heating or cooling the blood in cutaneous vessels locally leads to temperature change, ultimately affecting the heat-regulating centre in the hypothalamus. This will contribute to temperature regulation, as already explained.

As a consequence of the increased metabolic activity, capillary dilation and a rise in capillary pressure there is an increase in tissue fluid exchange across the capillary wall and cell membrane, all of which can contribute to increasing the resolution of chronic inflammation and rate of tissue healing.

The basic changes and their interactions are illustrated in a simple form in Table 7.5. Consideration of the therapeutic effects of cooling is given in Chapter 9 and of heating in Chapter 8.

Tissue damage due to excess local heat—burns

Burns are of considerable importance in medicine. Permanent skin damage or loss is a serious disability if anything more than a tiny area is involved.

It has been shown that skin temperatures over 45°C cause tissue damage but this depends on the length of exposure as well as the temperature. The sensation of heat gives way to one of pain at this same temperature; the pain increases in intensity with rising temperature. Both injury and the resulting pain are considered to be due to permanent damage to proteins in the basal skin cells. It is important to understand the relationship between time, temperature and the resulting damage. Thus skin temperature around 45°C can be tolerated for, perhaps, an hour or so before damage occurs but with higher temperatures the period shortens so that 50°C can be tolerated for about 1 min or so and 65°C about 1 s or so (Hardy, 1982). This refers to skin temperature.

Table 7.5 Physiological effects of local temperature change and their interactions

Cooling (fall in local tissue temperature)	Heating (rise in local tissue temperature)
Collagen extensibility reduced or unaffected	Collagen extensibility increased
Metabolism decreased	Metabolism increased ↓ Metabolic products ↓
Vasoconstriction of arterioles, venules and capillaries ↓ Vasodilation	Vasodilation of arterioles, venules and capillaries ↑ Axon reflex ↑
Nerve stimulation (Conduction decreased) → Via cutaneous receptors ↓	← Nerve stimulation
Blood cooled → regulates body temperature ← Blood heated by vasomotor control metabolism sweating	Hypothalamus
Viscosity increased	Viscosity decreased

(Blood flow increased — applies to the Heating column)

Many much hotter objects can be touched for short periods without causing a burn but they do not necessarily lead to sufficient heat transfer to raise the skin to the same temperature. Most people have experience of touching a very hot object, say a saucepan of boiling water with a temperature about 100°C, yet because the hand is removed very quickly no damage occurs, except a transient erythema.

This has important implications in the immediate treatment of burns. The damaged area should be cooled as quickly as possible. Cold water should be applied at once; a scalded hand should be plunged immediately into cold water.

REFERENCES

Barbour L. A., McGuire D. B., Kirchott K. T. (1986). Non-analgesic methods of pain control used by cancer outpatients. *Oncol. Nursing Forum*, **13**, 56–60.

Cetas T. C. (1982). Thermometry. In *Therapeutic Heat and Cold* (Lehmann J. F., ed.) Baltimore: Williams & Wilkins, pp. 35–69.

Fischer E., Solomon S. (1965). Physiological responses to heat and cold. In *Therapeutic Heat and Cold* (Licht S., ed.) Baltimore: Waverley Press, pp. 126–69.

Electrotherapy explained

Fox R. H., Woodward P. M., Exton-Smith A. N. *et al.* (1973). Body temperature in the elderly: a national study of physiological, social and environmental conditions. *Br. Med. J.*, **1**, 200–6.

Gammon G. D., Starr I. (1941). Studies on the relief of pain by counterirritation. *J. Clin. Invest.*, **20**, 13–20.

Hardy J. D. (1982). Temperature regulation, exposure to heat and cold and effects of hypothermia. In *Therapeutic Heat and Cold* (Lehmann J. F., ed.) Baltimore: Williams & Wilkins, pp. 172–98.

Holwill M. E., Silvester N. R. (1973). *Introduction to Biological Physics*. London: John Wiley.

Hubbard J. L., Mechan D. J. (1987). *Physiology for Health Care Students*. Edinburgh: Churchill Livingstone.

Kanui T. I. (1985). Thermal inhibition of nocioceptor-driven spinal cord nerves in rats. *Pain*, **21**, 231–40.

Lehmann J. F., de Lateur B. J. (1982). Therapeutic heat. In *Therapeutic Heat and Cold* (Lehmann J. F. ed.) Baltimore: Williams & Wilkins, pp. 404–562.

Lehmann J. F., Masock A. J., Warren C. G. *et al.* (1970). Effect of therapeutic temperatures on tendon extensibility. *Arch. Phys. Med. Rehab.*, **51**, 481–7.

Millard J. B. (1961). Effect of high frequency current and infra-red rays on the circulation of the lower limb in man. *Ann. Phys. Med.*, **6**, 45–60.

Sekins K. M., Emery A. F. (1982). Thermal science for physical medicine. In *Therapeutic Heat and Cold* (Lehmann J. F., ed.) Baltimore: Williams & Wilkins, pp. 70–132.

Swartz C. E., Goldfarb T. D. (1974). *A Search for Order in the Physical Universe*. San Francisco: W. H. Freeman.

Wadsworth H., Chanmugan A. P. P. (1980). *Electrophysical Agents in Physiotherapy*. Marricksville, NSW, Australia: Science Press.

Wright W., Johns R. J. (1961). Quantitative and qualitative analgesia of joint stiffness in normal subjects and in patients with connective tissue diseases. *Ann. Rheum. Dis.*, **20**, 36–46.

8.

Therapeutic conduction heating

GENERAL PRINCIPLES

It is intended in this chapter to describe those methods of therapeutic heating which involve the application of some heated substance directly to the surface of the skin. The transfer of heat therefore takes place by conduction but it must be recognized that there is also some transfer due to radiation; any hot body emits infrared radiation. (In fact in at least one text these treatment methods are referred to collectively as 'the infra-red energies'; Griffin and Karselis, 1988.) However, while it seems sensible to consider conduction methods separately from radiation heating by infrared (see Chapter 13), the effects of both are similar in that they cause superficial heating.

Therapeutic heating can thus be divided into:

1 *Superficial heating* due to heat conduction or infrared radiation being produced by hot packs and similar means, as described in this chapter, and infrared lamps, as described in Chapter 13.
2 *Deep heating*, also referred to as conversion or conversive heating, due to the conversion of energy passing through the tissues to heat, as with ultrasound (Chapter 6), shortwave (Chapter 10) and microwave diathermy

187

(Chapter 12). (Strictly speaking, infrared radiation is also conversion heating.)

The distinction between these two groups is important; the skin and subcutaneous fat act as a thermal barrier to conduction and much radiation heating, thus limiting the heating of deeper tissues; there are, of course, indirect effects on deeper tissues mediated through the nervous system or due to the heated blood being carried to other parts. In contrast, the conversive methods are able to generate heat in both superficial and deep tissues, as explained in Chapters 6, 10 and 13, much like metabolic heating.

Sources for therapeutic conductive heating are many and varied: the best known is the simple hot water bottle which exploits the heat energy that can be stored in water. Hot water is used in many methods of therapeutic heating, notably hot packs (hydrocollator packs), hot water baths (as contrast baths, whirlpool baths or as hydrotherapy in a large tank or pool); also various hot muds are largely hot water. Paraffin wax is an important form of conduction heating as is hot air or other vapour. Where the hot air is used to move a stream of fine solid particles against the skin surface the treatment is referred to as fluidotherapy. In these cases the heat is being transferred to the site by forced convection; transfer to the skin is by conduction, and some radiation. Table 8.1 summarizes the modalities and their methods of heat transfer.

When local heating is applied to the body it does not normally cause a rise in core temperature. As already explained, the heat added in one place is dispersed throughout the body—by conduction and convection—to be lost at other surfaces. Thus local temperature rises will be a balance between heat input and dispersion. As noted above, if the temperature is high enough to

Table 8.1 Methods of heating and their mode of action

Depth	Heating of tissues	Method of heat transfer to tissues	Modality
Superficial	Heat from outside leads to heating of tissues	Conduction with some radiation	Hot water bottle Hot pack— hydrocollator Hot water bath Hot muds, etc. Wax bath Electric heat pad
		Convection on to skin	Fluidotherapy Hot air (hairdrier) Hydrotherapy
Deep	Form of energy changed to heat in tissues = conversion	Radiation	Infrared radiation Microwave Shortwave diathermy
		Electric charge motion	
		Mechanical	Ultrasound

cause tissue damage, that is above 45°C, the time in which this damage occurs becomes shorter at higher temperatures. In the therapeutic situation such high skin temperatures are not applied so that after a local rise in temperature the dispersion mechanism can keep pace with the heat input. This allows local heat to be applied indefinitely without producing tissue damage.

The rate at which the local tissue temperature rise occurs depends on the heat introduced, both in terms of the temperature and the area of skin heated. It also depends on the thermal conductivity of the tissue involved. Fat and skin have a lower thermal conductivity than watery tissues and in general deeper tissues have higher conductivity (Sekins and Emery, 1982). It follows that heat flow in the tissues will be obstructed by the subcutaneous fat layer and will be assisted by vasodilation. Further, as the specific heat of water, hence of blood, is about twice that of fat it takes more energy to raise the temperature of blood. Because of this and the process of vasodilation the superficial tissues have more heat capacity. The major factor in dissipating heat in the tissues is forced convection by the venous blood and lymph carrying the heat away.

Local tissue heating is, of course, superimposed on the existing tissue temperature gradient which has been described in Chapter 7 in terms of temperature 'shells'. Application of heat to the surface will reverse this gradient locally (Fig. 8.1).

The rise in superficial tissue temperature does not occur instantly. As would be expected the skin temperature rises first, subcutaneous tissue temperature rises more slowly, and a very small change in superficial muscle temperature (of 1°C or so) takes as long as 20 or 25 min to occur. This is illustrated in Figure 8.2, which shows the temperature of various tissues against time: these

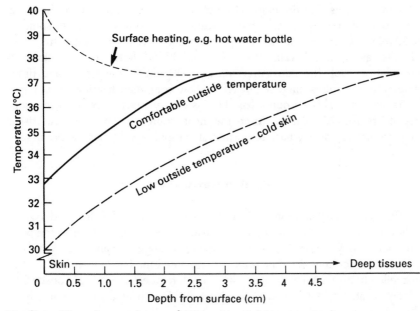

Fig. 8.1 Tissue temperature gradients.

Electrotherapy explained

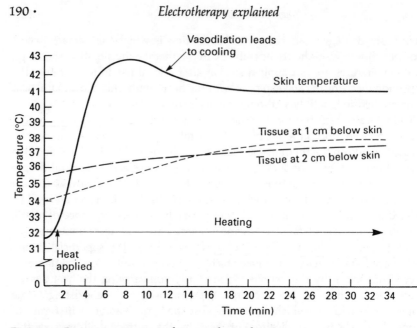

Fig. 8.2 Rise in temperature of tissues during heating.

data are based on studies by Lehmann *et al.* (1966) using the hydrocollator hot pack, and conform with others, e.g. Michlovitz (1986). The pattern would be similar whatever form of superficial heat were applied. Although the hot packs used cooled over the 30-min period, repeating the application every 10 min prolonged heating but made very little difference to the pattern (Lehmann *et al.*, 1966).

The marked rise in skin temperature of some 10°C contrasts with the trivial rise in deep-tissue (e.g. muscle) temperature of 1°C or so which takes some 25 or 30 min to achieve. The skin temperature may actually decrease after some minutes, as shown, because the increased blood flow due to cutaneous vasodilation cools the skin. After some 25–30 min these vascular and tissue temperature changes have stabilized so that continued heating leads to no further change. This accounts for the customary practice of applying such treatments for 20–30 min. After the heat source is removed the tissue temperatures fall slowly back to normal, skin more rapidly than deeper tissues.

Paraffin wax baths

Paraffin wax melts at around 54°C but this point can be lowered by the addition of mineral oil (liquid paraffin). Most wax baths are kept at temperatures between 42 and 52°C, often at the higher range for hand treatments and rather lower for the feet. The wax is maintained molten in stainless steel or enamelled baths which are electrically heated; temperature is kept constant by a thermostat. Some baths are contained within a heated outer water bath. There may be a fixed thermometer to check the temperature and a means of adjusting the thermostat setting to alter the temperature. Even if a thermometer is not an integral part of the bath the temperature of the wax must still be checked.

The more modern designs of wax bath can be adjusted for height. They are light, with a stainless steel bowl and outer fibreglass shell. Initial heating is quicker with this type because there is no waterjacket to be heated.

Method of application

The most widely used method of application is 'dip and wrap'. This can only be used for the extremities—hands, wrists, feet and ankles.

The area to be treated is inspected for contraindications. After washing and drying the part it is immersed for a second or so in the wax, withdrawn and allowed to cool for 2 or 3 s and then reimmersed. It is important to immerse the part briefly otherwise the outermost coating is melted off and the thickness of wax does not build. The procedure is repeated 6–12 times to produce a coating of wax 2 or 3 mm thick over the body part. The part is then put into a plastic bag or paper cover and wrapped in a blanket or towel to limit the rate of heat loss to the air. For any condition in which there is a proclivity for oedema the part should be elevated. Adequate elevation in which the part is kept above the level of the heart is of the utmost importance since otherwise the heating effect will tend to exacerbate swelling of the extremities.

The 'glove' of wax is normally left in place for some 15 min by which time the wax is completely solid although still malleable, so that it can be removed in one piece. To achieve higher skin temperature for longer periods the 'dip and leave in' method can be used. After a suitably thick layer of wax has been built up by a succession of dips the part is left in the wax bath for 15 or 20 min; this method can produce a much greater increase in tissue temperature (Abramson *et al.*, 1964), but it necessitates the hand or foot remaining dependent throughout the treatment, which is often deleterious.

A way of achieving the benefits of prolonged higher temperatures coupled with elevation is to place the wax-covered part in a loose-fitting plastic bag which is secured with a bandage around the wrist or ankle. The part is then elevated into a warm-air cabinet (simple heat cradle or infrared lamp will work); air temperature is about 70°C. This method can be combined with active exercise of the part while the limb is in elevation. The wax may fall away as it cools but a thin layer usually remains even as the fingers are moved. This method has been described for the treatment of post-traumatic osteodystrophy (Sudeck's atrophy).

If the part cannot be immersed in wax it is possible to coat the surface by either painting the wax on using a large brush, or ladling it over the part with a suitably large bowl placed beneath: the knees can be treated in this way. Alternatively, bandages of a suitable size and mesh can be soaked in the hot wax and then wrapped around the limb; additional wax can then be brushed over the bandage. These latter methods are useful if other ways of applying heat are not appropriate but are rarely used because of the inconvenience.

After use the wax is cleaned in a purifier and re-used.

Despite the fact that skin temperatures above 45°C can lead to damage it is possible to put the hand comfortably in a bath of wax at some 50°C. Water at the same temperature would be uncomfortably hot and ultimately cause damage. This is because the specific heat of paraffin wax is about 2.72 kJ/kg/°C, or less with added mineral oil, and therefore much lower than that of water at 4.2 kJ/kg/°C. Thus the amount of energy released by wax cooling 1°C is less than that of water. Perhaps more importantly, when the part is immersed in wax the cooler skin causes a thin layer of wax to solidify on the surface. Due to the relatively low thermal conductivity of wax this static layer acts to insulate the skin from the hotter surrounding wax: some air may be trapped between this solidified layer and the skin, adding to the insulating effect (Griffin and Karselis, 1988).

The wax transmits heat energy to the tissues by giving up energy as it solidifies—the latent heat of fusion—without any temperature change. This amount of energy is quite small: about 35 kJ/kg (Sekins and Emery, 1982). Although the temperature of the thin layer of wax on the tissues falls quite quickly on its outside surface the low thermal conductivity prevents much heat loss from the skin surface. It also prevents any evaporation of water from the skin thus further improving the insulating qualities. The net effect is to provide remarkably effective low-temperature heating of the part. When it is considered that the hand and foot have a relatively large ratio of surface area to volume and that the wax is applied evenly over all this surface, as well as the fact that there is relatively little subcutaneous tissue separating the small joints of the fingers and toes from the skin, it can be understood why such mild heating appears to be therapeutically effective. Certainly there is widespread approbation amongst patients who suffer with painful and stiff joints for this form of heat.

As a consequence of preventing water loss from the surface of the skin the wax treatment tends to leave the skin with more moisture hence feeling soft and pliable. This may be therapeutically valuable if the skin is dry. It is also claimed to soften adhesions and scars in the skin (Wadsworth and Chanmugan, 1980).

Contraindications and dangers

Wax is, of course, sterile as no organisms can live in pure oil. Wax should not, however, be allowed to enter an open wound since it will set in the tissues acting as an inert foreign body and delay healing. Large pieces of dirt in the wax bath may harbour organisms but it is extremely unlikely that these could ever lead to infection. Patients with skin infections of the part are not usually treated as heat may increase the inflammatory activity. Some individuals may become allergic to the wax with extended and prolonged treatments but this is rare. Acute dermatitis may be made worse by wax, or indeed any form of heat on the skin. Circumstances in which there is defective thermal sensation coupled with deficient cutaneous circulation, as occurs with recently healed skin grafts, should not be treated.

Wax is highly inflammable if it becomes overheated so it is a sensible precaution to have a fire blanket and suitable carbon dioxide or foam extinguisher available. Pouring water on blazing wax is ineffective because the wax floats on the water surface. Wax also renders the floor very slippery if spilt, so any spillage must be promptly dealt with.

Hydrocollator packs

These consist of a silicate gel, such as bentonite, enclosed in a cotton fabric container. This gel will absorb large quantities of water which, if it is hot, provides a considerable store of heat energy. The gel is contained in a set of separated fabric pockets, like a duvet, so that the whole pack is flexible and the gel confined. The packs are made in various sizes to fit different body areas. They are heated by being placed in a special tank of water warmed to 75–80°C by an electric heater controlled by a thermostat. The packs, supported on racks in the tank, take about 2 h to become fully heated from cold but rather less when being reheated.

The hot packs are wrapped in towelling before being applied to the part so that some four to eight layers, depending on towel thickness, intervene between the pack and the skin. This provides thermal insulation, largely because of the air in the towelling, so that although the pack is at about 75°C the skin temperature does not rise above 42°C or so. It takes some time (about 8 min: Lehmann *et al.*, 1966) for the skin temperature to reach its maximum. During this time the pack temperature is falling but the towelling and pack prevent the skin surface from losing heat so that the skin and superficial tissue temperature rises, as indicated in Figure 8.2. The towelling can be separated from the wet pack by a plastic sheet which prevents wetting of the towel and thus enhances the insulating effect; in this case less towelling may be used. If lower temperature packs (e.g. 65°C) are used less thickness of towelling is needed.

The packs are left in place for 20–30 min. If a fresh hot pack is used every 10 min the heating may be prolonged but there is no difference in the temperature reached in the subcutaneous tissues (Lehmann *et al.*, 1966). This is due to the control of heating exerted by the insulating effect of the fat layer and the heat removed by convection in the blood due to vasodilation, as already explained.

Other packs

There are various forms of hot moist packs which have been used therapeutically. A piece of absorbant lint or woollen material soaked in almost boiling water and then wrung out (using gloves) can be applied to the skin when the temperature has fallen to about 60°C. After about 5 min the pack will have fallen to skin temperature, at which point it is replaced. Such packs, often called Kenny packs, have been widely used in the past as a means of reducing the muscle soreness and tightness associated with poliomyelitis.

Mud packs (peloids), notably kaolin and peat, have been used as hot moist packs because it was considered that their chemical composition gave them specific therapeutic properties. This is no longer believed; in fact some peat may cause skin irritation, so it is now usual to apply cleaner and more convenient moist packs such as the hydrocollator type, described above.

Contrast baths

Contrast baths involve alternate immersion in hot and cold water producing marked hyperaemia of the skin. Such treatment will cause considerable sensory stimulation as the cutaneous hot and cold receptors are alternately activated. This stimulation is relatively vigorous because each time neural accommodation starts to occur the temperature stimulation is reversed. This strong sensory stimulation may act to suppress pain by means of the gate mechanism (see Chapter 3) and account for the subjective relief of pain that occurs in many patients receiving this treatment. It is also considered by many that contrast baths will help to reduce local oedema by promoting alternate vasodilation and vasoconstriction.

Method of application

Two suitably sized baths are filled, the hot at 40–45°C and the cold at 15–20°C (water from the cold tap is usually in this cold range). It is usual to start and finish with immersion in the hot water. The period of immersion in the hot water is longer—3 or 4 min—while immersion in the cold water is kept to 1 min. This cycle is repeated three or four times so that the whole treatment lasts anything from 15 to 25 min. An initial hot immersion of 10 min has been recommended to achieve hyperaemia (Lehmann and de Lateur, 1982).

During the treatment the hot water will cool and the cold will be warmed, partly due to the transfer of the warm/cold wet limb from one bath to the other. It is therefore usually necessary to top up both baths during treatment. This is not a problem that arises with large volumes of water. A thermometer should be available to check the water temperature.

Hydrotherapy

Warm water has been used for therapeutic purposes since ancient times particularly where the presence of natural warm water has provided an opportunity for the development of spas. In thermal areas in some parts of the world such as Iceland or New Zealand, the water appears as geysers or bubbles up in hot mud. Such sources often contain sulphur and other minerals. Ground water is forced to the surface after permeating deeply placed, and hence hotter, rock formations. Also in some limestone areas, e.g. the Mendips, water is carried deeply in porous rock to become heated; it emerges at Bath at about 44°C.

Swimming and exercising in warm water have beneficial effects which were often ascribed to the minerals dissolved in the water. As the whole body is immersed and the major therapeutic effect is considered to be due to the exercise rather than the water temperature, hydrotherapy is outside the scope of this book and other texts such as *Duffield's Exercise in Water* or *Hydrotherapy in Practice* by Davis and Harrison should be consulted.

Whirlpool baths

Whirlpool baths are stainless-steel tanks or baths of various sizes. The smaller ones are made to accommodate one limb, while larger ones allow the patient to sit. The 'whirlpool' refers to turbulence produced by an electric pump, or compressed air, which mixes air and water into a jetstream. This water agitation can be varied in force by controls on the pump (or turbine) and air pressure. The direction of the stream can be altered by changing the position of the output nozzle. A mixing tap allows any desired water temperature; temperatures between 36 and 41°C are usually employed.

The agitation of the water, the whirlpool effect, serves to stimulate the skin surface mechanically. This stimulation of large-diameter mechanoreceptors and thermoreceptors may account for the analgesic effects (Walsh, 1986), being due to the gate mechanism discussed in Chapter 3. The mechanical effect is further used in the cleaning of open wounds—gentle debridement of dirt and necrotic tissue. In circumstances where healing is slow, such as varicose ulcers, the mechanical effect is considered to provoke granulation tissue formation by increasing the local blood flow; this gives a gentle massaging effect. Although the water in these baths is changed for each patient it is often advisable to add an antibacterial agent to the water. Sodium hypochlorite (bleach) in 1 to 120 dilution is recommended (Walsh, 1986).

There is evidence that the temperature of the subcutaneous tissues rises with whirlpool bath treatment, like any other form of conduction heating (Borrell *et al.*, 1980), and thus there is a consequential increase in blood flow. There is also evidence that treatment in the whirlpool increases oedema; an increased tissue volume was found both in patients and in healthy subjects (Magness *et al.*, 1970). This is unsurprising since the extremities must be dependent during immersion in the warm water. If oedema is a likely problem it would be reasonable to modify the treatment so that it is followed by a period of warmth and/or exercise with the limb in elevation.

Treatment is usually given for a period of 20 min since longer treatments appear to give no greater benefit, at least in so far as tissue-heating is concerned. Prolonged immersion in hot water leads to temporary wrinkling of the skin which in healthy skin recovers rapidly on drying. However, repeated soaking tends to increase the risk of skin infection and exacerbate any infection already present; atrophic skin is particularly at risk.

Contraindications to treatment with hot water

There is very little chance of damage with these treatments since mild heat and simple, familiar materials are used. Local burns are only possible if very hot water is allowed to contact the skin; this could happen with the careless application of a hydrocollator pack or hot compress. With these treatments it is as well to be sure the patient has normal thermal sensitivity. Since local thermal regulation depends on the ability to increase cutaneous blood flow it is important to be aware of any ischaemic disease that might prevent an adequate vasodilatory response. This would apply to conditions in which the peripheral arteries were structurally damaged, such as arteriosclerosis or Buerger's disease, but not necessarily those due to vasospasm. If the whole body, or large segments, are immersed the heat loss mechanism of the body is affected because if the water temperature is above core temperature there is no way of losing heat from the areas under the water. Patients who have any deficiency of the cardiovascular or heat-regulating mechanism may be at risk in these circumstances.

Apart from the risks associated with excess heat there are some infections that are encouraged by wetness of the skin, notably certain fungal infections, the best known being tinea pedis (athlete's foot) and paronychia, which thrive in warm moist conditions. The presence of such conditions indicates that some form of dry heat would be more suitable or the part should be enclosed in a thin plastic bag, achieving the thermal effects without wetting the skin. Acute dermatitis or eczema may be exacerbated by immersion in hot or warm water or, for that matter, by any other form of heat. Similar considerations apply to inflammation of the skin due to radiotherapy or chemical irritants of any kind; in these circumstances the application of heat should be avoided.

The effects of heat and limb dependence have already been noted. Thus the presence of oedema can be seen as a contraindication in some circumstances.

Heated air treatment

Both simple hot, dry air and a mixture of air and water vapour are described as hot air baths. Small hot air cabinets—a metal box fitted with an electric fan or element heater, both thermostatically controlled—have already been mentioned in connection with wax treatment of the hand. They are useful for hand injuries with oedema and open wounds as the hand can be exercised in elevation and nothing but warm air comes in contact with the tissues. Temperature in the metal cabinet should be about 70°C, but because of the low thermal conductivity of air, the skin temperature is kept much lower.

Hot air cabinets, which contain thermostatically controlled heating elements and in which the whole body is enclosed, have been used in the past, notably in spas, to produce a small rise in general body temperature. Such treatment needs to be well controlled for the patient's safety: for example, adequate fluid replacement is important because of the losses due to sweating.

Small hand-held fan heaters, such as hairdriers, are occasionally used in order to dry and give mild heating to open wounds such as bedsores.

Hot moist air has been applied at spas in rooms with water vapour heated to various temperatures. There is also a device consisting of a cabinet enclosing the patient's trunk which provides thermostatically controlled moist air, continually humidified and circulated.

Fluidotherapy

Warmed air, thermostatically controlled, is blown through a mass of tiny cellulose particles (a powder) which become suspended in the moving air in a large metal cabinet. The effect is to produce a fluid-like mixture into which the distal part of the limb can be immersed through a hole in the box. The viscosity of the system is relatively low so that exercise can be performed in the moving particles—not unlike moving in warm water without the wetness. The air temperature can be regulated; treatment is usually given at anything between 38 and 45°C although somewhat higher temperatures can also be used. The amount of particle agitation can be varied and this determines the amount of skin stimulation. This treatment differs from hydrotherapy in that sweating can still act effectively as a heat loss mechanism.

Treatment is usually given for 20 min and is considered useful because it provides mechanical as well as thermal stimulation. To sterilize the powder and thus obviate any risk of cross-infection between patients an additional heater is used. Any open wound must be covered during this treatment to prevent the powder entering the tissues.

Electric heating pads

These vary from small pads about 30×30 cm to electric blankets. Electric resistance wire is contained in a suitable fabric and a set of resistances provided in a control unit so that the pad can operate at various temperatures. The resistance wire is heated and warms the fabric which when placed against the skin gives conduction heating. Such pads are often used as a convenient way of achieving muscle relaxation or relaxing muscle spasm prior to other treatments such as exercise or mobilization.

THE EFFECTS OF SUPERFICIAL HEAT ON THE TISSUES

The skin temperature rises rapidly where heat is being applied and the underlying subcutaneous tissue is also warmed to a lesser extent. The temperature of more deeply placed joints or muscle tissue is not raised directly by superficial heating, but see further comment below.

As has been explained, applying heat to the skin leads to reflex responses in order to dissipate the local heat. There is local skin vasodilation in the heated skin and subsequently vasodilation of skin vessels elsewhere to increase the body's heat loss. Thus when heat is applied to the skin surface, either as conduction heating or as radiation, little heating of the deeper tissues occurs because they are shielded by the thermal insulation provided by the subcutaneous fat and the fact that heat is removed in the increased skin blood flow.

However some conduction to the local deep tissues does occur and it is this that justifies the use of superficial heat for the treatment of such structures; for example, applying hot packs to the knee for the treatment of chronic arthritis. Further, it has been suggested, and supported by some evidence (Horvath and Hollander, 1949), that superficial heating of a joint may *decrease* the intra-articular temperature, and thus benefit an acute inflammatory arthritis. Other evidence and clinical experience do not accord with this suggestion.

A more recent study (Weinberger *et al.*, 1989) measured the intra-articular and skin temperatures of 5 patients with bilateral knee effusion. Hot packs at 42°C were placed on the right knee for 30 min and the temperature of both knees was recorded. Small but statistically significant rises in intra-articular temperature occurred in the treated knees a little later than the skin temperature rise. In the control knee there was no significant change in the intra-articular temperature but the skin temperature increased somewhat, although less than that of the heated knee. Other studies (e.g. Borrell *et al.*, 1980) have also found small temperature increases in joint structures due to superficial heating.

THE THERAPEUTIC USES OF SUPERFICIAL HEATING

Relief of pain

The various forms of superficial heating are widely used for pain relief; the mechanisms have been discussed in Chapter 7. Since the effects are largely confined to the skin it is reasonable to propose that the major pain-relieving effects are largely reflex as far as subcutaneous structures are concerned. Thus the stimulation of sensory receptors may activate the pain gate mechanism (see discussion in Chapter 3, p. 60). Muscle spasm, which is associated with pain, is also reduced by superficial heating (see Chapter 7). It is suggested that some pain reduction may be due to 'washing out' the pain-producing metabolites due to the increased circulation (Wadsworth and Chanmugan, 1980) but the major circulatory effect occurs in the skin rather than in the underlying structures in which the pain is usually located. Nevertheless there is a widespread acceptance of the efficacy of mild superficial heat as a means of pain relief despite a dearth of supporting clinical studies.

A rather unspecific sedative effect has been observed. During and after heat treatments patients have been found to sleep more readily. While this might be simply a consequence of pain relief it has been noted that skin temperatures rise just before the onset of sleep so that this sedative effect of superficial heat could be a reflex phenomenon (Lehmann and de Lateur, 1982).

Encouragement of healing

Mild superficial heating is used to encourage healing, not only in superficial injuries but also in more deeply placed lesions of, for example, ligaments or other joint structures. As already explained, marked skin heating will lead to only slight heating of the deeper tissues by conduction. Such heating could bring these subcutaneous tissues close to, or a little above, core temperature, which is the optimum for healing. It is suggested (Wadsworth and Chanmugan, 1980) that mild inflammation will benefit from temperature rises between 2 and 5°C which cause an increase of phagocytosis and encourage absorption of exudate. Chronic inflammatory states may benefit similarly. For these reasons superficial heat has been applied postoperatively and for many chronic inflammatory conditions, particularly the arthroses.

Increase of range of joint motion

There seems to be three mechanisms involved here. Firstly, the analgesic effect of heat allows greater tolerance of stretching. A comparison of stretching the hamstrings with prior superficial heating gave a greater increase of hip flexion than stretching alone (Michlovitz, 1986). Secondly, the viscosity of tissues will be reduced, which partly accounts for the reduction of joint stiffness that occurs with heating (Wright and Johns, 1961). Thirdly, increased collagen extensibility occurs at higher temperatures (Lehmann *et al.*, 1970). Heat is therefore used prior to passive stretching and/or exercise to increase joint movement or lengthen scars or contractures, for example in the chronic stages of rheumatoid arthritis or any condition in which fibrosis is a marked feature. Similarly, scars in the skin or subcutaneous tissues would benefit by heat prior to stretching.

Reflex heating

The cutaneous vasodilation that occurs in other parts as a consequence of local heating—illustrated by the skin temperature rise of the control knee described above—is sometimes called 'reflex heating'. It is, of course, due to reflexes mediated in the hypothalamus triggered both by the increased blood temperature and by stimulation of thermal receptors in the skin. This can be used therapeutically. If a proximal limb segment is heated the distal segment (and other parts) may show initial vasoconstriction followed by marked vasodilation. The initial constriction occurs to maintain normal blood pressure as vasodilation of the heated area occurs. The subsequent vasodilation, to lose heat, increases the skin blood flow. Thus injuries involving the skin of the extremities can be treated without heating or even touching the affected tissues. Similarly, if skin ischaemia is present the blood flow can be increased without risk.

Although temperature is the major factor controlling skin vasodilation it must be recognized that other factors contribute and are superimposed upon the vascular reflex. The onset of vigorous exercise will lead to some cutaneous vasoconstriction, for example (Johnson and Park, 1982).

Testing thermal sensation

This is necessary in the safe application of heat treatments. The customary method is to apply two test-tubes of water at 40–45°C and 15–20°C randomly to the area, asking the patient to identify which is which with the eyes shut. The temperature difference between the tubes falls during the test so that patients are actually discriminating between only a few degrees Celsius. (Any other method that requires the patient to distinguish small temperature differences is perfectly satisfactory.) Temperatures over 45°C or much below 15°C should not be used because these may test pain rather than thermal sensations.

Thus, in summary, superficial heat is used therapeutically for:

1 The relief of pain.
2 The relief of muscle spasm.
3 Sedation.
4 Encouraging and accelerating healing of injuries or mild or chronic inflammation.
5 Increasing the range of joint motion or lengthening scar tissue.

REFERENCES

Abramson D. L., Tuck S., Chu L. S. W. *et al.* (1964). Effect of paraffin bath and hot fomentations on local tissue temperature. *Arch. Phys. Med. Rehab.,* **45,** 87–94.

Borrell P. M., Parker R., Henley, E. J. *et al.* (1980). Comparison of 'in vivo' temperatures produced by hydrotherapy, paraffin wax treatment and fluidotherapy. *Phys. Ther.,* **60,** 1273–6.

Davis B. C., Harrison R. A. (1988). *Hydrotherapy in Practice.* Edinburgh: Churchill Livingstone.

Griffin J. E., Karselis T. C. (1988). *Physical Agents for Physical Therapists* 3rd edn. Springfield, Illinois, USA: Charles C. Thomas.

Horvath S. M., Hollander J. L. (1949). Intra-articular temperature as a measure of joint reaction. *J. Clin. Invest.,* **28,** 469.

Johnson J. M., Park M. K. (1982). Effect of heat stress on cutaneous vascular responses to the initiation of exercise. *J. Appl. Physiol.,* **53,** 744–9.

Lehmann J. F., de Lateur B. J. (1982). Therapeutic heat. In *Therapeutic Heat and Cold* (Lehmann J. F., ed.) Baltimore: Williams & Wilkins, pp. 404–562.

Lehmann J. F., Silvermann D. R., Baum B. A. *et al.* (1966). Temperature distribution in the human thigh produced by infra-red, hot pack and microwave applications. *Arch. Phys. Med. Rehab.,* **47,** 291–9.

Lehmann J. F., Masock A. J., Warren C. G. *et al.* (1970). Effect of therapeutic temperatures on tendon extensibility. *Arch. Phys. Med. Rehab.,* **51,** 481–7.

Magness J., Garret T., Erickson D. (1970). Swelling of the upper extremity during whirlpool baths. *Arch. Phys. Med. Rehab.,* **51,** 297.

Michlovitz S. L. (1986). Biophysical principles of heating and superficial heat agents. In

Thermal Agents in Rehabilitation (Michlovitz, S. L. ed.) Philadelphia: F. A. Davis, pp. 99–118.

Sekins K. M., Emery A. F. (1982). Thermal science for physical medicine. In *Therapeutic Heat and Cold* (Lehmann J. F., ed.) Baltimore: Williams & Wilkins, pp. 70–132.

Skinner A. I., Thomson A. M. (eds) (1983). *Duffield's Exercise in Water* 3rd edn. London: BaillièreTindall.

Wadsworth H., Chanmugan A. P. P. (1980). *Electrophysical Agents in Physiotherapy.* Marrickville, NSW, Australia: Science Press.

Walsh M. (1986). Hydrotherapy: the use of water as a therapeutic agent. In *Thermal Agents in Rehabilitation* (Michlovitz S., ed.) Philadelphia: F. A. Davis, pp. 119–39.

Weinberger A., Fadilah R., Lev A. *et al.* (1989). Intra-articular temperature measurements after superficial heating. *Scand. J. Rehab. Med.*, **21**, 55–7.

Wright V., Johns R. J. (1961). Quantitative and qualitative analysis of joint stiffness in normal subjects and in patients with connective tissue diseases. *Ann. Rheum. Dis.*, **20**, 36–46.

9. *Cold therapy*

Cold therapy, or cryotherapy, refers to the therapeutic use of local or general body cooling; this chapter is entirely concerned with the former. Cooling, as has already been explained, is simply the transfer of heat energy away from the body tissues. The result is to lower the local tissue temperature and provoke the thermoregulatory responses described in Chapter 7. Although cooling can be achieved in several ways, such as evaporating liquids or blowing cold air over the skin, the vast majority of cold treatments are given with crushed ice. Heat is thus transferred by conduction from the skin and the energy is used in changing the state of the substance from a solid to a liquid, i.e. by melting the ice.

Temperature changes in the tissues will depend on the amount of heat energy removed from the tissues and the rate of removal. Thus for a constant source of cooling the temperature drop in the tissues will depend on:

1 The temperature difference between the coolant and the tissues: the colder the application the greater the heat loss from the tissues.
2 The thermal conductivity of the tissues. This differs from one area to another. In general, water-filled tissues, such as muscle, have a high thermal conductivity compared to fat or skin (see Chapter 7). Thus the cooling of deep tissue depends on the nature of the overlying tissue. The normal layer of subcutaneous fat serves as thermal insulation so that heat loss through the tissues—or cold penetrating the tissues, which is the same thing—is largely dependent on the blood flow.
3 The length of time for which the cold is applied. The amount of energy loss is clearly dependent on time; temperature falls until the energy lost at the surface is balanced by heat energy supplied from the rest of the body, at which point the temperature becomes constant.
4 The size of the area that is being cooled. The larger the area, the more heat energy is lost.

While the skin temperature can be changed abruptly and markedly with the application of cold the deeper tissues are cooled much less and much more slowly. This has been demonstrated by several investigators. Figure 9.1

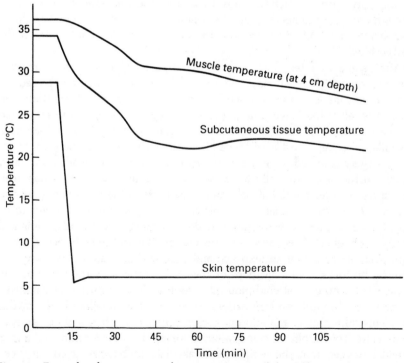

Fig. 9.1 Example of temperature changes in tissues of the calf on application of ice bags. Modified from Bierman and Friedlander (1940).

illustrates this point. In this example it takes some 30 min to lower the muscle temperature at a depth of 4 cm by 3.5°C or so. Muscle tissue at 2.5 cm can take up to 20 min or longer to drop 5°C (Palastanga, 1988).

PHYSIOLOGICAL CHANGES DUE TO COOLING THE SKIN

Putting ice on the skin surface leads to local changes at the cooled site and general systemic changes as the heat-regulating mechanism of the body is activated (see Chapter 7).

The local effects

There is immediate vasoconstriction of cutaneous blood vessels, shown by the blanching that occurs. This restricts the blood flow in the skin so that heat loss is minimized. The speed with which this vasoconstriction occurs indicates that it is a reflex in the autonomic nervous system, which is triggered by stimulation of the thermal receptors in the skin. There is also considered to be a direct effect of cold on the smooth muscle of the arterioles. In addition the precapillary sphincters, which are influenced by local hormones (e.g. serotonin and bradykinin), may be involved in local thermoregulation (Lee and Warren, 1978). This vasoconstriction leads to a dramatic decrease in blood flow through the skin, and hence limits the conduction of heat to the body surface. The increased blood viscosity, due to cooling, will also contribute to the slowed blood flow.

After some minutes the vasoconstriction may give way to a marked vasodilation which itself may last some 15 min before being replaced by another episode of vasoconstriction. This alternation of constriction and dilation is called the Lewis 'hunting reaction' (Lewis, 1930), in the sense that the vessel 'hunts' or oscillates about its mean position. This cold-induced vasodilation occurs most easily when the rest of the body is relatively warm and is largely confined to certain body areas. It occurs most readily and most rapidly in the face, especially the nose and ears, but also in the hands, feet, patella region, olecranon, buttocks and some parts of the chest wall (Fox and Wyatt, 1962). The explanation for this curious response to cold seems to be that it serves to protect the tissues from damage due to prolonged cooling and relative ischaemia. This idea is supported by the fact that it occurs most vigorously in areas that are exposed and in those regions on which pressure occurs—buttocks, anterior surface of knees and particularly the feet. Fox and Wyatt (1962) noted that cold-induced vasodilation was more readily induced in the lateral (weight-bearing) part of the sole of the foot than in the medial area. This response is variable from person to person. It tends to occur about 10 min after cold application and rather more rapidly, about 5 min, in the face. It will be noted that the peripheral areas that exhibit strong cold-induced vasodilation are well endowed with arteriovenous anastomoses in the skin, suggesting that these play a predominant role; however cold-induced vaso-dilation is variable and does not always show the clear-cut cycling effect.

The cause of this vasodilation is not yet completely elucidated. Originally an axon reflex mechanism involving a histamine-like substance (substance H) to cause local vasodilation was suggested (Lewis, 1930). As the increased blood flow washes out this substance the vessels constrict again thus continuing the cycle. Later suggestions include the possibility that as the temperature falls so smooth muscle activity is diminished and constriction is no longer possible. The consequent vasodilation rewarms the part, the smooth muscle recovers and it constricts again.

The foregoing explanation applies to the skin only, a region involved in thermal regulation. The response of muscle blood flow to cooling is less dramatic. It seems likely that cooling provokes vasoconstriction in all vascular smooth muscle and the increased viscosity certainly reduces the blood flow. There is, however, some evidence of reflex vasodilation of deep vessels (in the forearm) as a consequence of cooling the skin below 18°C and it is especially marked below 10°C.

Cooling a localized area of one forearm for 15 min has been shown to lead to a temperature drop not only in the underlying muscle, which reached maximum cooling about 18 min after cooling, but also in the same muscle on the other forearm (Wolf, 1971). The cooling of the contralateral forearm took much longer (42 min) to reach the lowest temperature. It is suggested that this effect might be therapeutically useful since it would allow some beneficial effects of muscle cooling to be achieved in, say, a hemiplegic patient by local icing of the unaffected side.

One striking feature of studies investigating muscle cooling is the length of time it takes to reach maximum cooling and the even longer period needed for rewarming. After heating, muscle temperatures rapidly return to normal because the vasodilation and lowered viscosity allow a high blood flow thus removing excess heat rapidly; after cooling the blood flow is diminished for the opposite reasons, so that muscle rewarming takes a good deal longer. The muscle is also shielded from warming from the surface by the subcutaneous fat layer.

The principal effect of cooling living tissue will be to reduce its metabolic rate in accordance with Van't Hoff's predictions discussed in Chapter 7. This will affect the activity of all tissues. Most evident will be the reduced oxygen uptake; in fact the erythema due to cold-induced vasodilation is distinguished from that due to heating due to its 'pinkness' because it contains less reduced haemoglobin. Thus cooling wounds probably does not benefit healing.

Cold applied to the skin provides a strong sensory stimulus by stimulating the cold receptors. This may be used therapeutically in the suppression of pain and treatment of hypertonicity. If the cold is sufficiently intense it reduces the conduction velocity of peripheral nerves. Synaptic transmission can also be delayed. All nerve fibres are not equally affected by cooling. As might be expected the small-diameter non-myelinated slow-conducting group IV C fibres are least affected; similarly, the B fibres, also small but myelinated and mainly preganglionic autonomic, are also little affected. The A delta fibres are the most susceptible to cold. These are small and thinly myelinated and are pain and temperature carriers (Table 9.1) (Douglas and Malcolm, 1955). This evidence was gained from studies on isolated animal tissues and it must be recognized that it may not apply to intact human tissues. Both motor and sensory nerve conduction velocities have been shown to be reduced (in the ulnar nerve) by cooling (Lee *et al.*, 1978). This study, in common with several others, showed that the effect of cooling lasted considerably longer than the application of ice.

Table 9.1   Peripheral nerve fibres affected by cooling

Most affected by cold		Moderately affected by cold	Least affected by cold
$A\beta(II)$	To intrafusal muscle fibres From low-threshold mechanoreceptors	$A\alpha$ Extrafusal muscle fibres Cutaneous, joint and muscle receptors	B Preganglionic efferent autonomic
$A\gamma$	To intrafusal muscle fibres		C Postganglionic efferent autonomic
$A\delta(III)$	Fast pain From high-threshold mechanoreceptors From thermoreceptors above 45°C		Slow pain, polymodal Nociceptors Thermoreceptors

Abramson *et al.* (1966) showed that cooling the forearm led to a marked fall in the motor nerve conduction velocity of the median and ulnar nerves and that these changes were strongly correlated with the tissue temperature fall. (Warming tended to raise the motor nerve conduction velocity to a peak at a temperature a little above core temperature and higher tissue temperatures had an inconsistent effect.)

Muscle strength is diminished by cooling the limb in water at 10–15°C, probably because of its effect on viscosity and metabolic rate, but there is evidence that the strength increases over the original value about an hour or so after cooling has ceased. Briefly applied cold, i.e. 5 min of ice massage, has also been found to increase isometric strength (Michlovitz, 1986; see discussion below).

Motor skills are diminished as a consequence of local cooling, again unsurprisingly since the loss of dexterity in cold hands is a common experience. This effect occurs at temperatures above those at which muscle strength is decreased. This effect could be due to diminished nerve conduction, especially sensory nerves.

In summary, the local effects of cooling include:

1 Immediate perception of cold—cold receptors are stimulated.
2 Immediate vasoconstriction of cutaneous vessels followed by cold-induced vasodilation in some areas, which may continue in a cyclical manner.

3 Reduced muscle blood flow.
4 Lowered metabolic rate, therefore less oxygen uptake.
5 Effects on peripheral nervous system with consequential reduction in pain and hypertonicity.
6 Slowed healing.

General effects of local cooling

Cooling applied to the skin immediately stimulates cold receptors which are more numerous than heat receptors in any given area of skin. Although some of these cold receptors will be firing at normal skin temperatures their activity increases greatly as cooling occurs, diminishing somewhat when cooling becomes steady, i.e. they show adaptation. Extreme cold is experienced as pain, involving pain receptors (see Chapter 7). Both pain and temperature neurons/synapse in the posterior horn of the spinal cord; the subsequent neuron ascends in the spinothalamic tract of the opposite side. Apart from a synapse in the thalamus with a neuron to the sensory cortex, giving awareness of cold, there are many collateral paths, particularly to the hypothalamus.

As explained in Chapter 7, the hypothalamus acts as a thermostat to maintain core temperature. The posterior hypothalamus is concerned with the response to body cooling, being affected by nervous input from the skin and probably other receptors as well as the blood temperature. To conserve heat the response, via the vasomotor centre, is cutaneous vasoconstriction. The skin blood flow can be increased by vasodilation much more than it can be diminished (Hubbard and Mechan, 1987) indicating that humans are better adapted to a hot environment; this is also evidenced by the efficiency of the human sweating response. The degree of general vasoconstriction that occurs is dependent on the extent of the cooling. Further, if the temperature drop is great enough shivering will occur. This increases metabolism, and hence heat production, by irregular muscle contractions. The resting metabolic rate can be doubled by shivering over periods of several hours and rather more over shorter periods (Hardy, 1982). However, it is expensive in physiological terms in that energy is being expended. As noted in Chapter 7, brown adipose tissue in neonates is able to produce heat by directly metabolizing but this does not seem to occur significantly in adults. Shivering in the muscles of mastication gives rise to the familiar teeth chattering with cold.

Awareness of cold leads to behavioural responses to maintain body temperature such as increased activity and putting on more clothes.

THERAPEUTIC USES OF COLD

Recent injuries

Cold is widely used in the treatment of recent injuries. If bleeding occurs cold serves to promote immediate vasoconstriction and makes the blood more viscid; both diminish the flow. Combined with pressure over the wound such treatment leads to haemostasis. However the cooling must not be so intense or so prolonged as to delay blood coagulation—clotting time is lengthened by cooling. If bleeding is occurring into the tissues, forming an intramuscular haematoma, for example, the same principle would apply but much longer periods of cold application would be needed to achieve cooling at depth, as noted earlier.

The immediate treatment of cutaneous heat burns requires rapid cooling of the area, as described in Chapter 7. Prompt cooling lowers the tissue temperature and thus limits tissue damage.

Soft tissue injuries of all kinds are almost universally treated by cold in the early stages. During this time the inflammatory changes occur in a well recognized sequence: the severity depends on the injury. Within hours, exudation of plasma into the tissues due to local vasodilation has occurred. This local oedema distorts the tissues which stimulates pain nerve endings. Pain is also produced by the action of local hormones, such as kinins and histamine, as well as other chemicals. The amount of pain will be related to the rate at which this oedema and chemical irritation occurs. Cooling will diminish the rate of swelling and production of irritants and so alleviate the pain. Compression and elevation of the part will also limit oedema formation. Thus the initial treatment of traumatic injuries can be defined by the acronym *ICE*, standing for ice, compression and elevation; the addition of rest, which is also highly appropriate in early treatment, turns the acronym into *RICE*.

The effect of cooling on metabolism is important in limiting the extent of the injury. Cell necrosis occurs over a period of several hours, releasing lysins and provoking local oedema. This leads to secondary cell damage which extends the area and severity of tissue injury. Therefore cooling in the early stages of injury, during the initial 2 h, will minimize secondary cell necrosis by reducing the metabolic rate (McLean, 1989). There is histological evidence that cooling can lessen the inflammatory reaction: experiments on pigs investigating the effects of ice on injured ligaments showed less inflammation when the ligaments were cooled compared to controls (Farry *et al.*, 1980). This study also showed that some swelling occurred in the subcutaneous tissues after removal of the ice in both injured and uninjured joints; the significance of this finding and whether it occurs in humans is not known.

Typical methods of treatment of an acute injury of an extremity, e.g. a sprain of the lateral ligament of the ankle, would involve the application of ice every 2–4 h during the first 2 or 3 days of the injury. This would be combined with rest, elevation and a suitable compression bandage.

Pain

Pain can be alleviated by the application of cold in several ways. The reduction of oedema and decreased release of pain-inducing irritants, mentioned above, is one. A direct effect on the conduction of pain receptors and neurons, reducing the velocity and number of impulses, is another. It is evident that this latter effect would only occur in the skin and then only if the temperature is much reduced. It is unlikely that the unmyelinated C fibres would be affected since they have been shown to continue to conduct at very low temperatures (see Table 9.1). The thinly myelinated A delta fibres which carry well-delineated 'fast' skin pain would be more susceptible. However, the pain due to tissue injury would be carried by C fibres and this is the pain that is usually being treated.

The immediacy of the effect of cold on pain suggests that it may act like other sensory stimuli on the pain gate mechanism (see Chapter 3) and since cold stimuli are quite intense they may lead to the release of endorphins and encephalins by the same mechanism (Palastanga, 1988). The fact that cold will effectively relieve pain, at least temporarily, has been supported by many studies, e.g. Benson and Copp (1974) and Parsons and Goetzl (1945).

Muscle spasm

Muscle spasm is linked to pain in that the pain of an injury appears to provoke muscle spasm as a protective measure. It has been suggested that the consequence of muscle spasm in causing tissue ischaemia may provoke further pain leading to a self-perpetuating cycle (Lee and Warren, 1978). There is therefore a reasonable expectation that the application of cold would reduce muscle spasm and so allow an increased range of movement.

Spasticity

Cooling has been used clinically for many years to reduce muscle spasticity. There is good objective evidence to support this, for example, cold producing a marked decrease in ankle clonus, described by Peterjan and Watts in 1962. The mechanisms by which the reduced spasticity may be brought about have been studied extensively (see reviews in Lee and Warren, 1978 and Lehmann and de Latour, 1982) without being fully elucidated. It is apparently not only the hyper-reflexia which can be affected but skilled activity of the upper limb has been shown to improve in hemiplegic patients after cooling in a 12°C bath (Hedenberg, 1970). Thus cryotherapy can lead to an improvement of neuromuscular function.

There would appear to be more than one mechanism by which cooling can affect spasticity, operating at two different sites, one in the skin and the other in the muscle itself. The immediate effect of stimulating cold receptors in the skin is to provide stimulation to the central nervous system. This is used therapeutically to facilitate muscle contraction—briefly stroking with ice over the appropriate dermatome, for example. Ice cube stroking over the biceps for 1–2 min has been shown to enhance the motor unit activity of subjects who had learned to activate a single motor unit with the aid of electromyogram biofeedback (Clendenin and Szumski, 1971). Cutaneous stimulation also appears to have reflex effects, diminishing gamma motor neuron activity or at least in some way diminishing the muscle spindle discharge, and so reducing spasticity. However it is not known how much of the effect is due to cold and how much to mechanical stimulation. It is also possible that sympathetic stimulation may contribute. Such effects would occur almost immediately as the skin temperature fell; a drop in muscle temperature would take longer, as already noted, but would last much longer (Peterjan and Watts, 1962). It has been suggested that muscle cooling might lead to reduced muscle spasticity by reason of the differential effect of cooling on the small myelinated fusimotor efferents and secondary afferents on the one hand, and the large thickly myelinated motor nerves to the extrafusal fibres on the other. It will be recalled that conduction in the former is more easily affected by cooling than in the latter (Table 9.1). Changes in the viscostatic properties of muscle tissue may also play a part since cooling makes the muscle—both intrafusal and extrafusal fibres—more viscid thus allowing less rapid stretching.

It must be recognized that there is a range of different responses to cooling; the responses of neurologically damaged patients are notably inconsistent (Urbscheit *et al.*, 1971). In order to ascertain the effectiveness of cooling as a means of reducing spasticity for any particular patient it would seem advisable to apply sufficient cold at least to reduce muscle temperature, i.e. for 25–30 min (Lehmann and de Lateur, 1982).

Muscle strengthening

There is evidence that cooling the skin surface can lead to greater strength of the underlying muscles, although there are also conflicting reports of a strength decrease following cryotherapy. Most investigators have concerned themselves with isometric strength. For example, Rajadhyaksha *et al.* (1982) found an increase of around 17% of the quadriceps after 30 min of ice applied to the anterior aspect of the thigh compared with a control group. Interestingly this was to some extent retained 24 h later.

The muscle strength increase has been ascribed to a facilitatory effect on the alpha motor neuron pool, at least in the short term. Sympathetic system stimulation has also been suggested as the mechanism for greater immediate muscle strength; cold stress has a potent effect on the sympathetic system and catecholamine release. If the muscle is cooled it will be more viscid and thus use more energy on contraction, resulting in weakness. This, it has been suggested, would account for the finding of lowered muscle strength on cooling. These contradictory findings may thus be reflecting a difference in the degree of cooling in different investigations.

Chronic inflammatory conditions

The value of cold therapy for acute inflammatory conditions is both rational and supported by clinical experience but this is not entirely the case with chronic inflammatory conditions. Many degenerative and chronic joint diseases have been treated successfully with cold therapy, including osteoarthrosis and chronic rheumatoid arthritis. Cold may well be beneficial in these conditions by virtue of its pain-relieving effect or because it may help to control such minor acute or subacute inflammatory changes as occur from time to time with degenerative joint conditions. Alternating hot and cold packs, or contrast baths, may be effective (Wadsworth and Chanmugan, 1980).

Chronic oedema and joint effusions

That cold treatment reduces chronic oedema is widely recognized. A recent study (Moon and Gragnani, 1989) has attempted to quantify this effect in 9 hemiplegic patients whose swollen hands were intermittently immersed in water at around 10°C for 30 min. Although hand volumes are variable, both between subjects and at different times in the same subject, there was a reduction in hand volume in all patients; it was statistically significant in 8 of them. During both treatment and measurement these hands were dependent; combining treatment with elevation may lead to even better results.

As well as interstitial oedema, inflammatory joint effusions are benefited by cooling. The application of ice and a compression bandage for an acute joint effusion are almost universally recognized treatments. The application of cold for obstructive oedema, such as that due to deep vein thrombosis, has a less rational basis and is not usually recommended.

Other therapeutic effects

Ice massage has been used in treatment of pressure sores, as have ice packs although the former is considered more effective (Lee and Warren, 1974). The beneficial effects are said to be due to the fact that cooling reduces vascular stasis.

Cooling is also used in conjunction with stretching in the later treatment of muscle tears and other athletic injuries and as prophylaxis against further injury. Cooling—using a vapocoolant spray—and stretching have been shown to be more effective than stretching alone in normal subjects (Halkovich, 1982).

In summary:

1 *Cold applied to recent injuries*
   a limits bleeding by vasoconstriction and increased blood viscosity;
   b limits pain by reducing the rate of oedema formation and production of pain nerve irritants;
   c reduces the metabolic rate and hence secondary cell necrosis.
2 *Cold for alleviation of pain*
   a acts as above;
   b reduces the conduction of some pain nerves in skin;
   c provides sensory stimulation, acting on the pain gate;

    d gives a strong cold sensation leading to endorphin release.
3 *Cold to reduce muscle spasm*
    a is linked to the effect on pain above.
4 *Cold to reduce muscle spasticity*
    a provides stimulation of cutaneous receptors and reflex inhibition of muscle activity;
    b affects the muscle spindle directly by more prolonged cooling;
    c increases viscosity which may diminish rapid stretch reflexes.
5 *Cold to facilitate muscle contraction*
    a provides brief stimulation of skin receptors—ice massage.
6 *Cold is also used in* chronic inflammation, effusion, muscle strengthening and stretching.

METHODS OF APPLYING COLD THERAPY

Cooling of the surface may be achieved in two basic ways: the application of a substance to a surface that is at a lower temperature, so cooling by conduction, or cooling by evaporating a chemical with a low boiling point from the surface. The former is by far the most widely used and the vast majority of cold treatments are given with melting ice. To achieve cooling over any but the smallest body region it is convenient and efficient to use flaked (or crushed) ice since this provides a large surface area of ice from which melting can occur. Ice blocks have the disadvantage of exerting local pressure which can impede circulation. Flaked ice is conveniently made in ice-making machines which produce a continuous supply of consistently sized flakes and store them in a large drained container. These machines work on the same principle as an ordinary domestic electric refrigerator and are usually plumbed in to the water supply.

Local immersion

This is the simplest method of all. It involves placing the part in a container of iced water—a mixture of water from the cold tap and flaked ice. The temperature can be controlled by varying the amount of ice used. At temperatures around 16–18°C continuous immersion can usually be tolerated for 15–20 min (Lee and Warren, 1978). At lower temperatures, such as around 10°C, continuous immersion is uncomfortable, so that intermittent application is usually given. This is done by leaving the part in the water for only 1 min or so at a time. Clearly such treatment can only be conveniently applied to the extremities—hand, forearm, foot and leg—which can be placed in a water bath. When the limb remains still in the water bath for relatively long periods it is necessary to agitate the water occasionally because the layer of water in contact with the skin tends to warm up; also the water temperature should be checked from time to time as it will gradually become warm and more ice may need to be added.

General immersion

A bath or tank is filled with sufficient cold water to allow the patient to sit waist- or chest-deep in the water. Water temperatures of 20–22°C are quite well tolerated for 10–15 min (Lee and Warren, 1978); lower temperatures would be tolerated for shorter periods. Such treatments are used to diminish spasticity.

Cold packs

Ice packs

Flaked ice is folded into damp terry-towelling or put into bags made of the same material and applied directly to the skin. They may be held in place by a plastic sheet wrapped around the part and the pack. A further towel or blanket is occasionally wrapped outside the plastic to decrease heat gain to the ice pack from the outside air. Cooling of the skin is quite rapid at first as the ice-cold water seeps through the towelling but after a minute or so the layer of water in contact with the skin tends to warm up somewhat so that these packs are quite tolerable for some 20 min. If the pack is removed after a few minutes and immediately reapplied with a fresh cold surface in contact with the skin, greater and more rapid cooling is achieved. However, rapid cooling can sometimes lead to skin damage (see below) so it is sometimes recommended that a thin layer of oil is smeared over the skin and separated from the towelling with paper. The aim is to provide some insulation to reduce the rate of cooling and to cause a rapid run-off of water from the skin.

Flaked ice may also be put in a suitably sized polythene bag; the top of the bag is tied to prevent water leaking out. This ice-filled bag can be moulded to fit the region to which it is being applied and a damp towel is used to separate the bag from the skin, with the skin oiled if there is thought to be any danger of cold injury to the surface. As the water from the melting ice is confined within the bag this is a clean and convenient method of application.

In all treatments with ice packs the bag should be removed after a few minutes to inspect the underlying skin to determine the response, and if it is considered abnormal the pack is not replaced.

Commercial cold packs

These are basically plastic, often vinyl, bags filled with a mixture of water and some substance that prevents the water freezing solid; thus the pack will remain flexible and can be moulded to the part. Silica gels are the most common.

Commercial cold packs are of various sizes but normally small enough to store in the freezer compartment of a domestic refrigerator. The pack will therefore be stored at a temperature below 10°C, often − 5°C or even − 12°C. It is important to be aware that initially these packs are at a lower temperature than ordinary ice packs and therefore have the potential to cool the skin very rapidly. However, their temperature rises rapidly on application and most of the cooling is due to melting ice which is at 0°C.

Depending on their size such packs may provide adequate cooling for about 20 min. As a precaution these packs can be applied over a wet towel to prevent ice burns (Harrison, 1978). As long as the towel remains wet as opposed to frozen it ensures that the surface in contact with the skin is not below 0°C.

Patients are sometimes advised to use bags of frozen peas as an ice pack for home treatment. Again the wet towel should be placed between the skin and the pack to avoid excessive cooling.

A totally different kind of cooling pack consists of chemicals which are mixed by breaking a container within the main pack; the resulting endothermic reaction causes strong cooling of the pack. These are, of course, one-use-only packs and are thus more appropriate for first-aid applications. If such a pack should accidentally be ruptured the contents should not be allowed to remain on the patient's skin since some are strongly alkaline and can cause skin irritation.

The only advantage of commercial packs seems to be convenience since it has been found that ice packs lower subcutaneous temperatures better than the chemical packs (McMaster *et al.*, 1978).

Ice towels

If a terry-towel is put into a mixture of flaked ice and water and then wrung out, much of the chipped ice will be found to adhere to the cloth. This can be placed over quite a large area to give immediate surface cooling. The ice towel will need to be replaced by another one after 2 or 3 min (or after 1 min in the case of the first towel) to give adequate cooling; say 20 min in total. It is a particularly useful technique for the treatment of muscle and allows movement and/or exercises to be performed while cold therapy is being applied.

Ice massage

This is used for two distinct purposes and thus involves two distinct techniques. Firstly, it can assist in the relief of pain by what has previously been called counter-irritant action. The second purpose is for muscle facilitation and involves brief stimulation of the skin dermatome supplied by the same nerve roots as those of the muscle.

The massage is given with a solid piece of ice, either as an ice cube wrapped in paper or cloth or an ice 'lollipop' on a wooden stick. This latter can be made quite simply by putting a wooden tongue depressor (spatula) upright in a small plastic cup of water in the freezer. Being larger, the lollipop lasts longer and is easier to handle than the usual size of ice cube.

The ice block is moved over the part using a slow circular motion for some minutes. During this time the patient will feel cold, burning and then aching sensations before the part finally becomes numb. This may take 5–10 min and is appropriate for pain relief. For neurological facilitation the ice should be applied only briefly, either dabbing for about 4 s at a time or short strokes applied over the dermatome.

Evaporating sprays

Spraying a rapidly evaporating liquid on the skin has the effect of using heat energy and hence cooling the surface. Ethyl chloride was originally used but it is highly inflammable and thus posed some risk. Other sprays, e.g. fluori-methane, are non-flammable. The liquid is sprayed on to the area to be cooled in a series of short strokes of about 5 s each with a few seconds' intervals between each. The nozzle of the spray is held about 45 cm from the skin surface and close to a right angle. Cooling from such sprays can be very rapid but does not last very long. If spraying near the face care should be taken to avoid the eyes and prevent the vapour from being inhaled.

Cold-compression units

Cold therapy combined with intermittent compression devices to a limb segment are available. Cold water is circulated in a sleeve which is put over the limb and part of it is inflated at intervals.

In summary, cold can be applied as:

1 *Conduction cooling*
   a Immersion
      i Local
      ii General
   b Cold packs
      i Ice packs
      ii Commercially made cold packs, either re-usable or disposable
   c Ice towels
   d Ice massage
      i Slow for pain relief
      ii Brief for muscle facilitation
2 *Evaporative cooling*
   a Evaporating spray

CONTRASTING HEAT AND COLD TREATMENTS

In the sense that heating the tissues adds energy whereas cooling extracts energy these are obviously opposite treatments. However, many conditions appear to benefit from either thermotherapy or cryotherapy. This is not a contradiction, for some of the effects are indirect and the total effect on the tissues is complex. The apparent paradox has spawned several studies of superficial heat and cold applied to the same condition for comparison. For example, a cross-over comparative trial on chronic rheumatoid arthritic knees (Kirk and Kersley, 1968) showed little objective difference but cold was associated with somewhat more pain relief. Pain thresholds in the shoulders of healthy subjects (Benson and Copp, 1974) were found to be raised by both heat and cold but significantly more so by the latter.

In summary:

1 Both heat and cold appear to be useful in relieving pain and muscle spasm.
2 Spasticity is reduced by cooling.
3 Recent trauma benefits from immediate cooling, reducing bleeding, rate of oedema formation and pain.
4 Later, the same injury will benefit from mild heating to increase metabolism and gently increase the healing processes. Cold has been shown to diminish healing.
5 The tendency to oedema is encouraged by heating but decreased by cooling.
6 Skilled movements are impaired by cooling.
7 Muscle activity can be facilitated by brief local cooling.
8 Joint stiffness is decreased by heating and increased by cooling.

DANGERS AND CONTRAINDICATIONS

There are two ways in which tissue injury might occur. Firstly excessive local cold can lead to damage in normal tissues and secondly some pathological conditions may predispose the patient to cold injury due to temperature falls that would otherwise be harmless. It must be said that in either circumstance damage is rare.

Excessive local cold on normal tissue

The mildest form consists of the appearance of erythema and tenderness of the skin a few hours after the application of ice, subsiding in a day or two; this is called an ice burn. A more severe form, an ice burn with fatty necrosis, shows bruising as well as more tenderness and can last up to 3 weeks (Lee and Warren, 1978). Such injuries are rare and are said to occur in areas which are underlain by thick subcutaneous fat and which have been cooled rapidly. Inadequately crushed ice can lead to a large piece being held against the skin for a long time, which increases the possibility of an ice burn.

With extreme cold freezing of the tissues can occur but this is extremely unlikely ever to occur with the treatment methods described above. What happens depends on the rate of cooling; if it is rapid ice crystals can form in the cells which may lead to cell death, whereas slower cooling tends to cause freezing of the extracellular fluid and withdrawal of water from the cells. This is referred to as 'frostbite' and only occurs if the body suffers extreme exposure; similar prolonged exposure to low temperatures without freezing the tissues, 'immersion foot' for example, can also produce severe tissue damage.

Certain pathological conditions

Cold sensitivity

Vasospasm.   Raynaud's phenomenon is a condition often associated with connective tissue disorders in which excessive vasoconstriction, triggered by cold, occurs in the digital arteries. Obviously cold treatment should not be used to provoke vascular spasm. Some other vascular conditions may have an element of vasospasm as well as obstruction, such as thromboangiitis obliterans (Buerger's disease), and therefore should not be treated with cold. With vascular disorders which are primarily obstructive, such as arteriosclerosis, cold treatments are considered unsuitable by many but the reasons are unclear. Since cold reduces the metabolic rate it is difficult to see what harm can occur as the tissues are already partly ischaemic; in fact cooling is temporarily beneficial in relieving pain.

Cryoglobinaemia.   An abnormal protein is present in the blood; it can form a precipitate at low temperatures blocking blood vessels and thus causing local ischaemia. Although not common, this condition can also be found in association with some of the connective tissue disorders such as systemic lupus erythematosus and rheumatoid arthritis.

Cold urticaria.   Cold causes the release of histamine from mast cells leading to a local weal and erythema and sometimes general (systemic) symptoms such as lowered blood pressure and raised pulse rate.

Cardiac disease

Coronary thrombosis and anginal pain have sometimes been provoked by cold leading to the suggestion that locally applied ice may cause reflex vasoconstriction of the coronary arteries and should therefore not be given to patients who have coronary artery disease. Injunctions to avoid ice treatment, especially of the left shoulder, for such patients have frequently been repeated but with little supporting evidence. The matter has been studied by electrocardiographically monitoring 25 patients who had known coronary artery disease while ice packs were applied to the left shoulder (Lorenze *et al.,* 1960). Only one of these patients showed changes in the electrocardiogram of any significance. It seems likely that any effect on the heart is due to greater demand due to increased blood pressure. Thus careful local cooling is reasonable for these patients but cooling large areas should be avoided (Lee and Warren, 1978).

Arterial blood pressure

Cooling larger areas, such as a limb segment, can lead to a transient rise in arterial blood pressure. This could well be dangerous for hypertensive patients or those with especially labile blood pressure. Monitoring the blood pressure during and for a short time after treatment would be advisable if large areas are to be cooled and there is uncertainty regarding the blood pressure response.

Sensory deficiency

It is sometimes asserted that ice should not be applied to areas with some sensory deficiency (e.g. Wadsworth and Chanmugan, 1980), but this seems illogical since cooling can lead to partial sensory loss anyway and it can be safely applied to an anaesthetic area (Lee and Warren, 1978). However, two points must be borne in mind. Firstly, the neurological effects of cooling, such as facilitation of muscle contraction, require intact sensory nerves; secondly, the normal circulatory response is altered if the autonomic nerves are affected so that tissue cooling occurs more rapidly and more deeply than normally. Therefore caution is required if skin with defective innervation is to be treated. In connection with this point thermal sensation testing is recommended by some as a necessary precaution prior to cryotherapy but assessing pain sensation (and/or the autonomic response) would seem more rational.

Emotional and psychological features

Some patients may have a strong aversion to cold in any form or to local cold applications in particular. This may be partly due to cultural factors since our language abounds with metaphors in which 'cold' has some unpleasant connotations, e.g. in cold blood, cold-hearted. There is an obviously physiological association with fear—cold feet and cold sweat. Both cold and fear stimulate the sympathetic system. There is also an emotional link:

> Pale grew thy cheek and cold,
> Colder thy kiss
> Truly that hour foretold
> Sorrow to this!

> Byron: 'When we two parted'

Even the medical term 'frozen shoulder' implies the concept of ice locking movable joints. The connection of cold with death is also well recognized. Thus the patient may exhibit a strong emotional disapprobation of cold which would make it inappropriate to use cryotherapy. It has been claimed that this is more likely to occur in elderly patients; this may be due to the fact that a greater range of skin temperature occurs in the elderly compared with young adults (Howell, 1982), presumably because the control mechanism is becoming less efficient in old age.

Hypersensitive areas

Assertions are sometimes made that certain parts of the body should not be treated with ice for reasons which are not made clear; for instance, the region of the ear because there may be some effect on the vagus nerve. However, there seem to be no reports or evidence of any deleterious effects. Similarly the medial aspect of the knee or the axilla in obese patients is said to be more susceptible to ice burns.

Precautions with particular cooling methods

It has already been noted that evaporating sprays can lead to rapid local cooling so that prolonged application can cause skin damage. Applications should therefore be restricted to sprays of about 5 s separated by 10 or 20 s intervals and the skin should be constantly inspected. Ethyl chloride is inflammable, so naked flames and heaters should be avoided; also the vapour should be kept clear of the eyes and not inhaled.

Ice bags—flaked ice in a plastic bag—can be kept in the freezer compartment of a refrigerator for home use; bags of frozen peas make a satisfactory and easily available substitute but it is important to understand that the temperature can be below 0°C in the freezer— −5°C or even −12°C. Therefore such packs should be separated from the skin by a wet towel.

If large areas of the body are to be cooled it is important to be aware of the systemic effects that can occur—the blood pressure rise already noted, as well as simple chilling of the patient leading to a possible drop in core temperature.

REFERENCES

Abramson D. I., Chu L. S. W., Tuck S. *et al.* (1966). Effect of tissue temperature and blood flow on motor nerve conduction velocity. *J.A.M.A.*, **198**, 156–62.

Benson T. B., Copp E. P. (1974). The effects of therapeutic forms of heat and ice on the pain threshold of the normal shoulder. *Rheumatol. Rehab.*, **13**, 101–4.

Bierman W., Friedlander M. (1940). The penetrative effects of cold. *Arch. Phys. Ther.*, **21**, 585–91.

Clendenin M. A., Szumski A. J. (1971). Influence of cutaneous ice application on single motor units in humans. *Phys. Ther.*, **51**, 166–75.

Douglas W. W., Malcolm J. L. (1955). The effect of localised cooling on cat nerves. *J. Physiol.*, **130**, 53.

Farry P. J., Prentice N. G., Hunter A. C., Wakelin C. A. (1980). Ice treatment of injured ligaments: an experimental model. *N.Z. Med. J.*, **91**, 14–16.

Fox R. H., Wyatt H. T. (1962). Cold induced vasodilation in various areas of the body surface in man. *J. Physiol.*, **162**, 289–97.

Halkovich R. (1982). Effect of fluori-methane spray. In *Proceedings of the IXth International Congress of World Confederation for Physical Therapy*. Stockholm, pp. 474–9. *International Congress (IXth) of World Confederation for Physical Therapy* May 23–28 (1982). Stockholm: Legitimerade Sjukgymnasters Ricksförbund.

Hardy J. D. (1982). Temperature regulation, exposure to heat and cold and effects of hypothermia. In *Therapeutic Heat and Cold* (Lehmann J. F., ed.) Baltimore: Williams & Wilkins, pp. 172–98.

Harrison M. A. (1978). Effects of ice treatment. *Physiother. Sport*, October.

Hedenberg L. (1970). Functional improvement of the spastic hemiplegic arm after cooling. *Scand. J. Rehab. Med.*, **2**, 154.

Howell T. (1982). Skin temperature gradient in the lower extremities of old women. *Exp. Gerontol.*, **17**, 65–7.

Hubbard J. L., Mechan D. J. (1987). *Physiology for Health Care Students*. Edinburgh: Churchill Livingstone.

Kirk J. A., Kersley G. D. (1968). Heat and cold in the physical treatment of rheumatoid arthritis of the knee. *Ann. Phys. Med.*, **IX**, 270–4.

Lee J. M., Warren M. P. (1974). *Cold Therapy in Rehabilitation*. London: Bell and Hyman.

Lee J. M., Warren M. P., Mason S. M. (1978). Effects of ice on nerve conduction velocity. *Physiotherapy*, **64**, 2–6.

Lehmann J. F., de Lateur B. J. (1982). Cryotherapy. In *Therapeutic Heat and Cold* (Lehmann J. F., ed.) Baltimore: Williams & Wilkins, pp. 563–602.

Lewis T. (1930). Observation upon the reactions of the vessels of the human skin to cold. *Heart*, **15**, 177–208.

Lorenze E. J., Carontonis G., DeRosa A. J. (1960). Effect on coronary circulation of cold packs to hemiplegic shoulders. *Arch. Phys. Med. Rehab.*, **41**, 394–9.

McLean D. A. (1989). The use of cold and superficial heat in the treatment of soft tissue injuries. *Br. J. Sports Med.*, **23**, 53–4.

McMaster W. C., Little S., Waugh T. R. (1978). Laboratory evaluation of various cold therapy modalities. *Am. J. Sports Med.*, **6**, 291–4.

Michlovitz S. L. (1986). Cryotherapy: the use of cold as a therapeutic agent. In *Thermal Agents in Rehabilitation* (Michlovitz S. L. ed.) Philadelphia: F. A. Davis, pp. 73–98.

Moon A. H., Gragnani J. A. (1989). Cold water immersion for the oedematous hand in stroke patients. *Clin. Rehab.*, **3**, 97–101.

Palastanga N. P. (1988). Heat and cold. In *Pain: Management and Control in Physiotherapy* (Wells P., Frampton V., Bowsher D., eds) London: Heinemann Medical Books, pp. 169–80.

Parsons C. M., Goetzl F. R. (1945). Effect of induced pain on pain threshold. *Proc. Soc. Exp. Biol. Med.*, **60**, 327–9.

Peterjan R. H., Watts N. (1962). Effects of cooling on the triceps surae reflex. *Am. J. Phys. Med.*, **41**, 240–51.

Rajadhyaksha V., Dastoor D. H., Shahani M. (1982). Influence of cooling of anterior aspect of thigh on maximal isometric tension of muscle quadriceps. In *Proceedings of the IXth International Congress of World Confederation for Physical Therapy*. Stockholm, pp. 494–8.

Urbscheit N., Johnston R., Bishop B. (1971). Effects of cooling on the ankle jerk and 'H' response in hemiplegic patients. *Phys. Ther.*, **51**, 983–8.

Wadsworth H., Chanmugan A. P. P. (1980). *Electrophysical Agents in Physiotherapy*. Marricksville, NSW, Australia: Science Press.

Wolf S. L. (1971). Contralateral upper extremity cooling from a specific cold stimulus. *Phys. Ther.*, **51**, 158–65.

10.

Electromagnetic fields: shortwave diathermy, pulsed electromagnetic energy and magnetic therapies

Electrotherapy explained

The use of magnetism in therapy
 Static magnetic fields
 Low-frequency magnetic fields
Effects and safety of electromagnetic fields

The title and indeed siting of this chapter may seem curious but the importance of electromagnetic phenomena and their relationships to other phenomena already considered and to be described in Section V provide justification.

NATURE

Electromagnetism is one of the four fundamental forces known to exist in the universe; it binds matter together at the atomic level. It accounts for the structure and behaviour of atoms with regard to both their chemical properties and also the production of electromagnetic radiations. The other forces are gravity—the most evident, and responsible for holding together the planets, stars and galaxies—and two additional ones deep within the atom. The strong force holds protons and neutrons together within the atomic nucleus and the weak force is responsible for the behaviour of subatomic particles in the nucleus.

Electromagnetic phenomena can be considered from three different aspects:

1 *Electrostatics* concerns the electric force between electric charges. There is an attraction between the negative charge of the electron and the positive charge associated with the proton and equally a repulsion of like charges. These forces act between any charges and their strength and direction can be described by drawing lines called lines of electric force. The area in which this force acts is called an electric field.
2 When charges move it is referred to as an *electric current*; the effects on the tissues have been discussed in Chapters 2 and 3. An inevitable consequence of constantly moving charges is the formation of a magnetic force at right angles to the direction of the charge motion. The area in which the magnetic force is evident, called the magnetic field, can be mapped in a similar way to the electric field by drawing lines to show direction. Such fields are familiarly demonstrated by using iron filings to form thousands of tiny magnets which fall in line with the direction of the magnetic force. Both electric and magnetic fields are customarily shown in terms of lines of force which represent the direction and magnitude—greater force with closely spaced lines—of the force.
3 If an electric charge is accelerated it causes the production of an *electromagnetic radiation* which radiates away from the moving charge and once generated is independent of the charge. These radiations include radio waves, visible light and X-rays (see Frontispiece), and are discussed in Chapter 11.

Thus in summary:

Where electric charges are:

1 Not moving there are electrostatic forces

2 Moving with a constant velocity there are magnetic forces.

3 Accelerating there is emission of radiations.

Notice that electric and magnetic fields as well as the emission of radiations can all occur at the same time.

The electric field, i.e. electric force, is measured in volts and the rate of motion of the charges, i.e. electric current, is measured in amperes. The current — flow of charges — might be the familiar current of electrons in a metal wire or movement of ions in a fluid or electrons orbiting an atomic nucleus. In all cases a magnetic field is generated at right angles to the flow of charges. Materials in which the atoms can be arranged in such a way that the magnetic forces are made to add together exhibit obvious magnetic properties. Nickel, cobalt and iron and their alloys including steel are all called ferromagnetic materials. All other materials exhibit only very weak magnetic properties but in all instances the effect is tiny, therefore magnetic fields can pass through the tissues without being altered. The tissues can be said to be 'transparent' to magnetic fields.

In Chapter 2 the effects on the tissues of a constant current were considered. Such currents are very small so that the magnetic field would be negligible. Magnetic fields, produced by large steady currents outside the tissues or by permanent magnets, are sometimes used therapeutically (see below) but there are no easily detectable effects on the tissues. In fact even very high-intensity magnetic fields do not seem to damage animal or human tissues. However, some birds appear to utilize the vertical component of the earth's magnetic field as a navigational method. Therefore there must be some physiological mechanism able to recognize these extremely weak magnetic fields. There is also some evidence that humans have some similar magnetic sense (Baker, 1981).

If the electric current is made to change, whether by becoming larger or smaller or changing direction, the consequent magnetic field follows exactly. Thus if the current was repeatedly reversed at, say, 50 cycles per second the resulting magnetic field would change in intensity and direction in the same manner. In the UK the mains current is such a current, evenly alternating at 50 Hz and has been described in Chapter 3 (therapeutically as diadynamic and sinusoidal currents). The changing magnetic field has important consequences.

As mentioned already, the motion of electric charges produces a magnetic force; these three components all act at right angles to one another. The reverse will also occur, that is movement of a magnetic force through electric charges will cause these charges to move in a direction at right angles to the direction of magnetic motion. This is often described in terms of electrons in a coil of wire being caused to move, i.e. a current flows when a magnet producing a magnetic field is moved closer. Such energy transfer is known as electromagnetic induction — because an electric force is induced in a conductor without contact—and is the basis of much modern use of electricity. It allows the conversion of electrical energy to motion, an electric motor, or the reverse, a dynamo or the change of electrical voltage, a transformer (see Appendix C).

It makes no difference in principle if the magnetic force is produced by electrons moving in a wire (forming an electromagnet) or electrons moving by orbiting atomic nuclei in ferromagnetic materials. The magnetic field produced by a current in a wire is vastly increased by applying it to a soft iron 'temporary' magnet.

The strength of the magnetic field is obviously dependent on the number of charges that move in a given region in a given time. Thus higher currents will give stronger magnetic fields and if the current is kept in a small area, by forming the wire into a coil, the magnetic field around the coil will be still stronger.

It is usual to think of electric currents being induced in wires, as described above, but a current will only flow if the charges—electrons or ions—are free to move. So in insulators polarization, that is distortion of the electron 'cloud' around the atomic nucleus, will occur (Fig. 10.3c). If the changing magnetic field induces currents in a solid block of conducting material instead of a wire the induced currents will follow paths at right angles to the magnetic field and hence parallel, but in the opposite direction, to the current inducing them. These are called 'eddy currents'. ('Eddy' simply because they are usually induced by a current in a coil and hence eddy in a circular, but opposite, direction.)

In Chapter 3 it was explained how varying electric currents passing in the tissues would affect excitable tissue, nerve and muscle. This included a wide range of currents of different pulse lengths and intervals, including alternating currents of 50 Hz and other frequencies. All of these will produce magnetic fields, albeit of low intensity when these currents are used therapeutically. If strong magnetic fields, generated outside the body, are passed through the tissues peripheral nerves can be stimulated by the induced currents in a similar way to nerve stimulation by faradic-type currents. This method has also been used to stimulate motor nerves in the motor cortex. Similarly low-intensity magnetic fields at these frequencies are sometimes used to encourage healing in ununited fractures or Perthes' disease (Harrison and Bassett, 1984). Other proposed effects of low-frequency magnetic fields will be discussed later.

If the alternating currents considered above are made to occur at higher frequencies, the rapid acceleration of charges causes a significant production of electromagnetic radiations, as already mentioned. As the frequency of the alternating current increases so the wavelength and frequency of radiations alters (see Frontispiece). This is more fully described in Chapter 11. The radiations emitted by the alternating current—often called an oscillating current at higher frequencies—are familiar as radio waves. All electromagnetic radiations have the same velocity of 3×10^8 m/s and differ from one another in their wavelength and frequency. At frequencies of several hundred kHz the radio waves produced have wavelengths of about 1 km; at frequencies of 1 MHz they have wavelengths of 300 m and at 10 MHz the wavelengths would be 30 m. The bands of radio wave frequencies around these three regions are called long, medium and shortwave bands respectively. Modern radio receivers usually give the frequencies rather than wavelengths. All radio frequencies in the range of 10–100 MHz are called shortwave and because the device for producing therapeutic heating is in this range it is called 'shortwave diathermy'. The first part of the name is unfortunate since it suggests that 'shortwave radio waves' are the effective therapy, which is entirely untrue. The radiations are largely irrelevant. It is the high-frequency oscillating currents generated in the tissues that cause the heating. Diathermy is a word, coined in 1907 from the Greek, meaning 'through heating' and this seems highly appropriate since it is an accurate description.

It may be wondered why heating should occur when high-frequency currents are passed through the tissues, since it was pointed out in Chapter 3 that therapeutic low-frequency currents produced negligible heating. The answer lies in the fact that much higher currents are being passed through the tissues with diathermy and, as also noted earlier, the heating would depend on the square of the current (heating $= I^2Rt$ where $I =$ current intensity, $R =$ resistance, and $t =$ time) so that a greater current would lead to very much greater heating. The low-frequency currents of Chapter 3 were mostly of a few milliamperes—or even a few microamperes—whereas diathermy heating might involve total currents of 0.5–1 A, although it is the current density (current per unit area) that matters.

The reason why large currents can be passed through the tissues if they are oscillating rapidly enough—i.e. have a high enough frequency—is that there is not enough time at each oscillation for nerve or muscle tissue to be affected. It will be recalled that excitable tissue is affected by altering the ionic balance across the membrane, as explained in Chapter 3. Currents need to pass for about 0.1 ms to stimulate a nerve with minimal current. Shorter current pulses will need higher currents. At the usual shortwave diathermy frequency of 27.12 MHz the current pulses would be less than 1/50th of a microsecond so that no effect on muscle or nerve can occur (Table 10.1).

PRODUCTION OF SHORTWAVE DIATHERMY

Since electromagnetic radiations are emitted in the radio and television bands certain specific frequencies have been allocated by international agreement for industrial, scientific and medical purposes to prevent interference with communications. These frequencies and their wavelengths are shown in Table 10.2. Of these the 27.12 MHz frequency is by far the most widely used because it has the widest frequency band; that is to say, the extent to which it is allowed to drift off the assigned frequency is much greater than the others. It would be more complex and expensive to achieve the required stability needed for the other two frequencies.

The source of the high-frequency current is an oscillator circuit, as described in Chapter 6, consisting of a capacitor and inductance whose dimensions are so arranged that they will allow electrons to oscillate at a frequency of exactly 27.12 MHz, the frequency of almost all shortwave machines. As explained in

Table 10.1 Effects of varying electric and magnetic fields on tissues

Electric field	Magnetic field
Direct current (constant unidirectional current; see Chapter 2)	*Steady magnetic field*
Causes continuous movement of ions	? No effect detected
→chemical changes in tissues	? Used in navigation
→tissue damage if more than a trivial current used	
No significant heating	
Therapeutically used for iontophoresis and effects of mild irritation	
Low-frequency varying current (currents with various pulse lengths and frequencies; see Chapter 3)	*Low-frequency varying magnetic field*
Causes nerve and muscle stimulation	Effects due to induced currents
No chemical changes if evenly alternating or very low intensity	? Therapeutic
No significant heating	
High-frequency currents (shortwave diathermy; see Chapter 10)	*High-frequency varying magnetic field*
Causes tissue heating due to large current because	Effects due to induced currents →heating
no nerve or muscle stimulation	
no chemical change	

Generate radiations
(radio waves)
No detectable effect on tissues

Note: High-frequency electron motion can cause microwaves and infrared radiations which cause heating when absorbed in the tissues; see Chapter 11. Some simplifications are made in this table—see later discussion on magnetic effects.

Table 10.2 Assigned frequencies and wavelengths

Frequency (MHz)	Wavelength (m)
13.56 ($\pm$ 6.25 kHz)	22.124
27.12 ($\pm$ 160 kHz)	11.062
40.68 ($\pm$ 20 kHz)	7.375

Chapter 6 the frequency (f) at which such a circuit will oscillate depends only on its electrical size, that is the product of capacity (C) and inductance (L): ($f = 1/(2\pi\sqrt{LC})$). In order to maintain the regular oscillation, electrical energy must be fed into the circuit in bursts at exactly the right moment in the cycle to make good the losses. Consider a simple pendulum. A regular change from potential to kinetic energy and from kinetic to potential energy occurs at a frequency determined by the length of the string (size of the system). If the pendulum is allowed to swing freely in air, the amplitude—but not frequency—of the oscillations will diminish due to friction until the pendulum eventually comes to rest. The oscillations are said to be damped and unsustained. The same happens in an electrical oscillating circuit. In order to maintain the amplitude of the 'swing', a 'push' must be given at the right time. This is achieved by means of an electronic switch—either a thermionic valve or a transistor—which is coupled to the circuit so that current is added in time with the oscillations (Fig. 10.1). Sometimes the circuit is in the form of a power oscillator in which the electrical oscillations are generated at the required power and frequency using a valve and a cavity (pot) resonator. This latter is an oscillating circuit whose large capacitance is provided by a metal box of precise dimensions enclosing the inductance. Such circuits are very stable oscillators and thus are less prone to cause interference to radio transmissions. The other common method involves the use of a transistor-controlled circuit often including a crystal for timing the frequency (see Chapter 6). This is a relatively low-power circuit and a separate amplifier circuit is used to increase the power to levels appropriate for therapy. Power is drawn from the mains with the voltage stepped up (to around 1000–2000 V) to operate the circuits.

The part to be treated is included in the 'patient' or resonator circuit which is coupled inductively to the oscillator circuit (Fig. 10.2). This involves a coil in each circuit being placed close together, forming a transformer, so that the magnetic field generated by the oscillator circuit induces a current in the resonator coil. Energy will be effectively transferred if the two circuits are in tune, i.e. have the same frequency. Since the frequency of both circuits is proportional to $1/(2\pi\sqrt{LC})$ it is only necessary to arrange it so that the product of capacity and inductance in one circuit is the same as the product of capacity and inductance in the other.

The capacity of the resonator circuit will vary because the tissues contribute to the capacity so a variable capacitor must be adjusted to bring the circuits into resonance. This tuning can either be done manually, using the excursion

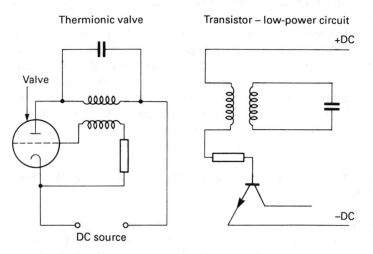

Fig. 10.1 Methods of boosting the oscillations.

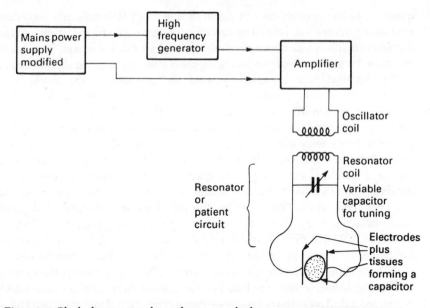

Fig. 10.2 Block diagram to show shortwave diathermy generation.

of a meter or brightness of a light to indicate maximum resonance, or automatically. In this latter case a motor drives the tuning capacitor and is itself regulated by the output from the resonator circuit. This automatic mechanism, another example of negative feedback, keeps the machine tuned even if the patient moves a little.

Once tuned, the heating of the tissues is controlled by regulating the output of the machine. This is done in different ways in different machines. Some vary the voltage to the oscillator circuit in a series of steps; others vary the coupling between the oscillator and patient's circuit, either by moving one of the coils or by moving a screen between the coils. In all cases the output is varied by a control on the machine marked 'intensity', 'output' or 'dose'.

The tissues may be coupled into the shortwave field in two ways: as part of the dielectric of a capacitor, as in Figure 10.2, or as part of the load of an inductance. In the first case the tissues are influenced by the oscillating electric field. This is called a 'condenser (capacitor) field method' or 'capacitive method'. In the second the tissues are subjected to an oscillating magnetic field which will induce oscillating currents in the tissues in the way described above (see Fig. 10.9). This is called inductothermy.

TRANSMISSION OF HIGH-FREQUENCY CURRENTS TO THE TISSUES

When the kind of low-frequency currents discussed in Chapter 3 are applied to the tissues it is necessary to apply conducting electrodes to the skin surface. Even with oscillations of about 1 MHz this method is still needed. Currents of megahertz frequencies heat the tissues they pass through and were used extensively by physiotherapists some 40 years ago and known as longwave diathermy, for the reasons given above. For higher frequencies, i.e. shortwave, the current can be passed through insulators as a displacement current and can thus be applied to the tissues with an air gap.

Effects of high-frequency currents on the tissues

The major effect of passing currents of sufficient intensity at frequencies above 1 MHz is to cause heating. The nature of heat was considered at some length in Chapter 7 and it will be recalled that heat is energy, basically the amount of random molecular and atomic motion in a material. Anything that increases the internal kinetic energy of matter causes heating, usually accompanied by a temperature rise in the material.

The tissues contain large numbers of ions, which are the charge carriers when a current flows in the tissues (convection current; see Chapters 2 and 3). If an electric field is applied first in one direction and then in the other the ions will be accelerated first one way then the opposite, colliding with adjacent molecules to give up some energy to them and so increasing the total random motion, that is heating. At the most commonly used therapeutic frequency of 27.12 MHz the movement is more of an oscillation about a mean position but the rapid acceleration affects nearby particles leading to significant heating (Fig. 10.3a).

The tissues are, of course, largely water. Water molecules behave rather differently because, although electrically neutral as a total molecule, they are polar, that is the ends of the molecule carry small opposite charges. Because of this they are sometimes called dipoles. When rapidly reversing charges are applied to polar molecules they will rotate to and fro (Fig. 10.3b). This rotational energy disrupts the motion of adjacent molecules causing more total random motion and hence heat.

Atoms and molecules which are not charged can also be affected by the rapidly oscillating electric field in that the paths of their orbiting electrons are distorted. As the electric field changes direction one side becomes more positive and the other more negative so the average position of the electron 'cloud' shifts, being attracted to the positive and repelled from the negative side (Fig. 10.3c). This does not cause motion of the molecule but the interaction with other neighbouring molecules leads to more random motion and therefore some heating. However, it must be appreciated that very little energy is converted to heat by this latter mechanism. As far as tissue heating is concerned it is the least important. Ionic movement is the most consequential as it is a very efficient converter of electrical energy to heat (Ward, 1986).

It follows from what has just been said that if high-frequency currents are applied through non-polar materials there will be little energy lost as heat. This explains why the plastic covers of the shortwave electrodes do not become hot; neither does the insulation of the wires, nor for that matter the air spacing between electrode and patient. The oscillating electrical force will

(a)

Ionic
motion

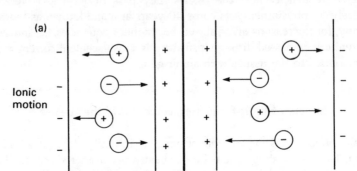

Positive and negative ions move to and fro under the
influence of an oscillating electric field.

(b)

Dipole
rotation

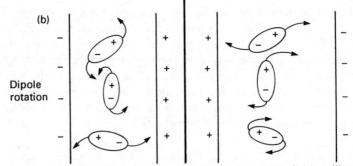

Polar molecules rotate to and fro as the electric field oscillates.

(c)

Electron
'cloud'
motion

'Molecular
distortion'

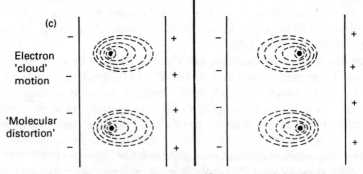

˙The paths of orbiting electrons are distorted first in one
direction then in the other as the electric field oscillates.

Fig. 10.3 The effects of oscillating high-frequency electric fields on the molecules and
ions of the tissues. (a) Ionic motion: positive and negative ions move to and fro under
the influence of an oscillating electric field. (b) Dipole rotation: polar molecules rotate
to and fro as the electric field oscillates. (c) Electron 'cloud' motion—molecular
distortion: the paths of orbiting electrons are distorted first in one direction then in the
other as the electric field oscillates.

readily pass through such insulators; the electron clouds distort to and fro in much the same way as electrons in a wire move to and fro at a low-frequency current, but of course with much less movement. As there are fewer collisions so there is little heating. Such currents are called displacement currents.

In summary: heat is generated in the tissues

1 Mainly by to and fro motion of ions—a high frequency convection current
2 To a lesser extent by dipole rotation—polar molecules rotating back and forth
3 Negligibly by electron cloud movement—molecular distortion.

PHYSIOLOGICAL EFFECTS AND THERAPEUTIC USES OF SHORTWAVE DIATHERMY

The therapeutic effects of continuous shortwave diathermy given at an intensity that causes detectable heating are usually considered to be solely due to the heating. The effects of heating and the therapeutic uses have already been considered in Chapter 7. The only difference to be considered when using shortwave diathermy is the site of heating in the tissues—the pattern of heating. A summary of the effects is given below.

Local tissue heating

Local tissue heating leads to a complex set of inter-related physiological responses, some of which are temperature-dependent physical changes (points 1–3 below), while others are physiological responses developed to protect the body from damage due to excess local heating (points 4 and 5 below). The direct effects are:

1 Increased metabolic activity of all cells.
2 Decreased viscosity of all fluids.
3 Increased extensibility of collagen.
4 Increased blood flow.
5 Effects on the nervous system.

Heating with shortwave diathermy can cause local temperature increases of a few degrees Celsius quite readily. Since the shortwave diathermy field is strongest in the superficial tissues heat is detected in the heat-sensitive nerve endings of the skin (see Chapter 7 and Table 7.4 for the physiological effects of temperature rise).

In summary, local heating with shortwave diathermy can be used to:

1 Accelerate the resolution of chronic inflammation.
2 Accelerate healing.
3 Relieve pain.
4 Reduce muscle spasm.
5 Increase the extensibility of fibrous tissue.
6 Control acute and chronic infection.

General effects

The local effects of heating cannot be isolated from the general effects which are concerned with maintaining a constant body temperature. As local heating occurs there is a constant loss of heat from the rest of the body. This is regulated by vasomotor adjustments under the control of the hypothalamus.

PRINCIPLES OF APPLICATION

To apply the capacitor field method either rigid metal plates enclosed in plastic or flexible metal sheets encased in thick rubber are used. The former are called rigid or plate electrodes or space plates and are positioned by means of supporting arms; the latter are flexible or malleable electrodes which can be positioned under the part to be treated with spacing provided by suitable material.

For inductothermy two methods are in use. A long tubular flexible conductor covered in thick rubber—called a cable or coil—can be plugged into the shortwave machine, providing an inductance in the patient's circuit. This may be wrapped around the part to be treated in a spiral manner or made into a flat helix—the so-called 'pancake' coil. The cable is separated from the skin by towel spacing. The varying magnetic field set up permeates the tissues inducing eddy currents. The second method involves a small flat metal coil enclosed in a plastic drum with a capacitor in parallel. This assemblage is called a monode. It produces a magnetic field and hence eddy currents like the hand-made coil.

While there is an undoubted distinction between the capacitative method and the electromagnetic inductive method it must be recognized that the application of any form of inductive coil, as well as causing heating due to magnetically induced eddy currents, has an electrostatic or capacitative field between each end, and indeed each turn, of the coil. In some configurations of the coil this appears to be the major method of heating (see Scott, 1965).

Heating pattern in the tissues—capacitor field method

Understanding and as far as possible controlling the distribution of the electric field of shortwave diathermy and hence the heating in the tissues is the central skill in the application of shortwave diathermy treatments. The electric field pattern, and hence the heating pattern, with various sizes, shapes and positions of electrodes relative to the tissues can be approximately predicted for homogeneous tissue. The tissues are, of course, far from homogeneous so that the field pattern is markedly altered by the nature and orientation of the tissue through which it passes. It was noted above, and illustrated in Figure 10.3, that a high-frequency alternating current would pass in the tissues as an oscillation of ions, a rotation of dipoles and electron 'cloud' distortion. The first depends on conduction whereas the others depend on the ease of polarization which is correlated with a property of insulators known as the dielectric constant. (The terms 'insulator' and 'dielectric' are often used for the same materials but it must be noted that they describe different properties. Insulation describes the resistance to current flow—the difficulty that charges encounter in moving through the material. The dielectric refers to the ease with which the effect of a charge can be passed through the material, i.e. the ease of polarization, measured by the dielectric constant.) The dielectric constant of air (and all other gases) is close to unity but substances that polarize strongly, such as pure water, have a high dielectric constant—water is 81.1. Most familiar insulators have low dielectric constants, e.g. polythene 2.3, oil 2.2, paper 3.7, mica 5.7, and glass approximately 9. See also Table 10.3 for the dielectric constants of some tissues.

If an electric field is applied across homogeneous material it will be uniform but if there is a boundary between materials with different dielectric constants and/or different conductivities the electric field is refracted at the boundary. This is much the same as the refraction that occurs when visible radiation (or any wave motion) passes from one medium to another.

In general, those tissues that have a high dielectric constant are good conductors, e.g. water and tissues with a high water content. The reverse is also evident; fat tissues have a low dielectric constant and low conductivity (Table 10.3). Notice that conductivity is the reciprocal of resistance, so when it is stated that fat has a low conductivity it is equivalent to asserting that it has a high electrical or ohmic resistance. Thus the electric field in the tissues tends to be refracted at various interfaces both at the surface and between various tissue layers. The overall effect is to spread the field within the tissues. For a fuller description and explanation of these factors see Ward (1986) and Guy (1982).

It will be obvious that the distribution of the electric field in the tissues will also depend on the size and position of the electrodes. Some simplified illustrations of the effects of different sizes and orientations of electrodes are shown in Figure 10.4. The shape of the tissues will also have an effect.

It is self-evident that for any given output of the shortwave source the larger the field the less energy is available per unit volume. Thus to provide

Table 10.3 Dielectric constants of some tissues

Tissue	Dielectric constant	Conductivity* $(\Omega m)^{-1}$
Skin, muscle and other tissues with high water content	113	0.6
Fat, bone and tissues with low water content	20	0.01–0.04

*Conductivity is the reciprocal of resistivity which has units of ohm-metre, so conductivity $\frac{1}{ohm.metre}$ or $(\Omega m)^{-1}$.

Dielectric constants and conductivities at 37°C with 27.12 MHz frequency. Modified from Guy (1982).

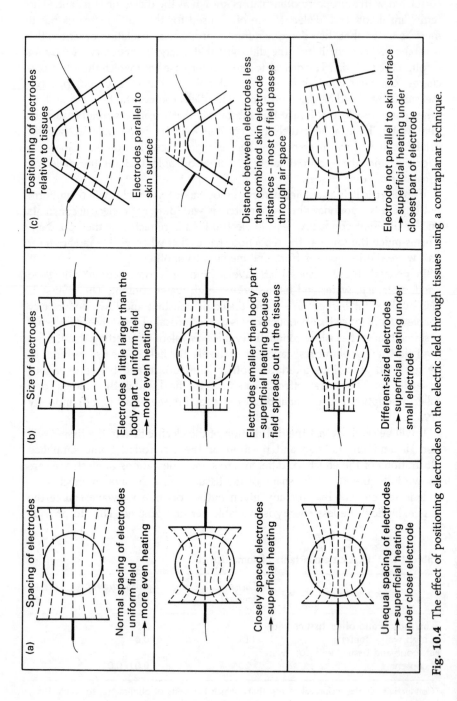

Fig. 10.4 The effect of positioning electrodes on the electric field through tissues using a contraplanar technique.

sufficient energy for heating in the tissues it is necessary to concentrate the field in the particular area to be treated. Equally it is important not to allow the field to be so concentrated as to produce excessive heating and hence damage. The following points should be considered in conjunction with Figure 10.4.

Spacing of electrodes

Within limits the widest possible spacing tends to lead to the most uniform field in the tissues. Close spacing leads to greater heating of the superficial tissues. The limits are set by the output of the machine and the size of the electrodes. In practical terms skin–electrode spacing of approximately 7 cm is about the most that will allow significant tissue heating with most machines. However, such large spacing will give greater dispersion of the field so that although it is more uniform, and thus the deeper tissues are *relatively* more heated, the losses are such that the deeper tissues can be less *absolutely* heated (Fig. 10.5). It has been suggested (Scott, 1957) that for most shortwave sources at maximum output, spacing of about 4 cm is the maximum that will give the greatest absolute heating of the deep tissues. Conversely, the minimum skin electrode distance is about 2 cm. As is evident from Figure 10.5 even the most uniform field will still generate more heat per unit area in the skin than in the deeper tissues. This ensures the safety of shortwave diathermy treatments since the skin is highly sensitive to temperature changes. Note that spacing refers to the distance of the metal electrode, not the plastic cover, from the skin.

Size of electrodes

It seems best to apply electrodes that are a little larger than the part to achieve

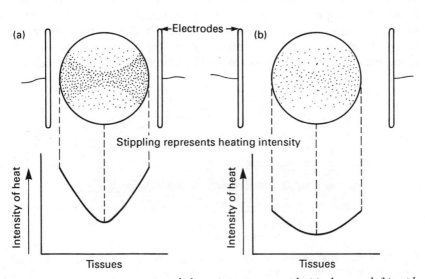

Fig. 10.5 Heating intensity (stippled area) in tissues with (a) close and (b) wide spacing.

a uniform electric field through the tissues. If one electrode is larger than the other the field tends to be concentrated on one side and dispersed on the other.

Positioning of electrodes relative to the tissues

When the electrodes are angled to each other with air between them the field tends to take the shortest pathway and passes largely between the nearest points. If a material of high conductivity, such as the tissues, is interposed the field will preferentially pass through the material which offers the least impedance. It is therefore important to position the electrodes parallel to the skin surface so that the skin–electrode distance is as constant as possible. Because of the low impedance of the tissues, if the electrodes are placed in the same plane, i.e. for coplanar treatments, then the field passes through the tissues and not through the air between the electrodes. However, if the distance between the electrodes is closer than the combined skin–electrode distances then the field will pass between the electrodes and not through the tissues.

Notice that close spacing of one electrode, uneven-sized electrodes and one electrode angled to the tissue surface all lead to much the same effect— superficial heating due to concentration of the field on one side.

Nature of the tissues and their relationship to one another

Much the most important factor affecting the pattern of the shortwave field through the body is the nature of the tissues and their relationship to one another. In circumstances where parallel paths are available, as in the coplanar treatment illustrated in Figure 10.6, the field passes predominantly through the tissues of high dielectric constant and conductivity—the water-filled tissues such as muscle and blood vessels. Thus when the shortwave field is passed through the long axis of a limb, as in Figure 10.8, there is marked heating in the vascular channels and muscle and negligible heating in the bone and fat. However, in order to reach these tissues the field must traverse the subcutaneous fat. It has been established that fatty tissue heats up much more

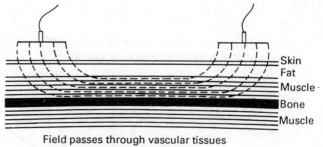

Field passes through vascular tissues
→ main heating in superficial muscle

Fig. 10.6 Coplanar technique. The electric field passes through vascular tissues, therefore the main heating is in the superficial muscle.

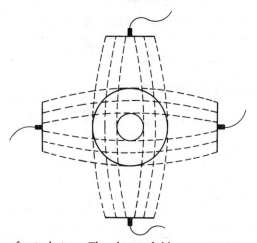

Fig. 10.7 Cross-fire technique. The electric field passes in tissues, avoiding the air-filled cavity. To heat walls fully, treat in one direction for half the treatment and in the other for the second half.

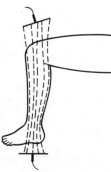

Fig. 10.8 Longitudinal application. The electric field concentrates in vascular channels and where the cross-sectional area is least, therefore there is greater heating in these areas.

than muscle tissue in the shortwave field (Schwan, 1965). This leads to most of the energy of shortwave treatments by those methods being absorbed in the subcutaneous fat, which is a considerable therapeutic disadvantage. The reason for this apparently anomalous behaviour is that fatty tissue consists of fat cells between which many vascular channels run; the field is concentrated into these narrow channels and this causes marked local heating (Scott, 1965; Ward, 1986).

Heating pattern in the tissues—inductothermy

Heating by inductothermy is due to eddy currents. The difference between inductothermy and the capacitor field method lies in the way energy is introduced into the tissues leading to a different pattern of heating. The

Electrotherapy explained

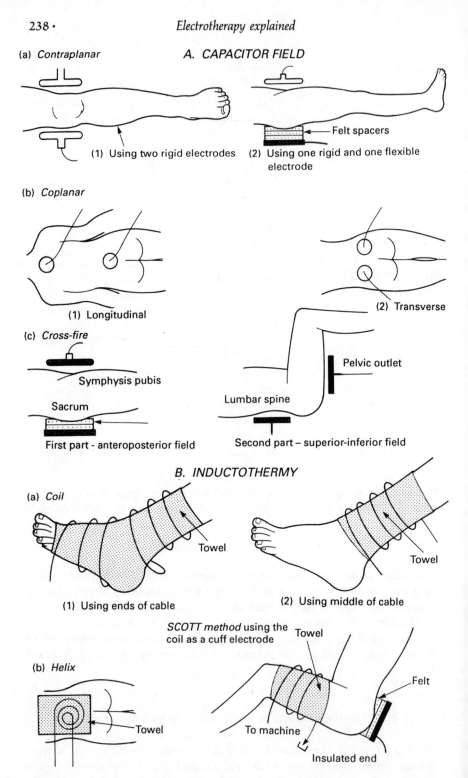

(a) *Contraplanar*   **A. CAPACITOR FIELD**

— Felt spacers

(1) Using two rigid electrodes   **(2)** Using one rigid and one flexible electrode

(b) *Coplanar*

(1) Longitudinal

(2) Transverse

(c) *Cross-fire*

Symphysis pubis

Pelvic outlet

Sacrum

Lumbar spine

First part - anteroposterior field   Second part – superior-inferior field

B. INDUCTOTHERMY

(a) *Coil*

Towel

Towel

(1) Using ends of cable   **(2)** Using middle of cable

SCOTT method using the coil as a cuff electrode   Towel

(b) *Helix*

Felt

— Towel

To machine

Insulated end

Fig. 10.9 Techniques of application of shortwave diathermy.

magnetic field can pass easily through the tissues. It is strongest close to the conductor and weakens as it spreads out. Therefore most of the heating occurs in the superficial tissues but not especially in fatty tissues as occurred in capacitative applications. The result is that proportionally more energy is absorbed in the superficial muscle underlying the fat and skin, hence more heating occurs in this region (Guy, 1982). However, in any configuration the cable will have some capacitative effects, i.e. an electric field, between different parts, especially between the two ends but also between each turn of the coil. These fields are quite important and account for much of the heating when shortwave is being applied with the cable (Ward, 1986). An electrostatic screen (called a faradic screen) can be used to eliminate the electric and leave only the magnetic field. When this is done experimentally, heating diminishes dramatically (Ward, 1986) showing that capacitative effects account for most of the heating. It has been recommended (Forster and Palastanga, 1985) that the ends of the cable would be preferred for treating high-impedance structures and the middle of the coil for superficial low-impedance tissues, e.g. muscle (Fig. 10.9).

In all these techniques the cable must be kept at a distance of 2–3 cm from the skin surface to give a sufficient spread of field. This is achieved partly by the rubber insulation of the cable and partly by applying the cable over a minimum of 1 cm thickness of towelling or other suitable material. The plastic casing of the drum electrode ensures suitable spacing but an additional air gap is also needed to achieve adequate-depth heating (Lehmann and de Lateur, 1982); 2 cm is an appropriate distance.

It is also important that adjacent turns of the coil are evenly separated from each other by insulating material to avoid overheating of the cable and spread the field. Wooden or perspex spacers are provided for this purpose.

Technique of application

1 The nature of the treatment should be explained to the patient.
2 The part to be treated should be adequately exposed. There are several reasons for this. Firstly, the area must be thoroughly examined for possible dangers and contraindications (see p. 242) prior to treatment and inspected afterwards. Secondly, clothes in the electric field can cause several problems:

   a They may be made of synthetic material or contain metal fastenings (see p. 243).
   b They may be damp or conceal dampness on the skin.
   c They may constrict circulation to the part.
   d They may obscure the field of vision for setting the skin–electrode distance correctly and for observing the visible effects of the heat.

3 Thermal sensation must be tested and recorded (see p. 200).
4 The part to be treated and indeed the whole patient must be supported in a

position that is safe, convenient and comfortable. Metal objects, synthetic materials and anything damp should be removed from the area of the field. Forster and Palastanga (1985) recommend a distance of at least 30 cm away from the electrodes. If the skin is damp it must be dried. Adequate support is particularly important if a manually tuned machine is used since any movement of the part disturbs the circuit tuning.

5 Traditionally the shortwave diathermy machine plus the electrodes to be used are tested by the physiotherapist prior to treatment. Apart from any safety considerations this has the added advantage of reassuring the patient, especially if it is a first treatment. This is normally done by placing one hand between the electrodes, with the usual air or felt spacing or winding the coil over towelling around one arm. The apparatus is then switched on and tuned and the output slowly increased until some heating is felt. A tuning indicator, usually a neon-filled tube, can also be used to demonstrate that tuning has occurred.

6 An appropriate method of treatment for the required effect is selected— capacitor field or inductothermy. The capacitor field method may be applied in different ways (Fig. 10.9):

   a *contraplanar*: electrodes are placed on opposite sides of the part, to treat deeply placed structures, e.g. joints.
   b *coplanar* (Fig. 10.6): electrodes are placed on the same side of the part to treat more superficial structures, e.g. the spinal musculature.
   c *cross-fire* (Fig. 10.7): half the treatment is given with the electrodes in one contraplanar position and for the second half the electrodes are repositioned at right angles. This technique is used for deeply placed organs in the pelvis and for air-filled cavities such as the frontal and maxillary sinuses.

   Additionally the type of electrodes are chosen—rigid or flexible— together with the appropriate size.
   The inductothermy cable can be arranged as:

   a a coil, wound round the circumference of a limb.
   b a helix, for a flat surface, e.g. the lumbar spine (Fig. 10.9) or incorporated in a monode.

   The electrodes are positioned relative to the tissues with appropriate spacing. Other parts of the body must be protected from the field set up from all aspects of the electrode and from the connecting leads. The leads must not be closer together than the terminals of the machine nor close to any conductor in which they could induce heating.

7 The patients must be given precise instructions about the degree of warmth that should be experienced and the warning that if it is hotter than is comfortable the physiotherapist should be notified immediately as failure to do so can result in a burn. They must also report where the heating is felt and any concentration of heat in one particular region. In

addition they should be instructed not to touch any part of the apparatus, not to move or fall asleep. The patient is the only source of knowledge of what heating is occurring so it is essential for the patient to understand and co-operate fully in order to regulate the heating.

8 The apparatus is then switched on, tuned and the heating adjusted to the appropriate intensity as indicated by the patient. As vasodilation takes place, heat is dissipated and the intensity may have to be increased. It is equally important not to turn the intensity too high before this has occurred.

9 If any pain or discomfort occurs during treatment the machine should be switched off at once. Pain could be due directly to the treatment, overheating or causing increased local oedema for example. It could also be due to the position of the patient. If the patient is left in the same position for a few minutes after the heat has been turned off, the pain will diminish or disappear only if heating is the cause.

10 At the end of treatment, which can last up to 30 min (Wadsworth and Chanmugan, 1980) the heating can be assessed to some extent by the presence and intensity of erythema on the skin and by palpating the skin and judging the increased surface temperature.

DOSAGE

If energy is added to the tissues faster than it is being dissipated the temperature must rise which causes vasodilation to increase heat removal until the heat gain and loss are once more in balance at a new, higher local temperature (see Chapter 7 and Fig. 10.10). It usually takes some 15–20 min for these vascular adjustments to occur and thus reach a steady state but it can be longer. This is the reason for applying such treatments for approximately or slightly longer than 20 min.

As the heating due to shortwave diathermy treatments can only be known from descriptions given by the patient, it is important to be able to communicate the amount of heating. Dosage can be described as shown in Table 10.4.

The therapeutic benefits of maximum tolerable heating must be weighed against the risks involved of tissue damage.

The term 'subthermal' or 'athermal' for imperceptible heating is best avoided as these words suggest that no local heating occurs because it cannot be felt.

It must be stressed that the perceptions of the patient are the only safe guide to the heating in the tissues. Similar energy inputs can lead to widely differing heat perceptions due principally to differences in blood flow (Scott, 1957).

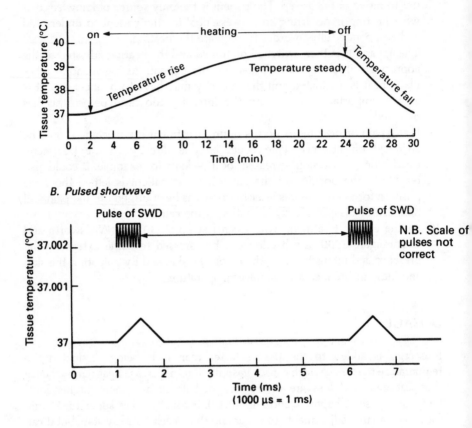

Fig. 10.10 (a) Continuous shortwave: as heat is added the local tissue temperature rises but at the same time the body's thermoregulatory system reacts, removing heat until a steady state is reached at a new higher temperature. (b) Pulsed shortwave: the small (negligible) temperature rise due to each impulse is dissipated during the pulse interval. *Note*: the different time and temperature scales of (a) and (b); pulse lengths and intervals are not to scale; the temperature changes shown in these figures are not based on actual measurements.

POTENTIAL DANGERS IN THE APPLICATION OF SHORTWAVE DIATHERMY

All the potential dangers inherent in any heat treatment must be taken into account (see Chapter 7).

In addition there are some specific considerations, as described below.

Table 10.4 Dosages of shortwave diathermy

Dosage	Description of heat to patient	Use
Maximum tolerable heating	As hot as you can bear	*With extreme caution* to increase extensibility of collagen fibres
Normal heating	Comfortable warmth	For chronic inflammation and long-standing conditions
Mild heating	Mild gentle warmth	↑
Minimal perceptible heating	So that you can only just feel the warmth	For acute conditions and where the effects of heating must be
Imperceptible heating	No feeling of warmth at all	carefully monitored

Burns

Burns can be due to:

1 The patient being unaware of the heat, defective thermal sensation or unconsciousness.
2 Concentration of the shortwave field happening so quickly that a burn occurs before the patient has time to react.

Concentration of the electric field

If there is a material of high dielectric constant/low impedance in the field, such as metal or moisture, this will concentrate the electric lines of force and a burn can result. All metals are relatively low-resistance conductors and even if enclosed in plastic, as in the armpieces of spectacles, will provide a low-impedance pathway. Similarly many pieces of metal are to be found in clothing, e.g. zip fasteners, hook-and-eyes, buckles, all of which can have the same effect. Whether significant field concentration will occur or not depends on the size, shape and orientation of the metal with respect to the field. A long slender pointed piece of metal like a key or silver propelling pencil with its long axis parallel to the lines of force of the field and touching the skin at its point would provide a conductor concentrating the current at the point of contact with the skin. Notice that although the metal itself would become warmed by the passage of the current it is where the metal touches the high-resistance skin that maximum heating, and hence the burn, will occur. Whether a burn occurs or not will depend on local field strength which is dependent on the output of the shortwave diathermy machine and to what extent the field is concentrated. Even something like an earring, although small, may cause burning because it has point contact with the tissues.

Metal implanted or accidently embedded in the tissues, such as fixation of fractures and metal arthroplasties, can lead to burning at the junction of the metal with the tissues for the reasons explained above. In these cases the patient would not feel any heat because there are no thermoreceptors in the tissues and the evidence of damage would be deep pain. Small round pieces of metal such as tooth fillings have little or no effect but large wire dental splints may be a risk, as are intrauterine contraceptive devices.

Water droplets on the skin, such as sweat or wet dressings, can also provide this low-resistance pathway and therefore carry the same risk.

Inadequate spacing of electrodes or leads so that they come in contact with the part, or uneven spacing so that one section of the skin–electrode distance is less than the rest will also cause concentration of the field.

Touching of the output cables by the patient or physiotherapist while the shortwave diathermy machine is in use at a high output setting can cause a severe burn caused by an electric arc breakdown through the cable insulation (Evaluation report, 1987).

Cardiac pacemakers

Another specific danger is to those patients who have cardiac pacemakers. These can be affected by all kinds of electromagnetic fields, transformers, electric razors; a number of cases due to shortwave diathermy have been reported (Jones, 1976). Demand-type (triggered) pacemakers can be affected and their rhythm altered or even stopped altogether. It is therefore important that patients with such pacemakers be kept away from shortwave diathermy machines.

Although not as critical, electronic hearing aids can be affected by the shortwave diathermy field.

Synthetic materials

These may have the following disadvantages (personal communication (AR) with UK Dept. of Health, Mann, 1989):

1 They do not absorb moisture as readily as natural materials.
2 They ignite more easily than natural materials and can produce large volumes of toxic fumes. (There have been a number of cases where shortwave electrodes or cables have overheated and caught fire.)
3 The material itself or any coating applied (e.g. for fire resistance) may alter the field either by absorbing energy or by concentrating the field. Contact lenses are safer removed if that region is being treated. Therefore such materials should not be in the shortwave diathermy field.

Distance from the shortwave diathermy machine

Delpizzo and Joyner (1987), quoting from the Canadian Department of Health and Welfare (DHW, 1983) state that the minimum distance that the operator should maintain from the shortwave diathermy machine is 1 m from the applicators and 0.5 m from the leads. Short excursions closer to the electrodes are permitted but only when necessary. These precautions are also recommended by the Australian National Health and Medical Research Council.

Obese patients

Because the subcutaneous fat layer is more easily heated than muscle (see p. 233) the power absorbed in the fat is almost eight times that absorbed in muscle (Delpizzo and Joyner, 1987). Capacitive electrodes should be avoided with obese patients (those who weigh 20% or more than normal body weight); a magnetic field output, e.g. a coil, is more suitable to produce deep tissue heating (Kloth *et al.*, 1984).

Pregnancy

A study of birth outcomes among physiotherapists in Sweden found a very slightly higher than normal incidence of stillborn or malformed infants born to those operating shortwave diathermy units (Kallen, 1982). Although no direct link has been found it is probably a wise precaution to avoid excessive exposure to shortwave diathermy during pregnancy and direct application to the area of the uterus.

Implanted slow-release hormone capsules

It is sensible to avoid treating the area where the capsule is implanted.

CONTRAINDICATIONS TO SHORTWAVE DIATHERMY

From the foregoing a list of conditions and circumstances in which the application of shortwave might be dangerous or damaging can be deduced.

1 Implanted pacemakers.
2 Metal in the tissues.
3 Metal on the surface of the tissues that cannot be removed, such as forms of external skeletal fixation or dental splints.
4 Impaired thermal sensation.
5 Patients unable to control their movements or whose co-operation cannot

be presumed, for example the very young or mentally unstable patients or those with uncontrolled movements due to disease.

6 The pregnant uterus.

7 Conditions in which haemorrhage is occurring or likely to occur. Any form of heat, by increasing the vasodilation and decreasing blood viscosity, might prolong haemorrhage but usually with other forms of heat this is confined to the surface. In the case of shortwave diathermy, heating can be induced in the deeper tissues so that enlarging haematomas or haemarthroses would be affected and therefore should not be treated. Similar concerns apply to treating the pelvis during menstruation.

8 Ischaemic tissues whose blood flow cannot be increased to dissipate heat and meet the demands of the increased metabolic activity. This would be most commonly found in the feet of patients with atheroma of the femoral and popliteal arteries. Heating ischaemic tissue is entirely inappropriate because it leads to increased demand on an already precarious circulation causing pain and possibly precipitating gangrene. Reflex heating of the proximal part, e.g. an inductothermy coil around the thigh, is safe and may have therapeutic value since it will provoke reflex vasodilation of the affected foot. However, this may only be moving a limited blood flow from one tissue to another and may have no long-term beneficial effect.

9 Malignant tumours should not be treated by any form of heat in case the increased metabolic rate leads to increased rates of growth or metastases. While this concept is much hallowed by repetition there does not seem to be clear supporting evidence for it. In fact for several years there have been trials using heat, including shortwave diathermy, to destroy tumour cells and thus halt growth. Heating alone has had limited clinical success but heating in combination with ionizing radiation or chemotherapy is apparently more promising (Oleson and Gerner, 1982). Similarly it is often recommended that possible precancerous tissues, such as those damaged by radiation therapy, should not be further stressed by heating since this might provoke malignant changes. Again, while it seems sensible to avoid heating damaged tissue there seems no direct evidence of carcinogenic effects.

10 Active tuberculous lesions should not be treated since heating may increase activity of the bacillus. Once again there seems to be no evidence on this matter but it certainly seems reasonable to avoid such lesions.

11 After venous thrombosis. Sites of recent thrombosis should be avoided in case heating loosens the clot leading to pulmonary embolism (Scott, 1957). When the vessel is fibrosed it is safe to treat.

12 While the patient is pyrexic any form of extensive heating should be avoided.

PULSED HIGH-FREQUENCY ELECTROMAGNETIC ENERGY—PULSED SHORTWAVE

The output of shortwave diathermy machines can be pulsed—applied in short bursts—in the same way as ultrasound (see Chapter 6). This modality is known, confusingly, by a profusion of slightly different names; well over 20 can be found! The first part of the title above is descriptive but lengthy; the second part is more widely understood. It has also been called 'pulsed electromagnetic field', 'pulsed high peak power electromagnetic energy', 'pulsed electromagnetic energy or PEME', 'pulsed shortwave diathermy', 'pulsed high-frequency current' and 'Diapulse'. This last, although a trade name, is widely used.

Development

In the early 1930s a doctor, Abraham Ginsberg, collaborated with a physicist, Arthur Milinowski, in some experimental work and developed a special shortwave therapy unit which was manufactured and called Diapulse. Gins-berg described this as an athermal shortwave apparatus. The Second World War interrupted development but in the 1950s the Diapulse Corporation began to market the machine. Reports on its clinical use and effectiveness began to appear over the next decade and by the mid 1970s other manufacturers were producing and marketing shortwave machines whose output could be pulsed.

Pulsed shortwave

Conventional shortwave apparatus generates a continuous output at 27.12 MHz, as described on p. 225, which produces heating in the tissues if applied at a suitable intensity. A typical paradigm is shown in Figure 10.10a. If the continuous oscillations are 'chopped up' into a series of very short bursts any trivial heating generated is dissipated during the long intervals between pulses, as illustrated in Figure 10.10b.

Production

Production of the oscillating high-frequency field for continuous shortwave diathermy has already been described on p. 225. By incorporating a timing circuit, the output can be turned on and off, allowing bursts of oscillations to be emitted for any length of time. Diapulse machines give 65 μs pulses but other machines give other pulse lengths and some allow a choice (Table 10.5). The rate at which the pulses are repeated, sometimes called pulse frequency, can also be varied and determines the pulse interval that is the pause between pulses. Each pulse is itself a series of oscillations. As the shortwave diathermy frequency is 27.12 MHz, in 1 s there are 27.12×10^6 cycles, and in 1 μs there are 27.12 cycles. A 65 μs pulse therefore contains 1762.8 oscillations. At 100 pulses per second each complete period lasts 10 000 μs (i.e. 10 ms). The first pulse would therefore be separated from the next by an interval of 9935 μs. This is illustrated in Figure 10.11. The duty cycle, i.e. the ratio of pulse length

Table 10.5 Examples of pulsed shortwave sources

Machine	Pulse width (μs)	Pulse frequency (Hz)	Method of altering intensity	Maximum output wattage	
				Peak power (W)	Mean power (W)
Diapulse	65	80, 120, 200, 300, 400, 500, 600	Six settings 1–6	975	38
Megapulse	20, 40, 65 100, 200, 400	100, 200, 400, 600, 800 also 1 in 3 and 2 in 3 intervals	No variation	500	160
Curapuls Ultramed	400	15, 20, 26, 35 46, 62, 82, 110, 150, 200	10 settings Continuously variable	1000	80

Diapulse: Diapulse Ltd., Diapulse International Sales Corp.
Megapulse: Electromedical Supplies (Greenham) Ltd.
Curapuls: Nomeq.
Ultramed: Bosch, Robert Bosch GmbH.

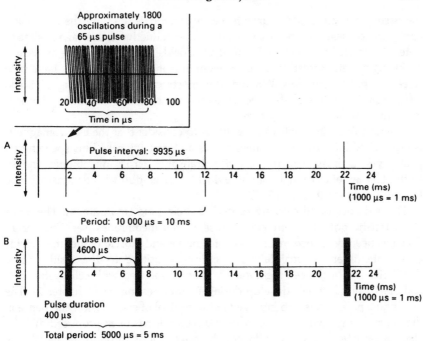

Fig. 10.11 Pulsed high-frequency oscillations. A = 65 μs pulses of 27.12 MHz oscillations repeated 100 times per second. Duty cycle = 0.65%. If peak power is 1000 W, mean power is 6.5 W. B = 400 μs pulses of 27.12 MHz oscillations repeated 200 times per second. Duty cycle = 8%. If peak power is 1000 W, mean power is 80 W. Inset: 1762.8 oscillations during a 65 μs pulse.

to total period, is in this case 0.65% and the mark space ratio is 1:152.9 (65:9935).

The energy introduced into the tissues can be varied in a similar way to that of a conventional shortwave source and is referred to as the intensity or output and measured in watts. There are two measures of power that can be considered: the power of each pulse—peak power or instantaneous power— which can be very high (975 W for Diapulse) and the average or mean power which is very much lower because of the pulse intervals, see Table 10.5. If the duty cycle for any given setting is known the average power is that proportion of the peak power (Fig. 10.11).

How pulsed shortwave is believed to work

It must be said that all explanations advanced to explain the mechanisms of pulsed shortwave are entirely speculative. In discussion of this issue a distinction is often made between the electric (capacitative) field, sometimes called the E field, and the magnetic field, sometimes called the H field. The electric field produces currents in the tissues which themselves cause magnetic fields and similarly, as already pointed out, the magnetic field passing through the tissues will cause eddy currents, i.e. an electric field. Using the coil in any configuration leads to both capacitative and inductive fields, again already noted. It is possible to eliminate the electric fields from a drum-type applicator by fitting a metal screen (a faradic screen) in front. Some machines have such screens, e.g. the Curapuls. Whether the effects caused by the magnetic field differ from those due to the electric field in the tissues is not known but it is thought to be important by some.

A simple but reasonable explanation is to consider that the electromagnetic energy 'stirs' ions, molecules, membranes and perhaps cells thus speeding up phagocytic activity, enzymic activity, transport across membranes and so forth. This would account for the evident acceleration of inflammatory and healing processes (Evans, 1980).

The activities of all cells are related to their ionic environment. There is a characteristic potential difference across all cell membranes (see Chapter 1). This has been described in Chapter 3 for nerve and muscle tissue; the outside of the membrane is maintained electrically positive to the inside. Some depolarization of the cell membrane is often associated with cell dysfunction and electrical potentials develop during wound healing (see Chapter 2). The membrane potential is also involved in the control of cell division and hence in the control of growth, development and repair. It has been proposed that the electromagnetic field could influence the flow of ions through the membrane and therefore restore the normal cell potential in some damaged cells: for discussion of this see Hayne (1984).

Some consider the pulsing to be an important feature; one of us has previously speculated on this (Low, 1978). As noted in Chapter 6, pulsed ultrasound has been shown to accelerate healing at different rates with different intensities and pulse lengths (Dyson and Pond, 1970). It is reasonable to suppose that both electromagnetic and mechanical pulsing have similar effects at a subcellular level, a piezoelectric link. Pieozelectric effects are known to occur in the tissues, for example, mechanical stress on bone leads to a redistribution of charges (Fukada and Yasuda, 1964). It is argued that the importance of pulsing may lie in the fact that brief pulses of high intensity will not necessarily have the same effect as an identical quantity of energy applied continuously. Compare the maximum peak power with the maximum mean power, shown in Table 10.5. An analogy might be drawn with hammering a nail into a piece of wood. Rapidly repeated gently tapping has no effect but the same total energy delivered as a few stout blows can drive the nail firmly into the wood. This suggests that there is a threshold which must be exceeded to produce an effect, and which is successful in brief bursts but could be excessive if uninterrupted.

The view of many, particularly in the USA, e.g. Lehmann and de Lateur (1982), is that there are no therapeutically specific effects due to pulsed shortwave. Beneficial effects are simply due to the recognized effects of very mild heating. A trial comparing continuous shortwave with pulsed electromagnetic energy (Wilson, 1974) on 20 matched pairs of patients with ankle sprains showed clearly superior results in those treated with pulsed energy. Unfortunately more total energy (22.5 W-h) was applied with continuous shortwave than with pulsed energy (15 W-h) which leads to the contention (Lehmann and de Lateur, 1982) that the greater total heating of continuous shortwave would be contraindicated for this acute condition. Thus the same results are subject to opposite interpretations. A pilot study comparing continuous with pulsed energy in the treatment of chronic low back pain (Wagstaff *et al.*, 1986) concluded that pulsed energy was more effective. There seems a dearth of other studies on this point but in any case it may be something of an otiose argument since heat is nothing other than random particle motion.

PHYSIOLOGICAL EFFECTS OF PULSED SHORTWAVE

There has been some research into the effects and efficacy of this therapy which can broadly be divided into experimental work in the laboratory and clinical research. Two main effects have been demonstrated in laboratory experiments, the acceleration of wound healing in animals (Cameron, 1961; Fenn, 1969) and the acceleration of nerve regeneration which has been convincingly demonstrated in rats (Wilson and Jagadeesh, 1976; Raji, 1984).

A number of careful, controlled clinical studies have demonstrated that various forms of pulsed shortwave will increase the rate of healing. Fifty boys undergoing orchidopexy were treated with pulsed energy or a dummy machine. The bruising and swelling of those receiving treatment were found to have resolved significantly faster (Bentall and Eckstein, 1975). A similar comparison of Diapulse with dummy machine was made of the healing rates of skin graft donor sites. Twice as many pulse energy-treated patients were healed in 7 days (Goldin *et al.*, 1981). Sprained ankles have been treated in at least three clinical trials. Twenty matched pairs of patients were treated, one of each pair with a dummy machine. After 3 days the treated patients were found to have less pain and disability (Wilson, 1972). Another trial on a much larger number of patients attempted to compare different machines—Diapulse and Curapuls—with a placebo and found some slight benefit from both sources but not as dramatic an effect as Wilson had found (Pasila *et al.*, 1978). A third study (McGill, 1989) of 37 patients (19 treated, 18 controls) found no significant difference between them (see discussion of these studies below). Various hand injuries have been successfully treated in a trial involving 230 patients (Barclay *et al.*, 1983) in which very significant reductions in swelling, disability and pain were found during the first 7 days. (This study has been criticized because there was no placebo treatment for the control group.) Increased rates of healing have also been claimed as a result of pulsed energy treatment after dental surgery (Aronofsky, 1971). As might be expected it has also been used in the treatment of sports injuries (Wright, 1973) and for chronic back pain (Wagstaff *et al.*, 1986).

In summary, the main effects of pulsed shortwave include:

1 An increase in the number and activity of cells in the injured region.
2 Reabsorption of haematoma.

3 Reduced inflammation.
4 Reduced swelling.
5 Increased rate of fibrin deposition and orientation.
6 Increased collagen deposition and organization.
7 Increased nerve growth and repair.

THERAPEUTIC USES

It seems that pulsed shortwave is an effective treatment for all tissue trauma, both accidental and postoperative, especially during the early stages, for up to about a week. Thus all recent injuries, such as the hand injuries and sprained ankles already noted, as well as acute traumatic synovites and haematomas could be treated.

Acute infections, such as paranasal sinusitis, as well as subacute and chronic infections which it has been claimed will benefit, are also suitable for treatment. From the experimental evidence quoted above there seems to be a reasonable case for the early treatment of peripheral nerve lesions. Pain due to a variety of conditions including degenerative arthritis and neurogenic pain (phantom limb pain, causalgia, Sudeck's atrophy etc.) and pain due to osteoporosis (Wilson, 1981) seem to improve, sometimes dramatically, with this treatment.

APPLICATION OF PULSED SHORTWAVE

Pulsed shortwave can be applied to the body tissues in the same way as conventional shortwave (Fig. 10.9) but several machines, e.g. Diapulse and Megapulse, limit the method of application to a drum-type electrode consisting of a flat helical metal coil contained in a plastic casing (Oliver, 1984). The pattern of effects in the tissues would be the same as described for heating the tissues with continuous shortwave. Thus one would expect the drum-type electrode to cause effects principally in the skin and superficial muscle tissues, having weaker effects as it spreads deeper and further into the tissues.

The patient is placed in a comfortable, supported position and the nature of the treatment explained. The drum-type electrode is placed close to, or just touching the skin over the area to be treated. The parameters of treatment which can be adjusted are selected and set and the machine is tuned, unless it is automatic.

DOSAGE

There is little evidence and even less agreement concerning the treatment parameters that should be used. The guidelines given in Table 10.6 have been recommended

Hayne (1984) suggested that one could compare the energy for different

Table 10.6 Suggested doses for pulsed shortwave

Source	Condition	Pulse width (μs)	Pulse frequency (pps)	Time (min)	Frequency of treatment
Hayne (1984)	Acute/superficial lesions	65	100–200	15	2–3 times daily
	Pain relief	65	200–300	20	Not stated
	Subacute/chronic and deep-seated lesions	65	300–400	Not stated	Not stated
Low (1988)	Acute conditions	40–65	400–600	20	3 times daily
				60	Once daily
	Pain relief	65	100–200	10–20	Once or twice daily
	Chronic conditions	400	400–600	30–60	Once daily
Megapulse instruction manual	Acute conditions	*Average power range* 0.25–3 W		10–20 depending on depth and area	Twice daily if possible
	Subacute (resolving) conditions	3–6.5 W			
	Chronic conditions	7.5 W +			
Curapuls instruction manual	Recent-onset	Intensity (pulse power): Almost always at maximum — Circuplode–8, Flexiplode–7	*Pulse frequency (pps)* Low, e.g. 46	10–15	Once or twice daily
	Later stages	Condenser electrodes–10. For extremely acute disorders select a lower intensity	Higher, e.g. 110		Three times a week

combinations of pulse widths and repetition rates by calculating the number of cycles of high-frequency energy for each. An alternative way of expressing the output is the average power in watts for each setting.

Others believe that short treatment times of 5–10 min are effective for all conditions. While an open mind must be kept on the matter, the evidence does seem to suggest that longer treatment times with high pulse repetition rates and short pulses are most effective. This is illustrated by the three studies on sprained ankles mentioned above:

1 Wilson (1972) treated for 1 h/day with 600 pulses/s, 38 W mean power, which led to a good result. After 3 days the treated group had improved about twice as much as the controls.
2 Pasila *et al.* (1978) gave 20-min treatments at 38 W mean power which led to the treated ankles doing marginally better than the controls.
3 McGill (1989) gave 15 min of 19.6 W with no significant difference between treated and control groups.

CONTRAINDICATIONS

Unlike continuous shortwave there is no significant heating with the low average power applied by the very short pulses so that there is no danger of a burn due to concentration of the field by metal or water; thus pulsed shortwave can be applied through wet dressings and in the presence of metal implants. However, it is important to realize that the treatment is relatively, not absolutely, athermic so that longer pulses given at higher frequencies can lead to heating and hence burning. Pulses of 100 μs or less at a few hundred hertz could not possibly produce significant heating.

There have been no damaging effects of any kind reported to date with pulsed shortwave. However, due to the unknown mode of action discussed above it is considered prudent to avoid rapidly dividing tissues, such as the fetus or the uncontrolled growth of precancerous tissues or neoplasms. Similarly the theoretical risk of reactivating encapsulated lesions suggests that tuberculosis should be avoided. It is recommended that seriously hyperpyrexic patients should not be treated.

As cardiac pacemakers could certainly be affected in the same way as described for continuous shortwave such patients should be kept clear of pulsed shortwave sources, although there seem to have been no injuries reported. Hearing aids and other electronic equipment, such as some modern telephones, can be affected and although not dangerous to the patient can be inconvenient.

LOW-POWER PULSED HIGH-FREQUENCY ENERGY

A number of devices are available which generate pulses similar to those just described but at a tiny fraction of the power. The Fel apparatus which was devised by a French physicist and the Therafield Beta and Q pulse are examples. They produce pulses of 27.12 MHz oscillations at various repeat rates but with about 0.5 W average power and 15 W peak power. There are some reports of their effectiveness in treating a variety of conditions, e.g. Debelle *et al.* (1977). These results were not substantiated in a rigorous controlled trial by Barker *et al.* (1985) involving ligament sprains.

Oedema and bruising were found to be less on the treated side during a controlled study of recovery after bilateral blepharoplasty (Nicolle and Bentall, 1982). All these sources apply energy to the tissues by means of an induction coil aerial placed on the surface of the skin. It has been claimed that the proximity to the tissues compensated for their low output. (For the blepharoplasty study the aerials were fashioned into spectacle frames worn over the dressings.) There are several reports of these low-power pulses being used successfully to encourage healing of skin wounds: it is possible to speculate that insufficient energy is reaching deeper structures to have any therapeutic effect.

Methods of application vary but usually the small induction coil is held in contact with the skin over the lesion by a bandage or Velcro strap. Length of treatment times suggested also vary a good deal but are often quite long, 1–2 h or even up to 6 h/day. The small battery-operated devices have been used for 16 h each day.

THE USE OF MAGNETISM IN THERAPY

It has already been explained that magnetic forces are an inevitable consequence of the movement of charges so that any electric current produces a corresponding magnetic field. Having discussed high-frequency electromagnetic energy in this chapter it seems appropriate to give a brief account of the use of static and low-frequency therapies.

There is no certainty about the way in which magnetic fields react with living tissue. As has already been noted, tissues are largely transparent to a magnetic field but varying fields will induce currents in any conductors, including the tissues, that they cross. Further, the living tissues contain many moving charges due to blood or lymph flow, cell movement, nerve impulses and so forth, which could interact with any magnetic field so that the concept of a static magnetic field is too simple.

It must also be recognized that all life forms occur in a permanent magnetic field—the earth's magnetic field—which varies from place to place and has other varying (mainly man-made) magnetic fields superimposed; see later discussion on this topic.

The inexplicable forces due to ferromagnetism have provided powerful suggestions of healing properties. Thus early in the 16th century Theophrastus Bombastus Paracelsus von Honenheim had apparently used iron rodlets to 'heal fractures and ruptures, pull hepatitis out, and draw back dropsy' among other wonders (quoted by Cameron, 1983). Later Mesmer used iron magnets for treatment and ever since there have been therapies based on some form of permanent magnet.

Static magnetic fields

The most recent form of these therapies is based on the fact that modern permanent magnets are much more powerful than earlier magnets. They are alloys of cobalt, nickel and various rare earths such as yttrium, that can be up to 15 times the magnetic strength of the older steel magnets. In one therapy, called biomagnetism, small (1.5 mm) magnets are stuck on the skin in the centre of an adhesive patch about 2 cm across, often over a trigger point. Biomagnetism is also called Taiki therapy and various other sizes of magnet are used. It is claimed to be effective in a variety of vaguely specified conditions (Holzapfel *et al.*, 1981) but there appears to be no definitive evidence.

Static magnetic fields are also provided by a flexible material containing magnetic strips of alternating polarity and covered with a thin metal foil. These are bandaged or stuck to the skin over the lesion to be treated and left in place continuously, but not for more than 1 week. The local magnetic fields provided by this material are said to be relatively large (Hayne, 1984). Various other versions of this material giving a static magnetic field have been developed with different configurations of the permanent magnets, e.g. Bioflex, a circular alternating polarity magnetic foil which can be used as a pad or a tunnel.

The mode of action of static magnetic fields is said to be similar to pulsed shortwave, only much slower because the tiny induced electric currents must reach a threshold before any biological process is affected (Hayne, 1989). The main therapeutic uses are said to be for circulation, analgesia and wound healing.

Low-frequency magnetic fields

A relatively powerful magnetic field set up in a large coil into which the part can be placed is provided by some machines, the Magnetron and Vitapulse for example. This field is oscillated, changing direction at various frequencies up to 50 Hz. Other pulsed devices use higher pulsing frequencies but much weaker magnetic fields and are placed in contact with the part to be treated. There is no objective evidence that clearly supports the therapeutic value of these therapies for many of the conditions for which they are recommended. However, there is evidence of the efficacy of pulsing low-frequency electro-magnetic fields in the treatment of ununited fractures (Bassett *et al.*, 1982) and Perthes' disease (Harrison and Bassett, 1984).

EFFECTS AND SAFETY OF ELECTROMAGNETIC FIELDS

For many years there has been concern that electromagnetic radiations might constitute a health hazard in some way. This has been engendered by the realization that exposure to all kinds of electromagnetic radiations has greatly increased over the whole world during the past hundred years or so. The basic argument is that up to this time living organisms had been exposed to natural background electric and magnetic forces over millions of years and would have evolved to tolerate and perhaps benefit from these forces. Suddenly over a few decades much greater electric and magnetic forces became a part of the environment. This is especially so close to high-voltage electric power transmission lines where the average magnetic field is somewhat higher than the average static earth magnetic field of about 0.5 gauss; the electric field close to the highest voltage lines can be 7–8 times greater than the typical natural field (Dowson, 1989). Radio waves at higher frequencies and microwaves at still higher frequencies also contribute, as do domestic appliances.

There have been a number of studies to establish whether there is any correlation between electromagnetic exposure and disease; in the main low-frequency electromagnetic energy has been considered because this would make by far the largest contribution to electromagnetic 'pollution'—if it is pollution. These studies can be classified into four groups:

1 Studies in the laboratory on animals and cell cultures exposed to controlled, artificially produced electromagnetic fields.
2 Similar studies of humans exposed to controlled electromagnetic fields.
3 Epidemiological studies of human populations exposed to electromagnetic fields, for example those living near power transmission lines.
4 Epidemiological studies of specific groups of people who are exposed to electromagnetic fields, e.g. in the electricity industry.

In the latter two groups several detailed studies have investigated the incidence of various cancers, especially in children, to ascertain whether there was an increase among those exposed to the higher electromagnetic fields. Some found no effect while others found a slight but significant correlation between disease and exposure to strong electromagnetic radiations. (For a further account see Dowson, 1989.) Some studies found increased risk of malignant disease among electrical workers, e.g. Milham (1982).

Suggestions have been made that exposure to strong electromagnetic fields might be associated with depression. In a study of patients committing suicide, no association was found between the relation of power lines to their place of residence (Reichmanis *et al.*, 1979). However, a later re-evaluation of the data measuring the electromagnetic fields found a significant relationship (Perry *et al.*, 1981). A study of workers at a Russian high-voltage electricity substation (Asanova and Rakov, 1966) found dysfunction of the (in particular, autonomic) nervous system associated with rather generalized complaints of headaches, insomnia, sluggishness, fatigue and other complaints in a high proportion of workers. This and other studies led to strict regulations concerning exposure of people to electromagnetic fields in the USSR. These are still the most restrictive in the world. This evidence has not been confirmed, although a recent study (Dowson and Lewith, 1988) found an association between recurrent headache and radiations from overhead high-voltage cables, especially at a particular distance of 60–80 m.

Numerous experiments have been done, mostly at low frequency, to define the effects of electric and magnetic fields on cells, tissues, organs, systems and even behaviour, in animals and humans. There is evidence for effects on the central nervous system, on fat and calcium metabolism and on circadian rhythm in humans and animals from electromagnetic fields of various strengths and frequencies amongst numerous others. For an extensive review see Sheppard and Eisenbud (1977); an earlier review and discussion by Presman (1970) or more recently, Becker and Marino (1982). Although much of these data are contradictory and confused it can be firmly stated that relatively weak electric and magnetic fields are able to evoke many neuro-physiological effects. It is repeatedly suggested by these experiments that electromagnetic energy has a communicating and controlling influence on biological systems when applied at low intensities, which is lost at higher intensities. Suggested mechanisms include causing conformational changes in molecules of cell walls and the stimulation of adrenocortical responses to stress.

In summary, at the present time there is no certain evidence of significant health damage from artificial electromagnetic fields. The beneficial effects of low-intensity fields are difficult to quantify. It is agreed by all that more research is urgently needed in this area.

REFERENCES

Aronofsky D. H. (1971). Reduction of dental post-surgical symptoms using non-thermal pulsed high-peak-power electromagnetic energy. *Oral Surg.*, **32**, 688.

Asanova T. P., Rakov A. I. (1966). *The State of Health of Persons Working in Electric Field of Outdoor 400 and 500 kV Switchyards. Hygiene of Labor and Professional Diseases 5.* Translation in special publication 10. Piscataway, NJ: IEEE Power Engineering Society.

Baker R. R. (1981). *Human Navigation and the Sixth Sense.* London: Hodder & Stoughton.

Barclay V., Collier R. J., Jones A. (1983). Treatment of various hand injuries by pulsed electromagnetic energy (Diapulse). *Physiotherapy*, **69**, 186–8.

Barker A. T., Barlow P. S., Porter J. *et al.* (1985). A double-blind clinical trial of low power pulsed shortwave therapy in the treatment of soft-tissue injury. *Physiotherapy*, **71**, 500–4.

Bassett C. A. L., Mitchell S. N., Gaston S. R. (1982). Pulsing electromagnetic field treatment in ununited fractures and failed arthrodeses. *J. Am. Med. Assoc.*, **247**, 623.

Becker R. O., Marino A. A. (1982). *Electromagnetism and Life.* New York: State University of New York Press.

Bentall R. H. C., Eckstein H. B. (1975). A trial involving the use of pulse electromagnetic therapy on children undergoing orchidopexy. *Kinderchirugie*, **17**, 380–2.

Cameron B. (1961). Experimental acceleration of wound healing. *Am. J. Orthop.*, **53**, 336–43.

Cameron H. U. (1983). Electromagnetic therapy: fact or fiction. *Mod. Med. N.Z.*, **16**, 17.

Debelle M., Lorthier J., Berghmans M. *et al.* (1977). Therapeutic effect of very low powered hertzian wave transmissions. *Brux-Med.*, **57**, 551–63.

Delpizzo V., Joyner K. H. (1987). On the safe use of microwave and shortwave diathermy units. *Aust. J. Physiother.*, **33**, 152–62.

DHW (1983). *Safety Code 25—Shortwave Diathermy Guidelines for Limited Radio-frequency Exposure.* Canadian Department of Health and Welfare, 83-EHD-98.

Dowson D. I. (1989). A review of epidemiological studies into the health effects of electromagnetic fields. *Compl. Hlth Res.,* **3,** 25–9.

Dowson D. I., Lewith G. I. (1988). Overhead high voltage cables and recurrent headaches and depression. *Practitioner,* **232,** 435–6.

Dyson M., Pond J. B. (1970). The effect of pulsed ultrasound on tissue regeneration. *Physiotherapy,* **56,** 136–42.

Evaluation Report: Shortwave Therapy Units (1987). *J. Med. Eng. Technol.,* **11,** 285–98.

Evans A. (1980). The healing process at cellular level: a review. *Physiotherapy,* **66,** 256–8.

Fenn J. E. (1969). Effects of pulsed electromagnetic energy (Diapulse) on experimental haematomas. *Can. Med. Assoc. J.,* **100,** 251–4.

Forster A., Palastanga N. (1985). *Clayton's Electrotherapy: Theory and Practice.* London: Baillière Tindall.

Fukada E., Yasuda I. (1964). Piezoelectric effects in cartilage. *Jpn. J. Appl. Physiol.,* **3,** 117–21.

Goldin J. H., Broadbent N. R. T., Nancarrow J. D., Marshall T. (1981). The effects of Diapulse on the healing of wounds: a double-blind randomised controlled trial in man. *Br. J. Plast. Surg.,* **14,** 267–70.

Guy A. W. (1982). Biophysics of high frequency currents and electromagnetic radiation. In *Therapeutic Heat and Cold* (Lehmann J. F., ed.) Baltimore: Williams & Wilkins, pp. 199–277.

Harrison M. J. M., Bassett C. A. L. (1984). Use of pulsed electromagnetic fields in Perthes disease: report of a pilot study. *J. Paed. Orthop.,* **4,** 579–84.

Hayne C. R. (1984). Pulsed high frequency energy—its place in physiotherapy. *Physiotherapy,* **70,** 459–66.

Hayne C. (1989). The healing fields. *Ther. Weekly,* March 16.

Holzapfel E., Crepon P., Philippe C. (1981). *Magnet Therapy.* Wellingborough: Thorsons.

Jones S. L. (1976). Electromagnetic field interference and cardiac pacemakers. *Phys. Ther.,* **56,** 1013–18.

Kallen B., Malmquist G., Moritz U. (1982). Delivery outcome among physiotherapists in Sweden. Is non-ionizing radiation a fetal hazard? *Arch. Environ. Hlth,* **37,** 81–4.

Kloth L., Morrison M. A., Ferguson B. H. (1984). *Therapeutic Microwave and Shortwave Diathermy.* HHS Publication FDA, 85-8237. US Dept. of Health and Human Services.

Lehmann J. F., de Lateur B. J. (1982). Therapeutic heat. In *Therapeutic Heat and Cold* (Lehmann J. F., ed.) Baltimore: Williams & Wilkins, pp. 404–562.

Low J. L. (1978). The nature and effects of pulsed electromagnetic radiations. *N.Z. J. Physiother.,* **6**(4), 18–22.

Low J. L. (1988). Shortwave diathermy, microwave, ultrasound and interferential therapy. In *Pain: Management and Control in Physiotherapy* (Wells P. E., Frampton V., Bowsher D., eds.) London: Heinemann, pp. 113–68.

Mann J. (1989) Department of Health Procurement Directorate, London.

McGill S. N. (1989). The effect of pulsed shortwave therapy on lateral ligament sprain of the ankle. *N.Z. J. Physiother.,* **16,** 21–4.

Milham S. (1982). Mortality from leukaemia in workers exposed to electrical and magnetic fields. *N.Z. J. Med.,* **307,** 249.

Nicolle F. V., Bentall R. A. C. (1982). Use of radio-frequency pulsed energy in the control of post-operative reaction in blepharoplasty. *Aesth. Plast. Surg.,* **6,** 169–71.

Oleson J. R., Gerner E. W. (1982). Hyperthermia in the treatment of malignancies. In *Therapeutic Heat and Cold* (Lehmann J. F., ed.) Baltimore: Williams & Wilkins, pp. 603–35.

Oliver D. E. (1984). Pulsed electro-magnetic energy—what is it? *Physiotherapy,* **70,** 458–9.

Pasila M., Visuri T., Sundholm A. (1978). Pulsating shortwave diathermy: value in treatment of recent ankle and foot sprains. *Arch. Phys. Med. Rehab.*, **59**, 283–6.

Perry F. S., Reichmanis M., Marino A. A., Becker R. O. (1981). Environmental power frequency magnetic fields and suicide. *Hlth Phys.*, **41**, 267–77.

Presman A. S. (1970). *Electromagnetic Fields and Life*. New York: Plenum Press.

Raji A. M. (1984). An experimental study of the effects of pulsed electromagnetic field (Diapulse) on nerve repair. *J. Hand Surg.*, **9B**, 105–11.

Reichmanis M., Perry F. S., Marino A. A., Becker R. O. (1979). Relation between suicide and the electromagnetic field of overhead power lines. *Physiol. Chem. Phys.*, **11**, 395–403.

Schwan H. P. (1965). Biophysics of diathermy. In *Therapeutic Heat and Cold* (Licht S., ed.) Baltimore: Waverly Press.

Scott, B. O. (1957). *The Principles and Practice of Diathermy*. London: Heinemann Medical Books.

Scott B. O. (1965). Shortwave diathermy. In *Therapeutic Heat and Cold* (Licht S., ed.) Baltimore, Maryland: Waverly Press Incorporated.

Sheppard A. R., Eisenbud M. (1977). *Biological Effects of Electric and Magnetic Fields of Extremely Low Frequency*. New York: New York University Press.

Wadsworth H., Chanmugan A. P. P. (1980). *Electrophysical Agents in Physiotherapy*. Marricksville, NSW, Australia: Science Press.

Wagstaff P., Wagstaff S., Downey M. (1986). A pilot study to compare the efficacy of continuous and pulsed magnetic energy (shortwave diathermy) on the relief of low back pain. *Physiotherapy*, **72**, 563–6.

Ward A. R. (1986). *Electricity Fields and Waves in Therapy*. Marrickville, NSW: Science Press.

Wilson D. H. (1972). Treatment of soft tissue injuries by pulsed electrical energy. *Br. Med. J.*, **2**, 269–70.

Wilson D. H. (1974). Comparison of shortwave diathermy and pulsed electromagnetic energy in treatment of soft tissue injuries. *Physiotherapy*, **60**, 309–10.

Wilson D. H. (1981). PEME: the new beam for fractures. *World Med.*, 97–8.

Wilson D. H., Jagadeesh P. (1976). Experimental regeneration in peripheral nerves and the spinal cord in laboratory animals exposed to a pulsed electromagnetic field. In *Proceedings of the Annual Scientific Meeting of the International Medical Society of Paraplegia. Part III: Paraplegia.* pp. 12–20.

Wright G. G. (1973). Treatment of soft tissue and ligamentous injuries in professional footballers. *Physiotherapy*, **59**, 385–7.

11.

Electromagnetic radiation

NATURE

As described in Chapter 10, apart from the weak and strong nuclear forces which hold the nuclei of atoms together, the only other fundamental interactions in the universe are gravity and the various aspects of electromagnetism. It is electromagnetism that is responsible for the structure, behaviour and chemical properties of the atom, and for electromagnetic radiations. Electromagnetism can be considered to have three aspects: electrostatic, magnetic and radiation (see Chapter 10).

Electromagnetic radiations are waves in the sense that they consist of regular sinusoidal variations of an electric and a magnetic field at right angles to one another. They are similar to sound and ultrasonic waves, considered in Chapter 6, in that they exhibit the features of energy transmission by any wave motion, but they differ from sonic waves in two important respects. Firstly, the wave is a variation in the strength of electric (and magnetic) fields and is thus independent of the atoms and molecules through which it passes, although it may give energy to them. Sonic waves on the other hand are variations in the position (e.g. compression) of the atoms and molecules of the material through which the wave passes (see Chapter 6). Secondly, electromagnetic waves are transverse waves, that is the variation occurs at right angles to the direction of travel. This is unlike the compressions and rarefactions of sonic waves which are longitudinal, i.e. in the direction of travel of the wave.

All electromagnetic waves have a constant velocity in space. When no matter is present they travel at a speed of 300 000 000 m/s (3×10^8 m/s) in a straight line—to be strictly accurate 2.9979×10^8 m/s. When radiations pass through matter the velocity is decreased somewhat but for most of the radiations the effect of air is trivial.

As these waves are simply regular variations in intensity of the electric and magnetic fields they can be described in terms of the number of times in each second they repeat that change, that is the frequency in hertz (Hz). Similarly, the distance between any point of the wave and the place where that point is repeated, say crest to crest, can be described as the wavelength, in units of length such as metres, millimetres or nanometres. The waves vary sinusoidally with both time and distance. This can be understood by considering the familiar experience of standing knee-deep in the sea. A photograph taken looking out to sea would show a series of waves spaced apart, that is the height of the surface of the sea varies with distance at a single instant of time. The cold seawater regularly falling to the ankles and rising, breathtakingly, up the thighs makes the observer vividly aware of the variation over time in one place.

These three factors, the velocity, the wavelength and the frequency are inter-related in that the speed of movement of the wave in one direction, the velocity (v) depends on both the wavelength (λ) and the frequency (f): $v = f\lambda$. This relationship is obvious when it is realized that the speed of travel of any cyclical motion depends on the length of the cycle and the number of repetitions per unit time. Consider a 5-year-old boy walking hand in hand with his father; both travel at the same velocity, covering the same distance in the same time; the boy takes many small steps (of high frequency, short length) while the father takes fewer longer strides (of low frequency, large length).

In spite of their constant velocity, electromagnetic radiations, differing only in wavelength and frequency, have very different interactions with matter and are therefore recognized in totally different ways. The list or spectrum of radiations, shown in the Frontispiece, extends from those with the longest wavelengths and lowest frequencies to those with the tiniest wavelengths and enormous frequency. They include radio waves, microwaves, infrared radiations, visible and ultraviolet radiations, X-rays, gamma and cosmic rays. The small range of radiations which are able to stimulate the retinal cells of the eye are recognized as visible light and so are by far the most familiar and best studied. In fact, much of the behaviour of electromagnetic radiations is understood and illustrated by reference to experiments done with light. Table 11.1 shows the electromagnetic spectrum.

The names given to the various radiations reflect their historical discovery and uses. Thus radio waves (also called hertzian waves) are divided into long-, medium- and short-wave bands in connection with radio and television broadcasting (see Chapter 10). Microwaves are also known as radar radiations. The naming of infrared, below the red, and ultraviolet, beyond the violet, are self-explanatory of their relationship to the colours of the visible spectrum. X-rays are also known as Roentgen radiations.

There is only an arbitrary division between one kind of radiation and the next, except for the limits of the visible spectrum which can be defined fairly precisely by what the human eye can and cannot see. The naming covers wide bands of radiations so that different effects may be due to different frequencies of the same radiation, thus long ultraviolet (UVA) has rather different effects in the skin from ultraviolet B (UVB).

Table 11.1 The electromagnetic spectrum

Radiation	Subdivisions	Wavelengths	Photon energies
Radio waves	Long-wave	3–1 km	
	Medium-wave	600–180 m	
	Short-wave and		4.1×10^{-11} eV
	television	30–3 m	to 1.2×10^{-2} eV
Microwaves		1 m–1 cm	
Infrared	Long	100 μm–2000 nm	1.2×10^{-2} eV
	Short	2000–770 nm	to 1.8 eV
Visible	Red	750–650 nm	
	Orange	650–600 nm	
	Yellow	600–550 nm	
	Green	550–500 nm	1.8–3.1 eV
	Blue	500–470 nm	
	Indigo	470–440 nm	
	Violet	440–400 nm	
Ultraviolet	A	400–315 nm	
	B	315–280 nm	
	C	280–100 nm	3.1–124 eV
	Short 'vacuum'	100–10 nm	
X-rays	Soft	10–0.1 nm	
	Hard	0.1–0.01 nm	124 eV to 124 MeV
Gamma		0.01 pm	

In many cases the wavelengths given are examples and do not define the limits of the particular subdivision.
Photon energies from Hay and Hughes (1972).
Note: nm or nanometre $= 10^{-9}$ m; pm or picometre $= 10^{-12}$ m (see Appendix E).

It will be evident that the magnitude (by analogy with water, the height of the wave) can vary. This is called the amplitude and is the strength of the electric and magnetic fields. This is not the only way in which the energy varies. It can be seen from the Frontispiece that those radiations which have the most vigorous effects on matter are those with the shortest wavelengths and highest frequencies, like X-rays and gamma rays; the energy increases with frequency. This occurs because radiations are made up of discrete units of energy called quanta which cannot be subdivided. The energy of 1 quantum of radiation depends on the frequency of that radiation multiplied by a constant. This latter, called Planck's constant, is equal to 6.626×10^{-34} joule seconds (Js). The energy of 1 quantum is called a photon. Quantum (or photon) energies are also expressed in electron-volts (eV), especially in connection with radioactivity. The electron-volt is the energy gained by an electron when it is accelerated through a potential difference of 1 V; it is equal to 1.602×10^{-19} J. Table 11.1 gives the electron-volt energy of each group of radiations.

It is important to understand this mechanism because it determines how electromagnetic radiations interact with matter. For example, it accounts for a threshold effect: radiations less than a certain frequency have no effect no matter how great the intensity applied but above that frequency the effect increases directly with intensity. Thus photographic film is not affected by any of the longer wavelengths, such as radio or microwaves or long infrared, no matter how intense, but it is blackened by any short wavelength (high-frequency) from somewhere in the short infrared onwards, even at very low intensities. The reason for this is that there is not enough energy in each quantum of low-frequency long-wavelength radiation to cause ionization of the silver halide molecule (a chemical change) that causes the photographic film to blacken.

Ionization means that an electron has been separated from its atom. Radiation that has this effect is called ionizing radiation. Atoms can be thought of as a positively charged nucleus with a number of rapidly orbiting electrons maintained in orbit by both the electrostatic attraction of the negative charge (electron) for the positively charged nucleus and the forces due to the electron motion. Electrons occupying different orbits have different energy levels and by giving energy to the atom an electron can be made to occupy higher energy levels; the atom thus absorbs a precise amount of energy. Similarly, when electrons are made to jump from a high energy level to a lower one a precise amount of energy, due to the difference in levels, is released. This is emitted in the form of electromagnetic radiation. The wavelength or frequency of this radiation depends on the energy difference. The transition between two energy levels by one electron can be made to occur due to the absorption of 1 quantum of radiation at a particular frequency and can cause the emission of 1 quantum of radiation of a particular frequency.

As noted earlier, electromagnetic radiations are produced whenever electrons are accelerated or decelerated. Radio waves, for example, are produced by high-frequency oscillating currents, as described in Chapter 10. It was seen in Chapter 7 that heat is molecular motion and if the rotational and vibrational movements of molecules are increased by heating, the changing electron motion leads to the emission of infrared radiations. Thus, any moderately hot body emits infrared radiation (also considered in Chapter 7). With greater heating more nuclear and atomic vibration will occur leading to the emission of radiations with shorter wavelengths and higher frequencies and thus carrying more energy. The emitted photons will have a range of different wavelengths with the shortest wavelength produced depending on temperature. Thus at higher temperatures some shorter wavelengths are produced. For example, at around 400°C the shortest wavelength emitted from a heated solid is in the infrared region but at about 700°C some radiations in the red visible region are emitted. Thus the solid glows *red-hot*. Still further temperature rises lead to even more vigorous vibration of atoms with the emission of photons with still shorter wavelengths, including the whole of the visible spectrum so that the object appears *white-hot*; this can occur at temperatures around 1500°C.

A second way in which visible radiations can be produced occurs when, for example, atoms and ions are made to collide in a low-pressure gas giving energy to an outer electron which subsequently returns to a lower energy level, causing the emission of a photon of energy characteristic of that particular transition energy. Therefore particular atoms produce radiations of particular wavelengths. This forms a line spectrum which is characteristic of the particular atoms. Sodium, for example, produces typical yellow lines giving the familiar yellow light of sodium-vapour street lighting. Ultraviolet radiations are produced in a similar way but involve higher energies and therefore shorter wavelengths. X-rays are produced when high-energy transitions are made to occur either when orbiting electrons jump between inner orbits or when rapidly moving electrons are abruptly decelerated. Gamma radiations are emitted from the nuclei of certain radioactive atoms.

In summary then, electromagnetic radiations consist of trains of waves given out whenever constant motion of an electron is changed. They consist of energy in the form of oscillating electric and magnetic fields perpendicular to one another and to the line of travel, emitted in 'packets' called quanta, each with an amount of energy that is proportional to the frequency. Thus electromagnetic radiations can be considered both as a wave system and as a stream of energy particles—photons. This wave-particle duality, as it is called, is no contradiction. It is simply that the two aspects of radiation are best modelled and described each in its own way. The terms 'electromagnetic radiations' and 'electromagnetic waves' are therefore used synonymously.

FEATURES OF ELECTROMAGNETIC RADIATION

Rectilinear propagation

Electromagnetic radiations travel in straight lines in space. This is clearly evident with visible radiations since shadows are formed where the light path is interrupted by an object. Radiations are emitted from their source in all directions so that if the source is relatively small the radiations will spread out equally in all directions with the result that the energy passing through a unit area per unit time—the intensity—will decrease with distance. This is illustrated in Figure 11.1. The relationship between the distance from the source and intensity of radiation is expressed in *the inverse square law* which states that the intensity of the radiation from a point source is inversely proportional to the square of the distance from the source: $I \propto 1/d^2$, where I = intensity and d = distance. This is, of course, only strictly true if there is no scattering or absorption of the radiations but for many radiations it is effectively true in air and of great practical importance (see later discussion on the application of infrared and ultraviolet). The consequence is that small changes of distance will cause large changes of intensity, as shown in Figure 11.1. Doubling the distance between the source and the irradiated surface will reduce the intensity to one-quarter; tripling the distance would reduce the intensity to one-ninth and so on. Similarly, halving the distance will quadruple the intensity.

Polarization

A beam of radiations contains millions of quanta per second which are in random planes to one another but all perpendicular to the line of travel. If

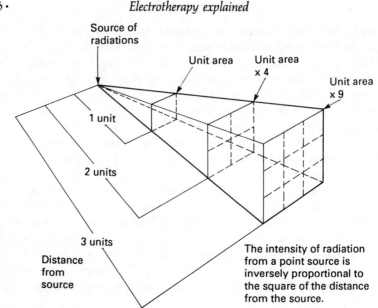

Fig. 11.1 The inverse square law. The intensity of radiation from a point source is inversely proportional to the square of the distance from the source.

radiations are passed through material which allows the passage of only those quanta whose electric (and magnetic) fields are in one particular plane it is called polarized radiation. Polarized light can be achieved by passing unpolarized light through certain mineral crystals, or more usually through a material called Polaroid which is made with long-chain molecules all in the same orientation (White, 1974).

Phase difference and coherence

Radiations emitted from a source consist of random bursts of radiation because each atom or molecule of the source acts independently so that the varying electric and magnetic fields are not 'in time' or 'in step'. It is possible to make all the emitting atoms radiate in phases by stimulating light emission in a special way in a device called a laser (discussed in Chapter 14). When this occurs the radiation is said to be coherent.

INTERACTIONS OF RADIATIONS WITH MATTER

Electromagnetic radiations travel unhindered in space (and to a large extent, for most radiations, in air) but on meeting matter several possible interactions can occur:

1 The electromagnetic radiations can pass unaffected through the material, i.e.

they are said to be *transmitted*. When they pass into the material they are said to penetrate.

2 The radiations may not enter the material at all, being turned back or *reflected*.

In both these cases as there is no energy lost to the material there is no effect on the material.

3 Radiation energy may be *absorbed*; if it is to have any effect it must be absorbed. This is Grotthus' law.

In real situations all three happen together so that some radiations are transmitted right through, some are reflected and some absorbed. The amount of each depends on the wavelength or frequency of the radiation and the nature of the material. Often one aspect predominates, for example light will be mainly transmitted through panes of window glass but it is evident that some of the light is reflected (if this were not so the glass would be invisible), also some is absorbed. In the case of a shiny metal surface reflection of visible radiations predominates.

Radiations entering a new material, a new medium, may be bent at the surface—a process called refraction—and transmitted at some angle to the original line.

Reflection of radiations

When electromagnetic radiations pass through matter they interact with the electric fields of the atoms and molecules and this determines their velocity in that particular material. Specifically, it is the dielectric constant and conductivity of the material that is involved. At the junction of two kinds of matter, say glass and air, the electromagnetic waves have to change velocity as the velocity is less in glass. The wave will not change in frequency so that only part of the wave energy can be transmitted; the rest is turned back or reflected. The amount of reflection depends on the radiation, the angle of incidence and the nature of the surface. The direction of the reflected radiation depends on the angle of the incident radiation. For a beam of radiation impinging on a plane surface the angle of incidence is equal to the angle of reflection (Fig. 11.2). Further, the incident and reflected beam are in the same plane as the 'normal', a line which is perpendicular to the surface at the point of incidence; i.e. in Figure 11.2 they all lie in the same plane of the page. These are the laws of reflection and are well understood in connection with visible radiation but are equally valid for other electromagnetic radiations, e.g. microwaves bouncing off a flat metal sheet in a microwave oven or, for that matter, any other wave system such as sonic waves, as described in Chapter 6.

The reflection of visible radiations from matter is, of course, central to human perception of the visible world. The recognition of colour and form is due to the reflection of radiations from objects (except when the object is

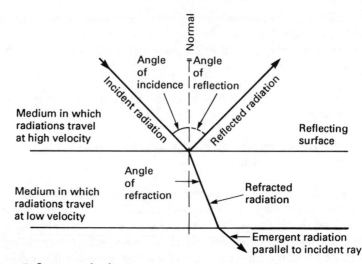

Fig. 11.2 Reflection and refraction.

emitting visible radiations of its own). The retinal cells of the eye are sensitive to extremely low energy levels and are able to detect a few photons and discriminate between colours with wavelength differences of only a few tens of nanometres.

The relationship between the amount of any given radiation reflected and the amount that penetrates any particular surface depends on the angle at which it strikes the surface — the angle of incidence. This can be understood in terms of photons having a greater chance of penetrating if they meet the surface at right angles — as a dart is more likely to penetrate if it strikes the board at right angles and more likely to bounce off if it strikes a glancing blow. Further, if a beam strikes a surface at right angles the area covered is the cross-section of the beam but if angled to the surface the area covered increases so that the intensity on unit area decreases. This can be easily demonstrated by shining a torch vertically down on to the floor and comparing the circle of light with the larger oval produced when the torch is shone at an angle. This *cosine law*, as it is called, states that the amount of radiation penetrating a surface is proportional to the cosine of the angle of incidence of the radiation (Fig. 11.3a). If the radiations are applied perpendicular to the surface the angle of incidence is 0°; the cosine of 0 is 1 which gives the maximum penetration. At an angle of incidence of 45°, cos 45 = 0.7, indicating that penetration is 70% of maximum. If the radiations are parallel to the surface, i.e. there is an angle of incidence of 90°, there will be no penetration of the surface because the cosine of 90 is 0. From Figure 11.3a and Table 11.2 it can be seen that small changes of angle from the perpendicular make very little difference; thus errors of 15 or 20° in the placing of lamps are insignificant but at large angles the absorption falls off markedly. (This is why people lie down on the beach to achieve a good suntan because when standing the sun's ultraviolet radiation strikes the body at a large angle of incidence.)

A further important consequence of this is the effect of parallel radiation on

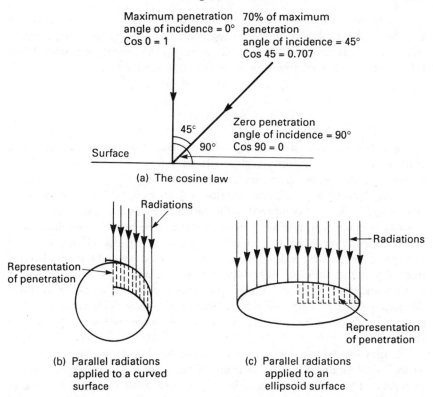

Fig. 11.3 Ratio of reflected and penetrating radiations. (a) The cosine law; (b) parallel radiations applied to a curved surface; (c) parallel radiations applied to an ellipsoid section.

Table 11.2   Table of cosines

Angle	Cosine
0°	1.0
15°	0.966
30°	0.866
45°	0.707
60°	0.5
70°	0.342
80°	0.174
90°	0.0

a curved surface. It will be evident that penetration will diminish around the sides of a circular surface as the angle of incidence increases and the cosine of the angle decreases (Fig. 11.3b). To achieve uniform irradiation it is necessary to apply radiations from two directions at right angles. If the surface is elliptical in section (Fig. 11.3c) the angular changes between radiation and surface are small except at the very edge of the ellipse. Thus parallel radiations applied to such surfaces give almost uniform penetration over much of the area. Since the trunk and some limb segments of the body are approximately ovoid in cross-section most of the body is more or less evenly irradiated in just two positions, i.e. sunbathing lying down prone and supine.

Refraction

When radiation meets a boundary with a medium in which it travels at a different velocity its velocity will be altered and it will be refracted or bent unless the radiation is perpendicular to the boundary (Fig. 11.2). The part of the wave front of any radiation entering a medium in which it travels more slowly will be delayed compared to the part of the wavefront still in the high-velocity medium. This will cause the wave front to be turned through an angle which depends on its relative velocities in the two media. (The velocity of waves in a medium depends on the nature of the medium and the wavelength/frequency of the wave: this is equally true of sonic waves, as noted in Chapter 6.) Consequently radiations of different wavelengths can be made to travel different paths by being refracted to different degrees. This is how a glass prism can be used to separate the different wavelengths of the visible spectrum.

The glass–air interface is, of course, used to bend visible radiations through lenses in all kinds of optical instruments, microscopes, magnifying lenses, cameras and so forth. The specialized transparent tissues forming the lens of the eye works in the same way. It is seen in Figure 11.2 that the refracted radiation is bent towards the normal as it enters a medium in which it travels more slowly: similarly the reverse is true. Thus visible radiations emerging from glass into air will be refracted away from the normal. In the case of, say, a parallel-sided block of glass the emergent ray is parallel to the incident ray but displaced sideways (see Fig. 11.2). Increasing the angle of incidence at the dense–less dense interface increases the angle of refraction. At a certain angle of incidence, called the critical angle, the radiation will travel parallel to the surface. At any greater angle the radiation would be reflected back into the glass, an effect called total internal reflection.

Reflection and refraction have been described largely in terms of visible radiation but it must be understood that these are general principles which apply to all electromagnetic radiations, albeit to different degrees with different radiations and media. Microwaves are reflected from metal surfaces, thus enabling the position of aircraft and ships to be monitored by radar. Long radio waves can be reflected by an ionized layer in the outer atmosphere. Ultraviolet radiations are retained in curved quartz rods (applicators) by total internal reflection.

Absorption and penetration

The relationship between the amount of an electromagnetic radiation that is absorbed and the distance it penetrates any given material is of the greatest importance. For a homogeneous material the amount of any given radiation absorbed will be a fixed proportion of the total radiation present at that point. Thus the amount of radiation penetrating and being absorbed will fall exponentially with the depth of penetration in the same way as sonic waves, described in Chapter 6. In order to describe this pattern of absorption in a convenient way a single figure is used which may be either the 'penetration depth' or the 'half-value depth'. The former is the depth penetrated at which approximately 63% of radiation has been absorbed (37% remaining), and the latter the depth at which 50% has been absorbed. This concept is illustrated in Figure 11.4. Different frequencies/wavelengths of radiation have different penetration depths in any particular material, thus materials of a particular nature and thickness can be used as filters. This filtering effect is applied in many situations, e.g. filtering out the short ultraviolet (UVC) radiations but leaving the longer ultraviolet rays for some treatments or filtering out all the UVR but leaving visible radiations, as in protective ultraviolet goggles (see Chapter 15). A global example of this is the filtering of radiation from the sun by the earth's atmosphere. The sun, which is at a very high temperature, emits all kinds of radiation, some of which falls on the earth's atmosphere, to be reflected, absorbed or penetrate to the surface of the earth. Almost all of the short ultraviolet radiations below 300 nm are absorbed by ozone in the upper atmosphere with oxygen and nitrogen also absorbing some visible and ultraviolet radiations. Water vapour and carbon dioxide absorb much infrared radiation. All of these absorb certain wavelengths particularly strongly (Holwill and Silvester, 1973). The net effect of atmospheric filtration of solar radiation is to allow a band of radiations to penetrate to the earth's surface from about 300 nm in the ultraviolet band to 2000 nm in the infrared, with a peak around 650 nm (see Fig. 15.2). Destruction of atmospheric ozone due to the release of chlorofluorocarbons will allow the penetration of more short ultraviolet rays and the continued release of carbon dioxide and other gases will increase absorption of infrared radiation contributing to global warming—the 'greenhouse effect'.

The concept of absorption described above and in Figure 11.4 is also important in considering the effect of radiations on the tissues. The penetration and absorption of the different modalities will be considered in the appropriate chapters but Figure 11.4 illustrates the generalized concept: some infrared and visible radiations may have half-value penetration depths of less than 1 mm while some microwaves have a half-value depth of several centimetres. It must, however, be emphasized that the tissues are not homogeneous so that absorption in the tissues is much more irregular than Figure 11.4 suggests.

Scattering

Radiations passing in non-homogeneous matter may be partly scattered, that is the direction of some radiations is altered, effectively reducing the depth of penetration. The scattered radiation may travel in a different direction and be absorbed at some point away from the main beam of radiation. Scattering is

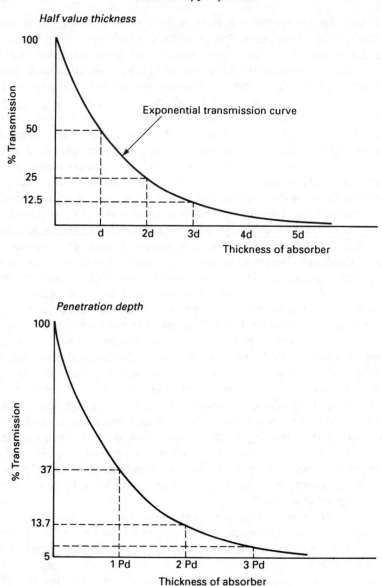

Fig. 11.4 (a) Half-value thickness. The intensity decreases by the same fraction in equal units of distance. The distance *d* is the half-value distance for intensity to decrease by half its previous value. (b) Penetration depth is the distance over which the intensity is reduced by a factor of $1/e$. e is a constant: 2.7, therefore $1/e = 0.37$. So penetration depth is the distance over which the intensity falls to 37% of its original value.

due to reflection and refraction from small particles and shorter wavelengths are more affected than longer ones. (For given particle size, scattering is inversely proportional to the fourth power of the wavelength—Rayleigh's law.) The shorter wavelength, e.g. the ultraviolet rays, are strongly scattered in the skin decreasing their penetration (Nightingale, 1959).

Other interactions

Some high-energy radiations such as ultraviolet or X-rays can be absorbed by certain crystalline substances to be re-emitted at longer, visible wavelengths. This process is called fluorescence.

The photoelectric effect occurs when photons fall on a suitable material causing the release of electrons which constitute a current that can be measured. This effect can be used to measure radiation, mainly visible, ultraviolet and X-rays. For infrared and other longer wavelength radiations the photon energies are insufficient so that such radiation is usually measured in other ways.

REFERENCES

Hay G. A., Hughes D. (1972). *First Year Physics for Radiographers*. London: Baillière Tindall.
Holwill M. E., Silvester N. R. (1973). *Introduction to Biological Physics*. London: John Wiley.
Nightingale A. (1959). *Physics and Electronics in Physical Medicine*. London: G. Bell.
White D. C. S. (1974). *Biological Physics*. London: Chapman and Hall.

12.

Microwave diathermy

INTRODUCTION

Microwaves are electromagnetic radiations that lie between radio waves and infrared (see Frontispiece). They are considered to be those wavelengths between 1 m and 1 cm, hence from 300 MHz to 30 GHz in frequency. Three particular frequencies are allotted for medical use in Europe (Table 12.1), while the 2450 and 915 MHz frequencies are allocated for medical use in the USA. Of these the 2450 MHz frequency is much the most widely available but is, perhaps, not the most satisfactory for therapeutic heating for reasons considered below. The heating effect of microwaves has become well known since the development of microwave ovens. They are also used in communications as 'line-of-sight' telephone links and, of course, in tracking ships, aircraft, rockets and satellites as radar. Although microwaves were first artificially

Table 12.1 Frequencies and wavelengths of microwaves used in medicine

Frequency (MHz)	Wavelength (cm)
2450	12.245
915	32.79
433.9	69.14

Europe uses all three; the USA the top two frequencies.

274

generated in the late 1930s it was the urgent need for powerful radar equipment during the Second World War that stimulated the development of generators which became increasingly available for medical use during the subsequent two decades.

Microwave radiation behaves like other electromagnetic radiation, described in Chapter 11, in that it is reflected and refracted at interfaces and will be absorbed or penetrate material to varying degrees depending on the nature of the materials. It also exhibits rectilinear propagation, a necessary feature for its use as radar. The fact that microwaves can be directed on to and will penetrate the tissues to some extent and yet be strongly absorbed by water and hence highly vascular tissue such as muscle makes it an effective method of tissue heating.

PRODUCTION OF MICROWAVES

It will be recalled from Chapter 10 that high-frequency oscillating currents will produce electromagnetic radiations of radio frequencies which can be radiated from suitable antennae as radio and television transmissions. At higher frequencies it becomes impossible for the electrons in the electric circuit to oscillate sufficiently rapidly because of the time needed for them to pass through a valve or transistor. For the higher frequencies of microwave at relatively high power a device called a magnetron is used. (Although the magnetron was invented in 1920 by A. W. Hull it was the development of the multicavity magnetron by R. T. Randall in the UK in 1940 which made the generation of higher-wattage microwave energy possible.) In principle the magnetron is like a large thermionic valve with a central heated cathode surrounded by a block of metal in which a number of 'cavities' have been cut and through which a strong magnetic field is applied. The metal block is positively charged attracting electrons emitted by the cathode which are whirled spirally at very high velocities by the axial magnetic field. When these pass over the openings they cause oscillating currents in the cavities whose frequency is determined by the dimensions of the cavity. These currents are collected and fed along a coaxial cable to the antenna or emitter which radiates microwaves. The coaxial cable consists of a central conductor surrounded by insulation which is itself surrounded by a flexible metal tube or sheath and external insulation. This provides conductors with a suitable capacitance and is made to a length which, connected to the emitter, conveys microwaves of a given frequency with maximum efficiency. The antenna, which is simply a suitable-sized and shaped piece of wire, is mounted in front of a metal reflector so that a beam of microwaves is emitted in one direction (Fig. 12.1).

The output of microwave energy can be controlled by varying the power supplied to the magnetron. Machines have an intensity control and the output is indicated on a meter which, of course, gives no reliable indication of the heating of the tissues. The frequency of the microwaves produced depends on the structure of the magnetron and is therefore fixed. There will also be a means of switching the mains power on and off and suitable indicator lights.

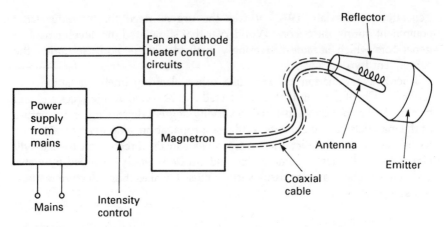

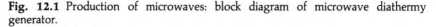

Fig. 12.1 Production of microwaves: block diagram of microwave diathermy generator.

On some machines a delay switch may be fitted to allow time for the magnetron to reach its proper working temperature.

Some machines have a switch that enables the output to be disconnected while leaving the magnetron heater circuit on—a standby switch. Thus successive treatments may be given or adjustment of the emitter made without having to switch off the magnetron and wait for it to warm up again.

The emitter, also called a director or applicator, gives out a beam of microwaves which diverges somewhat because it is technically difficult to produce a completely uniform beam (Ward, 1986). The effect of this divergence is to reduce the intensity of radiations considerably with distance (see the inverse square law, Chapter 11; Guy, 1982).

THE PHYSIOLOGICAL EFFECTS OF MICROWAVES ON THE TISSUES

When the electromagnetic energy of microwave radiation is absorbed in the tissues it provokes ionic movement, rotation of dipoles and electron orbit distortion (as already described for shortwave diathermy in Chapter 10) which leads to heating. The amount of heating will be proportional to the amount of absorbed radiation.

The effects of heating on the tissues have been fully considered in Chapters 7 and 8 so that it is sufficient here to summarize the local effects as causing:

1 Raised metabolic rate.
2 Increased blood flow.
3 Decreased blood and tissue viscosity.
4 Increased extensibility of collagen.
5 Effects on nerves, leading to pain relief.

Since microwaves are being applied from outside the tissues and 'beamed in' and are strongly absorbed by water it would be expected that heating would be greatest at the surface and diminish exponentially with depth (see Fig. 11.4). While this is a useful simple generalization it needs further elucidation.

The pattern of heating in the tissues

In Chapter 11 it was noted that when any radiation meets the surface of a different medium it may either be reflected or penetrate. Those radiations that do penetrate will only have an effect if they are absorbed (Grotthus' law); thus they will be ineffective if they pass right through. In the case of microwaves there is considerable reflection at the air–skin boundary and at skin–fat and fat–muscle boundaries in the tissues. The percentage of microwave radiation (at 2450 MHz) reflected varies with thickness of fat and skin from 50 to 75% (Scowcroft *et al.*, 1977). (Tissue thickness makes a great difference at this frequency. Some radiations that are reflected from the fat–skin interface and other interfaces in the tissues can be radiated out of the body.) At the other frequencies in therapeutic use some 60–70% of the energy is reflected but it is much less affected by variations in skin tissue thickness (Ward, 1980).

The relationship between the amount of radiation absorbed and that which penetrates is shown in Figure 11.4 as an exponential relationship in which the half-value depth for microwave is often given as 3 cm (penetration depth 4.3 cm). This smooth change would only be true if the tissues were homogeneous, which they are definitely not. Calculations can be made for an approximate model of the tissues, consisting of a 2 cm layer of fat over muscle and bone, by using the dielectric constants and conductivities of these tissues to give a pattern of heating, shown in Figure 12.2. This pattern occurs because the rate of absorption of microwaves is much lower in fat (half-value about 3.5 cm) and higher in the vascular muscle tissue (half-value about 0.7 cm). There is also reflection from the fat–muscle and fat–bone interfaces causing standing waves which lead to 'peaks' in the middle of each tissue layer (Fig. 12.2). These theoretical patterns, calculated by Ward (1980) are likely to be much less clearly defined in real tissue because of the irregularities of the interfaces, the heat-distributing effects of the blood flow, especially in muscle tissue, and also the effects of conduction. These calculations do not give actual temperature changes, just the relative energy absorption. When the same calculations are made for microwaves at 915 MHz (Fig. 12.2b), the relatively better heating of muscle compared to fat is strikingly illustrated; microwaves of lower frequencies penetrate further. For this reason, and due to unpredictable reflection from the surface, noted earlier, it is considered by some that 915 MHz (and 434 MHz which gives a similar pattern) are more suitable frequencies for therapeutic heating than the widely used 2450 MHz. While these patterns are predictions, the particular heating of the superficial musculature is supported, at least under some conditions, by experiments in which human tissue temperatures were measured (Lehmann and de Lateur, 1982). Although it is not shown in Figure 12.2, the skin would be heated to a

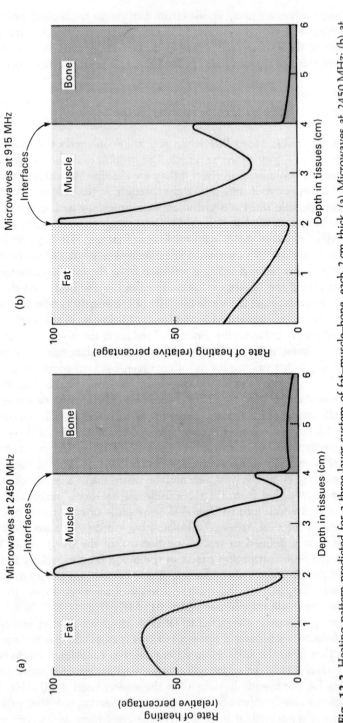

Fig. 12.2 Heating pattern predicted for a three-layer system of fat–muscle–bone, each 2 cm thick. (a) Microwaves at 2450 MHz; (b) at 915 MHz.

greater degree than the deeper tissues. This ensures the safety of microwave treatments since excess heating will be felt by heat receptors in the skin.

In summary then, therapeutic microwave radiation is largely absorbed in the first few centimetres of tissue traversed and especially in muscle. It is evident that microwave heating would be suitable for superficial muscle heating or for heating articular structures close to the surface, such as the wrist joint or anterior aspect of the knee, but it is not likely to affect deeply placed structures covered with muscle tissue like the hip joint. Perhaps it should be emphasized that heating patterns are highly irregular and probably vary considerably from patient to patient. A comparison might be made with ultrasound (see Chapter 6) which has similar penetration but is usually applied with a continuously moving treatment head which evens out the distribution of energy in the tissues.

So far, only the depth of heating has been considered but the distribution of energy over the surface is also important. This will depend on the size and shape of the emitter. Circular emitters usually give a somewhat ring-shaped pattern (but if close it may be more or less circular). Other emitters are available which are rather longer in one direction and give an oval pattern; still other emitters of apparently similar shape may give the greatest output at the central axis, diminishing outwards. This is often the situation in practice since many body areas are convex so that the centre of the area is nearest to the emitter. Some emitters are designed to focus the radiation into the tissues and thus achieve better depth of heating. All the emitters described so far are distance emitters, that is, they are applied to the tissues with an air gap. It is also possible to have contact emitters which, as their name suggests, are applied directly to the tissues.

Microwaves are markedly reflected from skin and in Chapters 6 and 11 it was explained that reflection depends on the different impedances encountered when waves—whether sonic or electromagnetic—pass from one medium to another. To achieve better transmission to skin and to enable the emitter to be made much smaller a suitable ceramic dielectric material is used. This will enable a better match to be made between the applicator and the tissues. These contact emitters can be made quite small, 1.5 or 3.5 cm diameter, and will radiate microwaves directly into the tissues away from the surface of the emitter. Other small emitters can be placed in body cavities—rectum, vagina and external auditory meatus—emitting radially to heat the walls of the cavity.

As microwave transmission is better with these contact emitters the power that can be applied may be limited to a low level (25 W); see later comment on cooled emitters. Small contact emitters are not widely used; they have been described as ineffective (Forster and Palastanga, 1985) and if hand-held are considered potentially hazardous (Scowcroft *et al.*, 1977), but no evidence is given. Special sandbags can also be used with some distance emitters to prevent the microwave radiations diverging so far and so giving greater intensity. They act like the ceramic dielectric emitters.

THERAPEUTIC USES

The indications are those of heating. Like shortwave, some debate surrounds the issue of whether there are any specific effects of microwave other than heating. There is no clear evidence of any effect except heat, but that does not mean that low-dose treatments giving imperceptible heating are ineffective. Thus the position is the same as that of shortwave—all the proven effects can be accounted for by the heating effect. In the case of pulsed shortwave the discussion centres on whether the effects are specific to the pulsing parameters or simply due to very low-intensity heating (see Chapter 10). Microwaves can also be pulsed and the effects are claimed to be the same as pulsed shortwave. However, there seems to be no evidence concerning pulsed microwave, in contrast to the case of pulsed shortwave where the evidence for accelerated healing is quite extensive.

Perhaps the particular pattern of heating due to microwave—the skin and superficial muscle are heated while the subcutaneous fat is largely avoided— could be considered specific since it contrasts with the usual pattern of shortwave heating (see Chapter 10).

The microwave heating of these largely superficial tissues is localized and can lead to:

1 *Pain relief*: this has been discussed in connection with heating in Chapter 7 and any pain relief due to microwave would be a consequence of the mechanisms already described:

    a Pain gate mechanism.
    b Accelerated removal of irritants due to blood flow increases.
    c Associated relief of muscle spasm.
    d Possible sedative effect.

2 *Reduction or relief of muscle spasm* due either to a direct effect on the muscle spindle mechanism (see Chapter 7) or to pain relief.
3 *Accelerated healing* due to increased metabolic activity and blood flow, applying to both post-traumatic healing and recovery of chronic inflammatory changes.
4 *Softening of collagenous tissues*, scar tissue or other fibrosis. This may require relatively high temperatures, necessitating great care.
5 *Microwave heating of muscle tissue*: one of the major uses of microwave therapy is for heating muscle tissue to achieve, amongst other things, an increase in intramuscular blood flow. This, it is believed, only occurs if the temperature is significantly raised. It has been shown in dogs that 15 min of microwave can cause a considerable rise in intramuscular temperature followed by an 85% increase in blood flow (Richardson, 1954). This increased flow only occurred after a critical threshold temperature had been reached. It has already been pointed out that 915 MHz microwave is much more efficient at heating the deeper tissues than the more usual 2450 MHz microwave (Fig. 12.2). Heating is, of course, limited by the skin surface

heating so that greater total heating and thus deep heating can be achieved if the heated surface is deliberately cooled. This can be done by passing cold air over the skin surface. Therapeutic applicators have been made which work at 915 MHz; these have contact emitters which contain a dielectric material with apertures through which cooling air is blown. As the emitter is used in contact with the skin the amount of scattered radiation is also diminished. These are considered by some to be an efficient way of generating even heating in the deep tissues. However with the thermal receptors in the skin deliberately cooled there is an increased risk of a burn, and extreme caution is required with this technique.

6 *Cancer therapy*: microwaves have also been utilized to provide heating in some cancer therapy (Oleson and Gerner, 1982).

PRINCIPLES OF APPLICATION

The patient should be positioned so that the part to be treated is comfortably supported and sufficiently exposed. Microwave should not be applied through clothing or where there is metal in the field. The nature of the treatment should be described to the patient, explaining how the microwave energy is dissipated in the body so that only a small temperature rise will occur, unlike the situation of a microwave oven in which the temperature can be made to rise to cooking levels because the heat and reflected microwaves cannot escape. The thermal sensitivity of the skin to which the microwaves are to be applied should be tested, as described in Chapter 7. The choice of emitter is dictated by the size of tissue area to be treated. The power should be switched on, the machine given time to warm up after which it can be left on a standby switch. The emitter should be positioned so that the radiations strike the surface at right angles, bearing in mind that as distance emitters have diverging beams, only the axial radiations will be strictly at right angles while the peripheral radiation will strike at small incident angles. While this may not make much difference (see cosine law, Chapter 11) when the emitter is 'square on', slight angling of the emitter increases the already considerable reflection from the skin surface, making the treatment ineffective.

The distance between the emitter and the skin determines both the area treated and the intensity because of the diverging beam. Thus if a small area is to be treated the emitter should be placed close to the skin, say 2–5 cm, and the appropriate heating regulated with the intensity control on the machine. If larger areas are to be heated the spacing can be increased, to 10 or 15 cm, and the intensity control advanced to give sufficient heating. Distances of about 10 cm are commonly utilized for most treatments.

The degree of heating required must be described to the patient, as for shortwave (see Chapter 10). Like other heat treatments the only information about the intensity and site of heating in the tissues is derived from the patient's sensations. The meter only indicates the output of the machine so it is essential to have the patient's full co-operation. He or she must also be warned to call if the heating becomes more than a comfortable warmth or if discomfort

Electrotherapy explained

or pain is felt, and to remain still. The patient is given a pair of microwave goggles (see below) if radiation could enter the eye.

DOSAGE

Treatment is usually given for 20 min as this is considered to be the optimum time (Wadsworth and Chanmugan, 1980) because the vascular adjustments have become 'steady' by this time. However, it is evident that the deeper tissues take rather longer to reach a maximum steady temperature (de Lateur *et al.*, 1970). At depths greater than 2 cm the temperature is still rising after 10 min (Boyle *et al.*, 1950). If significant muscle heating is required it would be reasonable to apply the microwave treatment for rather longer, say 30 min.

The intensity is regulated by the patient reporting the sensation of heat. It seems to take an absorbed dose of some 200 mW/cm^2 to give detectable heating (Knauf, 1968).

POTENTIAL DANGERS

Microwaves produce heating in the tissues so there are the same risks of damage due to overheating as with all other heat treatments (see Chapters 8, 10 and 13). However, some points need to be considered specifically in connection with microwaves.

Effects of metal

As microwaves are strongly reflected from metal surfaces any metal placed on the tissue surface will act as a shield preventing radiations reaching the underlying tissues; this may lead to ineffective treatment. Metal may also distort and concentrate the microwave field causing local overheating which could be dangerous. If metal is so placed that it could reflect microwave energy into the tissues it is again possible that overheating could occur. If, for example, the hand is rested on a metal surface and microwave radiation applied some would pass through the hand and be reflected back into it again. With normal sensory awareness there is no reason why this should lead to burning but it would be an undesirable and uncontrolled pattern of heating. Metal embedded in the tissues, due to accident or surgery, could also cause reflections in the tissues which might lead to overheating. Since there are no heat receptors in the deep tissues the patient would only be aware of deep pain when the damage had occurred. Such an effect does not seem to have been reported and would probably only be likely with superficially placed metal. However it is generally advisable to avoid treating the region of metal implants with microwaves. It should be noted that the reason for avoiding them is rather different than in shortwave applications (see Chapter 10).

Cardiac pacemakers

These could be affected if microwaves were directly applied to the region (see Chapter 10) but there is little, if any, risk from scattered radiation.

The eyes

Due to its structure (a water-filled sphere) the eye selectively absorbs microwaves and is not easily able to dissipate heat and thus can become overheated. Although cataracts in laboratory animals have been produced with high doses of microwaves there is no evidence that they have been caused in humans (Lehmann and de Lateur, 1982). It is considered wise to avoid exposing the eyes directly to high doses of microwave energy. If the treatment is such that radiation may enter the eye, when treating the anterior aspect of the shoulder with a distance emitter for example, the patient should be given goggles which are impervious to microwaves. Such goggles are of two kinds—either a metal mesh which reflects practically all microwave radiation but allows sufficient light between the mesh to see clearly, or a thin layer of metal supported on glass which again reflects microwave radiations but interferes little with visible light. However it is difficult to make goggles totally effective because of diffraction (Delpizzo and Joyner, 1987). It is important that microwave goggles do not become confused with ultraviolet goggles in busy physiotherapy departments as they can look similar but have different functions. Closing the eyes would not prevent the transmission of microwaves, but would diminish them.

The testes

While quite small temperature rises can interfere with spermatogenesis in mammals, which is why the testes are located outside the abdominal cavity, there is no evidence that mild heating has any damaging effect although marked heating can cause damage, albeit reversible. It is felt that heating of $100 \, mW/cm^2$ could possibly produce testicular damage in humans (Watson, 1971); therefore direct irradiation of the testes should be avoided and care taken to prevent large amounts of reflected or scattered radiation reaching the region.

The testes are more susceptible because of their exposed position and possibly their structure. The same does not apply to the deeply placed ovaries which are unlikely to be heated by microwave treatment.

General safety with microwaves

Patients undergoing microwave treatment are in a controlled situation, their thermal perception is checked and dosage regulated. For uncontrolled exposure fairly low levels of microwaves are recommended (Medical Research Council, 1971). Thus standards have been set for exposure of the public to microwave. These vary a good deal from one part of the world to another. In the UK the Medical Research Council has set $10 \, mW/cm^2$ as a safe level for continuous exposure and for higher doses it considers that the total should not exceed $1 \, mW\text{-}h/cm^2$. The Standards Association of Australia recommend a lower limit of $1 \, mW/cm^2$ at 2450 MHz (Delpizzo and Joyner, 1987). In the USSR and other Eastern European countries the permitted exposure is even lower, no more than $1 \, mW/cm^2$ for exposures of 20 min each day, for example (Watson, 1971). These low permitted exposure levels are based on statistical evidence of rather vague disorders—insomnia, depression, headache, heart rhythm changes, buzzing in the ears etc.—in factory workers exposed to low-level microwave emission (Watson, 1971). These results do not seem to have been found elsewhere; therefore this evidence for some athermic effect is not generally accepted. The question of whether microwave radiation has non-thermal effects on body tissue is central to this matter but the weight of evidence suggests that all the effects are due to thermal reasons (Scowcroft *et al.*, 1977) (Cf. the discussion on pulsed shortwave in Chapter 10.)

Measurements made by the National Radiological Protection Board on typical physiotherapy treatments with microwave indicate that the safe level of radiation is not exceeded under almost any conditions at more than 1 m in front or at the side of the emitter and 25 cm behind the emitter (Health Equipment Information, 1980; Fig. 12.3). If powers of more than 100 W are used the dimensions of the zones are increased, e.g. for 200 W it is increased to 1.4 m. However it must be noted that many emitters give out a very irregular beam of microwave radiation (Brown and Johnson, 1975). In order to obtain effective heating for treatment purposes these levels must be exceeded at the treatment site. However for the short times involved in treatment there is no evidence of hazard to the patient.

Scowcroft *et al.* (1977) recommend that treatment should be avoided through Micropore dressings as local heating has been known to occur, possibly due to interface effects. They also suggest that all physiotherapy departments should have access to a microwave power monitor.

CONTRAINDICATIONS

1 Diminished thermal sensation.
2 Defective arterial circulation,
3 Acute inflammation.
4 Recent haemorrhaging.
5 Metal in the area under treatment.
6 Malignancy.
7 Implanted cardiac pacemakers.
8 Intrauterine devices when using a vaginal electrode—a practice not

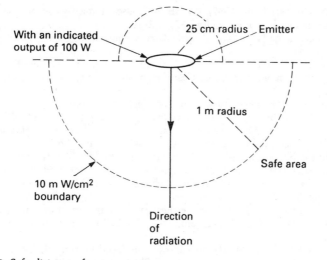

Fig. 12.3 Safe distances from a microwave source.

recommended by the preliminary report of the Chartered Society of Physiotherapy working party (Scowcroft *et al.*, 1977).
9 Eyes and testes, due to poor heat dissipation.

In summary, microwave safety has provoked a good deal of concern, much of it emanating from a failure to understand the nature of microwave energy. Microwave absorption leads to heating and if the heating is excessive a burn can result in the same way—but not due to the same mechanism—as from any other form of heat. Investigation of microwave burns in living tissue, in piglets, showed a characteristic pattern called 'layered tissue sparing' in which the skin and muscle tissues were burned but the intervening subcutaneous fat was relatively spared (Surrell *et al.*, 1987). This is in conformity with the pattern of microwave heating described earlier and with what would be expected. Non-thermal (low-dose) effects of microwave have not been established but there is sufficient uncertainty to warrant caution. Treatment with microwave as a form of therapeutic heating is safe provided the modality is understood and the precautions already described are followed.

REFERENCES

Boyle A. C., Cook H. F., Buchanan T. J. (1950). The effects of microwaves: a preliminary investigation. *Br. J. Phys. Med.*, **13**, 2–8.
Brown B. H., Johnson S. G. (1975). Microwave diathermy (treatment note). *Physiotherapy*, **61**, 117.
de Lateur B. K., Lehmann J. F., Stonebridge J. B. *et al.* (1970). Muscle heating in human subjects with 915 MHz microwave contact applicator. *Arch. Phys. Med. Rehab.*, **51**, 147–51.

Delpizzo V., Joyner K. H. (1987). On the safe use of microwave and shortwave diathermy units. *Aust. J. Physiother.*, **33**, 152–61.

Forster A., Palastanga N. (1985). *Clayton's Electrotherapy: Theory and Practice*. London: Baillière Tindall.

Guy A. W. (1982). Biophysics of high frequency currents and electromagnetic radiation. In *Therapeutic Heat and Cold* (Lehmann J. F., ed.) Baltimore: Williams & Wilkins, pp. 199–277.

Health Equipment Information (1980). No. 188, September. London: DHSS.

Knauf G. M. (1968). Biological effects of microwave radiations. *Arch. Ind. Hlth*, **17**, 48.

Lehmann J. F., de Lateur B. J. (1982). Therapeutic heat. In *Therapeutic Heat and Cold* (Lehmann J. F., ed.) Baltimore: Williams & Wilkins, pp. 404–562.

Medical Research Council (1971). *Recommendation MRC 70/1314*. January 8.

Michaelson S. M. (1982). Bioeffects of high frequency currents and electromagnetic radiations. In *Therapeutic Heat and Cold* (Lehmann J. F., ed.) Baltimore: Williams and Wilkins, pp. 278–352.

Oleson J. R., Gerner E. W. (1982). Hyperthermia in the treatment of malignancies. In *Therapeutic Heat and Cold* (Lehmann J. F., ed.) Baltimore: Williams & Wilkins, pp. 603–35.

Richardson A. W. (1954). Effects of microwave-induced heating on the blood flow through peripheral skeletal muscles. *Am. J. Phys. Med.*, **33**, 103–7.

Scowcroft A. T., Mason A. H. L., Hayne C. R. (1977). Safety with microwave diathermy: preliminary report of the CSP working party. *Physiotherapy*, **63**, 359–61.

Surrell J. A., Alexander R. C., Cohle S. D. *et al.* (1987). Effects of microwave radiation on living tissues. *J. Trauma*, **27**, 935–9.

Wadsworth H., Chanmugan A. P. P. (1980). *Electrophysical Agents in Physiotherapy*. Marricksville, NSW, Australia: Science Press.

Ward A. R. (1986). *Electricity Fields and Waves in Therapy*. Marrickville, NSW, Australia: Science Press.

Watson P. (1971). Microwave—their effects and safe use. *N.Z. J. Physiother.*, **4**, 20–24.

13. Infrared and visible radiations

INTRODUCTION

The spectrum of visible colours is found in a narrow band of wavelengths between 390 and 760 nm (see Frontispiece and Table 11.1). These wavelengths have enormously important biological effects. Photosynthesis in plants depends heavily on radiations in the red end of the spectrum and, most obviously to humans, the changes wrought in the cells of the retina allow colour to be distinguished. In fact this band of radiations is employed for the sense of sight by all animals with only minor differences of wavelength range. Infrared radiations are those of longer wavelength than the red end of the visible spectrum extending to the microwave region. It will be noticed that the boundary region between microwaves and infrared radiations—wavelengths of a few millimetres—is claimed by neither. This is simply due to these radiations not being typical; there is no hiatus in this region. Thus infrared radiations are said to extend from 760 nm to about 1 mm (Harlen, 1982)— 0.1 mm in Table 11.1 or 0.4 mm in other sources.

Infrared radiation can be subdivided into three regions—A, B and C

Electrotherapy explained

Table 13.1 Classification of infrared (IR) radiation

Type	Wavelengths	Former classification	Wavelengths	
IR A	760–1400 nm	Near IR	760–1500 nm	used in
IR B	1400–3000 nm	Far IR	1500–15 000 nm	therapy
IR C	3000 nm–1 mm			

(Harlen, 1982)—of which the first two are utilized therapeutically and correspond approximately to an older classification of 'near' and 'far' infrared (Table 13.1).

Infrared radiations are produced in all matter by various kinds of molecular vibration. Molecules altering shape due to some of the atoms moving apart and closer together without breaking free from one another can cause infrared emission. The various states of vibration and rotation that a given molecule may have can be altered by absorbed heat leading to the emission of many different wavelengths of infrared radiation. The result is that any heated body emits infrared radiations; indeed any material that is at a temperature above absolute zero emits infrared. Although the radiations will be of a whole range of different frequencies, the frequencies at which maximum radiations are emitted are proportional to temperature, thus the higher the temperature the higher the frequency and hence the shorter the wavelength. This has been described in Chapter 11, where the visible effect of increased heating leading to first red heat then white heat was considered. The fact that the wavelength of maximum production of radiation is inversely proportional to the absolute temperature of the source is called Wien's law. Thus for the human body with a skin temperature of around 30°C (303K; see Chapter 7) the peak emission is around 9500 nm in the long infrared region. At the higher temperature generated by a tungsten filament light bulb the peak emission is about 960 nm, i.e. in the near infrared, with plenty of emission in the visible region (see Fig. 14.3).

The shorter, visible radiations not only cause molecular and atomic motion but can also break chemical bonds when they are absorbed. It is this that provokes chemical changes in the retinal pigments which are detected in the optic nerve as sight. These and other chemical changes do not directly result in heat, unlike the atomic and molecular motion induced by infrared.

PRODUCTION OF INFRARED

As any heated material will produce infrared radiations, the wavelength being determined by the temperature, if near infrared is to be produced efficiently the material must not be oxidized (burnt) by the higher temperatures used. The most convenient method is to heat a resistance wire by passing an electric current through it. An ordinary household electric fire can be made of a coil of suitable resistance wire, such as nickel-chrome alloy, wound on a ceramic insulator.

Therapeutic infrared lamps

Different kinds of infrared lamps are used for therapy. One type is made in a similar way to an electric fire. In these heaters the wire glows red thus giving some radiations in the visible region but peak emission in the near infrared. The ceramic material, being heated to a lower temperature than the wire, gives only infrared and no visible radiations. Some infrared lamps for therapy have the wire embedded in the insulating ceramic (or porcelain or fireclay) so that no visible radiations are given out. The heater wire can also be mounted behind a metal plate or inside a metal tube which do not become red-hot but emit infrared in the same way. As such a lamp becomes hotter all the parts— the emitter, the metal plate on the end of the emitter, the protective wire mesh and the reflector—become heated giving off a range of wavelengths from near to far infrared.

The infrared emitter is placed at the focus of a hemispherical or parabolic reflector to reflect the radiations into an approximately uniform beam. Due to the relatively large size of the emitter compared to a conveniently sized reflector, and to prevent the risk of 'hot spots', the beam is made to diverge somewhat. The reflector and emitter are mounted on a strong, firmly supported metal stand which can be adjusted to alter the height and angle of the reflector/emitter. When such lamps are switched on they require some time to warm up because of the thermal inertia of the considerable mass of metal and insulating material that has to be heated; thus small lamps may take about 5 min but larger ones may take up to 15 min to reach maximum emission (Forster and Palastanga, 1985). Therefore before it is needed for treatment this type of lamp must have been switched on a sufficient time.

In spite of the fact that lamps with an exposed coil will give off a red glow they are collectively designated as 'non-luminous' sources to distinguish them from those that emit visible as well as infrared radiations; these are called 'luminous' lamps.

Luminous generators (incandescent lamps) consist of a tungsten filament in a large glass envelope which contains inert gas at low pressure. Part of the inside of the glass bulb is often silvered to provide a reflector. These lamps work on the same principle as a simple electric light bulb; the filament is heated to a high temperature (around 3000°C) by the current passed through it and so gives off a continuous spectrum in the infrared and visible regions. Oxidation of the filament does not occur because there is no oxygen present, only a trace of some inert gas. The peak emission occurs at near 1000 nm but radiation extends from the far infrared throughout the visible to the ultraviolet (see Fig. 14.3). These latter radiations are absorbed by the glass and are not therefore transmitted by the lamp (Ward, 1986). Sometimes the glass is reddened, absorbing some of the green and blue rays to give a red visible emission; this is believed to make little difference therapeutically (Lehmann and de Lateur, 1982). Luminous generators are sometimes called 'radiant heat' generators, indicating that heating is by both infrared and visible radiations.

The power of these sources varies. The smaller lamps, both luminous and non-luminous, are usually 250 to 500 W; large non-luminous ones are often either 750 or 1000 W while the larger luminous lamps are from 600 to 1500 W. Generally, the larger lamps are used to treat extensive areas but the same effect can be achieved by mounting three smaller luminous bulbs, which can be separately controlled in one holder. In this way a large area can be covered with all the bulbs in use and a small area using only one or two. In the interest of safety, large lamps are fitted with wire-mesh screens over the front of the reflector to prevent accidental contact with the hot emitter. The screen will also diminish any remote risk of the hot emitter element falling out on to patient or operator. (The fitting of these heating elements is of a screw-type or sometimes a special bayonet fitting as opposed to the ordinary two-peg bayonet fitting of household light bulbs. These are not easily dislodged by accident.)

Non-luminous infrared lamps emit most energy in the long infrared region, mainly around 3000 to 4000 nm, with only about 10% in the short infrared region between 1500 nm and the visible (Wadsworth and Chanmugan, 1980). Luminous lamps, on the other hand, emit about 70% in the short infrared with about 5% visible and the rest long infrared; also about 1% ultraviolet which is absorbed by the glass of the bulb (Wadsworth and Chanmugan, 1980).

ABSORPTION AND PENETRATION OF INFRARED AND VISIBLE RADIATIONS

Infrared radiations, up to about 20 000 nm, striking the body surface at or near the perpendicular, are effectively all absorbed (Ward, 1980). At exactly what depth the radiation is absorbed depends strongly on wavelength. Confusion sometimes arises because there is failure to recognize that the term 'penetration depth' has a defined meaning—the depth at which approximately 63% of the radiation energy has been absorbed—and is not the depth to which all radiations penetrate, or the depth beyond which none penetrate (see Chapter 11 and Fig. 11.4).

For most of the long infrared radiations penetration into the tissues is negligible. Around 3000 nm the penetration depth is about 0.1 mm while the longer infrared is largely absorbed by the water on the skin surface. Very long infrared—10 000–40 000 nm—has, like microwave, penetration depths of several centimetres. The short infrared and red end of the visible spectrum behave rather differently with gradually increasing penetration depths from 3000 to near 1200 nm. At around 1200 nm the penetration depth is of the order of a few millimetres (Ward, 1980) becoming less again in the visible range such that the red radiation penetrates well but the blue end is strongly absorbed (Table 13.2). This is demonstrated by putting a torch in the mouth and noting that only red light is transmitted through the cheek. It must be realized, however, that only a minute proportion of the original radiation is actually penetrating. The penetration depth also varies greatly with different relative thicknesses of skin and subcutaneous tissues which helps to account for the variation in quoted figures. Thus various sources give penetration depths of 1–2.5 mm (Laurens, 1933) or 0.36 mm (Nightingale, 1959) for near infrared. Modern sources suggest 1–2 mm (King, 1989) 2.5–5 mm (Gourgou-

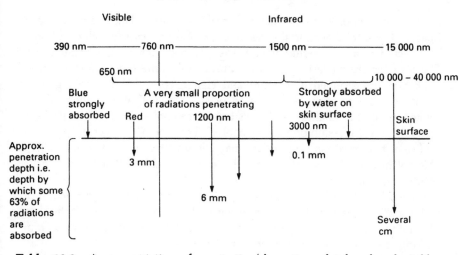

Table 13.2 A representation of penetration/absorption of infrared and visible radiations (not to scale).

liatos, 1990) for red light and near infrared, while infrared around 1200 nm has about twice this penetration depth.

Thus infrared radiation is characterized by being strongly absorbed near the skin surface; little radiation is reflected and only a small band of radiations, from 1500 nm in the near infrared to 650 nm in the visible, penetrates the tissues, and then only to a minor degree. The effect will therefore be marked heating of the skin. Some of this heat will be conducted to the subcutaneous tissues. This is the same as the situation of surface conduction heating, described in Chapter 8, and distinct from the diathermies (shortwave, microwave and ultrasound) which are able to pass the thermal barrier of the subcutaneous fat tissue.

PHYSIOLOGICAL EFFECTS

As a consequence of heating with infrared radiations local cutaneous vasodilation will occur. This is due to the liberation of chemical vasodilators, histamine and similar substances, as well as a possible direct effect on the blood vessels. The vasodilation starts after a short latent period of 1–2 min (Crockford and Hellon, 1959) and appears to be largely due to arteriolar vasodilation. This is evident from the nature of the erythema which develops with an irregular patchy appearance (quite unlike the erythema due to ultraviolet irradiation in which the capillaries are directly affected). The irregular margin of the erythema shows where some arterioles have dilated engorging the capillaries they supply while adjacent ones are unaffected. The rate at which the erythema develops and its intensity are related to the rate and degree of heating; for normal individuals heating the skin to about core temperature (37°C) over some 20 min will lead to very mild erythema; heating to around 42°C will lead to marked erythema. Reflex dilation of other cutaneous vessels will also occur in order to maintain a normal body heat balance, as discussed in Chapter 7. For mild heating the vasodilation of other parts, which could only be detected by a skin thermometer, is likely to begin after some 10 min or so. The local erythema lasts for some considerable time (about 30 min) after irradiation has stopped (Crockford and Hellon, 1959). With prolonged or intense heating sweating will start to occur. This will absorb some of the applied infrared irradiations and leads to surface cooling as it evaporates; see Chapter 7 for discussion on thermal control. This does not necessarily lead to inefficiency since cooling the surface may allow better penetration (Fig. 13.1). Thermal heat receptors will be stimulated in the skin so that the patient is aware of the heating.

Excessive and prolonged infrared application can cause the destruction of erythrocytes, releasing pigments and causing brown discoloration of the skin. This rarely occurs as a sequel to normal treatment; it usually results from prolonged exposure of the legs to domestic fires.

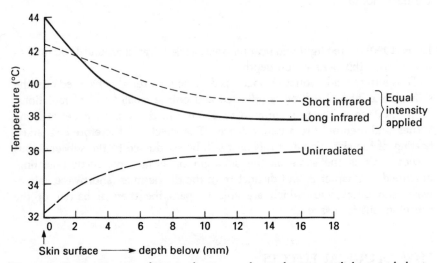

Fig. 13.1 Temperature gradient in the tissues due to heating with long and short infrared radiation. Modified from Nightingale (1959).

THERAPEUTIC USES OF INFRARED

Pain

Infrared is used therapeutically to relieve pain. The mechanisms by which this occurs could be the stimulation of sensory nerves in the skin leading to pain suppression by the pain gate mechanism (see Chapter 3) and also to a sedative effect (see Chapter 7 for discussion). Other suggestions that the increased blood flow may remove pain-provoking chemicals or that muscle spasm may be diminished and so reduce pain have also been advanced (Wadsworth and Chanmugan, 1980; Forster and Palastanga, 1985).

Muscle spasm

This is probably reduced as a consequence of the decreased pain, as there can only be very trivial direct muscle heating and only for the most superficial muscles. Muscles do seem to relax more readily with warmth and as pain and muscle spasm are so interdependent reduction of one leads to reduction of the other.

Acceleration of healing and repair

Application of infrared radiations to the surface of open wounds such as pressure sores or ulcers will dry the surface thus diminishing bacterial activity. It will also increase the superficial blood flow at least in the surrounding skin and increase all metabolic activities in the superficial tissues heated (Van't Hoff's law; see Chapter 7). Thus increased phagocytosis will occur with other defence and repair processes. Infrared is also used to encourage drainage and accelerate healing of skin abscesses and carbuncles. Red visible radiations have been reputed to accelerate wound healing for many years and there is some experimental evidence for this (see Chapter 14).

Prophylaxis of pressure sores

Infrared applied to areas of skin subjected to prolonged pressure or friction has been suggested in order to promote a greater blood flow in the skin and thus decrease the risk of skin breakdown. Since the vasodilation effect is temporary—it lasts perhaps 30–60 min after the application—it would need to be repeated at intervals.

Oedema of the extremities

Infrared has been recommended for the treatment of chronic oedema of the hand and foot (Wadsworth and Chanmugan, 1980). This must be given with the part in elevation since, as noted in Chapter 8, the application of superficial heating will tend to increase oedema if the part is dependent. Vessel dilation induced by heating will allow increased rates of fluid exchange and thus may help to increase the reabsorption of exudate. This effect is limited because infrared heats the superficial tissues and because it is usually only applied to one aspect at a time. Combining infrared radiation from several aspects with conduction heating, placing the elevated hand in a hot-air cabinet for example, is likely to be a more effective treatment. Heating the whole hand exploits the large surface area to volume ratio of the hand. Such heating arrangements coupled with active exercise are valuable in the treatment of hand injuries in general and those with an element of neurogenic pain, such as Sudeck's atrophy (post-traumatic osteodystrophy) in particular.

Skin diseases

Fungal infections which are difficult to control and thrive in moist conditions, e.g. paronychia, are sometimes treated with regular infrared therapy, usually as a home treatment. The proper application may be taught to the patient by the physiotherapist. The thorough drying of the skin surface coupled with local vasodilation seem to be the effective factors.

Infrared radiation has also been used in the treatment of psoriasis on the grounds that moderate hyperthermia can affect cell replication and therefore could benefit a hyperproliferative disease like psoriasis. Note that psoriasis is commonly and effectively treated with ultraviolet (see Chapter 15). A study involving a small number of patients (12) consisted of treatment with 30 min of infrared applied to both sides of the body at the highest tolerable temperature. Treatment was given 3 or 5 times per week for about 1 month and resulted in some remission for 8 of the 10 patients who completed the treatment (Westerhof *et al.*, 1987). Other methods of locally heating psoriasis, including conduction heating and ultrasound, have been described (Orenberg *et al.*, 1980).

As a precursor of other treatment

Infrared treatment is often used prior to other forms of treatment, e.g. muscle stretching, joint mobilization, massage or traction, in the belief that it will assist muscle relaxation and diminish pain. It is also used prior to exercise therapy for the pain-relieving effect and because it may contribute to muscle 'warm-up'. There is no evidence that muscle temperature or blood flow is increased to any significant extent by infrared radiation, unlike the diathermies.

Heating with infrared is also used prior to electrical stimulation, testing or biofeedback to warm the skin, making it more vascular and hence a better conductor; this is best before wetting the skin to lower its electrical resistance further.

EFFECTS AND USES OF VISIBLE RADIATIONS

Visible radiations are, by definition, able to stimulate the retinal cells of the eye. It is hardly surprising that simple exposure to light is considered to have some therapeutic effect. Some forms of depression have been found to be more evident during the darker winter months (seasonal affective disorder) and successful treatment consists of exposure to bright fluorescent lighting for a period every day (Wehr *et al.*, 1985).

The bile pigment, bilirubin, formed by the breakdown of haemoglobin can reach high levels in the blood of newborn babies leading to brain damage. This is called neonatal jaundice and is successfully treated by exposing the baby to blue light—ordinary fluorescent tubes may be used—in the region of 400–

450 nm. Any ultraviolet radiation is screened out. The beneficial effect seems to be due to the conversion of bilirubin to compounds which can be easily excreted.

Colour therapy, in which particular colours are applied or viewed for particular conditions, has a long history as alternative medicine in various forms. While there is no direct evidence of significant therapeutic effect an interesting association has been shown using electromyographic activity between viewing red light and greater maximum voluntary (hand-grip) contraction (Hasson *et al.*, 1989). It is speculated that seeing red light leads to arousal in the central nervous system and/or sympathetic stimulation (red for danger) and that the use of red in the treatment environment may increase muscle tone. Although blue light has been considered to have a calming effect, the study quoted above found no significant difference between the blue light and the controls.

CHOICE OF LUMINOUS (RADIANT HEAT) OR NON-LUMINOUS SOURCES

From the foregoing it is evident that the luminous (radiant heat) source is a more efficient tissue-heating source since it penetrates further (because peak emission is in the near infrared) and therefore the energy is distributed in a larger volume of tissue. Non-luminous radiation, on the other hand, with peak emission around 4000 nm is absorbed almost entirely in the skin. As the total heating is limited by the sensation felt by the patient, and thermal sense organs are close to the skin surface, it is evident that the non-luminous radiation will reach the limit of tolerable heating with a lower intensity than the luminous. These ideas are illustrated in Figure 13.1. It follows that if the desired effects are due to heating, the luminous near infrared source is preferred but if sensory stimulation is considered to be important then the non-luminous is most satisfactory. It is possible to achieve more even, deeper penetration by cooling the surface with a draught of cool air but the risks of burning may also be greater. Compare the similar mechanism for microwave (Chapter 12).

APPLICATION OF INFRARED RADIATION

If a non-luminous lamp is chosen it should be switched on up to 15 min before application to allow time for it to reach its maximum emission.

The patient is placed in a suitable, well supported position with the area to be treated exposed. The nature and effects of the treatment are explained to the patient, the skin to be treated is examined and the thermal sensation tested. If the eyes could be irradiated they are shielded. The lamp is positioned so that the radiations strike the surface at or near right angles to achieve maximum penetration, as described in Chapter 11. It is recommended (Wadsworth and Chanmugan, 1980) that the lamp is never positioned directly over the patient in case it tips over on to the patient or the element falls out. Both are unlikely with properly maintained lamps and reasonable care in positioning. Modern lamps are fitted with a protective mesh across the front to prevent contact with the bulb or element. The lamp is sited at an appropriate distance: about 60–75 cm for large 750 or 1000 W lamps and about 45–50 cm for the smaller ones. The luminous lamp is now switched on.

The heat sensation is described to the patient who is asked to indicate the amount of heat and the area in which it is felt. The intensity of heating is controlled by altering the position of the lamp, or on some by altering a resistance and hence the current to the luminous element. In spite of the reflector, radiations diverge considerably so that small changes of distance lead to quite large changes of intensity on the skin surface, described in Chapter 11 as the inverse square law. Adjustments are made to achieve the appropriate mild or moderate heating as reported by the patient. The patient is warned to report immediately if heating becomes more than a comfortable warmth as otherwise a burn could occur, and also not to touch any part of the lamp or to move during treatment.

Once the correct skin temperature is achieved the treatment is usually continued for about 20 min; it should be checked periodically as many lamps increase in output gradually over this time and may need to be adjusted. The 20-min treatment length is determined by the fact that it takes about this time for the vascular adjustments, noted above, to become complete.

At the end of treatment the skin should feel mildly or moderately warm and a moderate erythema should be evident. Skin temperatures of 36–38°C would be considered a mild treatment; the more usual moderate warmth gives skin temperatures of 38–41°C. The intensity of erythema does not necessarily parallel the skin temperature: some vasolabile individuals show a vivid erythema at quite moderate skin temperatures.

DANGERS WITH INFRARED TREATMENT

Burns

The most obvious danger is of a heat burn which occurs if the patient is unaware of the heat by reasons of defective sensation or reduced consciousness. Rarely, a mentally abnormal or perhaps masochistic patient may stoically tolerate painful and damaging levels of heat. Occasionally patients accidentally touch the hot element if there is no protective guard. These dangers can be avoided by careful application, adequate warnings to the patient and checking the effects on the skin (which is easily visible with this treatment) several times during the application. The suggestion, which is sometimes made, that the patient could be burnt if he or she fell asleep during treatment is more dubious. People have slept in front of powerful sources of infrared (open coal fires, gas and electric fires) over the centuries without being burnt except when consciousness was impaired, by alcohol or an epileptic episode, for example.

Burns can, of course, arise if the infrared lamp sets fire to some combustible material. Highly inflammable materials should not be in the region. Poor positioning of the lamp can lead to blankets or pillows being charred, but these should be of low flammability and thus relatively safe.

It has been suggested (Wadsworth and Chanmugan, 1980) that metal on the surface could cause a burn in the underlying skin. This will only be a danger if the metal itself becomes heated to the point at which contact with it is injurious. This is unlikely with the intensity and duration of most infrared treatments but it is a precautionary measure to remove surface metal from the area being irradiated. Additionally metal will reflect radiations and for that reason will lead to irregular application of infrared.

Skin irritation

Most acute inflammatory skin conditions are made worse by heating. Some chemical irritants on the skin have their effects increased by heating, sometimes to the point of irritation or inflammation. For this reason liniments which cause mild erythema (rubifacients) should be removed prior to treatment.

Lowered blood pressure

As infrared treatment causes marked cutaneous vasodilation it may lead to temporary lowering of blood pressure, particularly in elderly people who have less effective vasomotor control. This may lead to faintness especially on standing up immediately after treatment. It may also cause headache.

Areas of defective arterial blood flow

Areas in which the arteries and arterioles cannot respond by adequate vasodilation to the demands of additional heating should not be treated. Such areas would be those affected by arterial disease such as atherosclerosis, arterial injury or after skin-grafting. The possible result of heating such tissue would be tissue necrosis (gangrene).

Cataracts

Prolonged and extensive exposure to infrared, such as occurs in furnacemen, has been associated with the development of cataracts. This is not a significant danger for the usual lengths of treatment time. However, infrared applied to the eyes causes surface drying, hence irritation, and should be avoided.

Dehydration

Prolonged and intensive treatment to large body areas could cause sufficient sweating, leading to dehydration if the water is not replaced.

CONTRAINDICATIONS

1 Impaired cutaneous thermal sensation.
2 Defective arterial cutaneous circulation.
3 Patients whose level of consciousness is markedly lowered by drugs or disease.
4 Acute skin disease—dermatitis or eczema.
5 Skin damage due to deep X-ray therapy or other ionizing radiation.
6 Patients whose blood pressure regulation is defective.
7 Acute febrile illness—additional heating is not helpful and possibly dangerous to patients whose heat regulation system is under stress.
8 Tumours of the skin may be stimulated to increased growth.

REFERENCES

Crockford G. W., Hellon R. F. (1959). Vascular responses of human skin to infra-red radiation. *J. Physiol.*, **149**, 424–32.
Forster A., Palastanga N. (1985). *Clayton's Electrotherapy: Theory and Practice* 9th edn. London: Baillière Tindall.
Gourgouliatos Z. (1990). Application of the Monte Carlo model in the investigation of the direct penetration of light produced by single and multiple wavelength diode cluster probes. The 4th International Biotherapy Laser Association. Seminar on Laser Biomodulation, Guy's Hospital, London.
Harlen F. (1982). Physics of infrared and microwave therapy. In *Physics in Physiotherapy* (Docker M. F., ed.) London: Hospital Physicists Association Conference report series 35, p. 18.
Hasson S. M., Williams J. H., Gadberry W., Henrich T. (1989). Viewing low and high wavelength light. Effect on EMG activity and force production during maximal voluntary handgrip contraction. *Physiother. Canada*, **41**, 32–5.
King P. R. (1989). Low level laser therapy—a review. *Laser in Medical Science*, **4**, 141–150.
Laurens H. (1933). *The Physiological Effects of Radiant Energy*. New York: Chemical Catalog.
Lehmann J. F., de Lateur B. J. (1982). Therapeutic heat. In *Therapeutic Heat and Cold* (Lehmann J. F., ed.) pp. 404–562. Baltimore: Williams & Wilkins.
Nightingale A. (1959). *Physics and Electronics in Physical Medicine*. London: G. Bell.
Orenberg, E. K., Deneau D. G., Farber E. M. (1980). Response of chronic psoriatic plaques to localized heating induced by ultrasound. *Arch. Dermatol.*, **116**, 893–7.
Wadsworth H., Chanmugan A. P. P. (1980). *Electrophysical Agents in Physiotherapy: Therapeutic and Diagnostic Use*. Marrickville, NSW: Science Press.
Ward A. (1980). *Electricity Fields and Waves in Therapy*. Marrickville, NSW, Australia: Science Press.
Wehr J. A., Rosenthall N. E., Sack D. A. (1985). Role of light in the cause and treatment of seasonal depression. *Photochem. Photobiol.*, **41** (suppl), 45.
Westerhof W., Siddiqui A. H., Cormane R. H., Scholter A. (1987). Infrared hyperthermia and psoriasis. *Arch. Dermatol. Res.*, **279**, 209–10.

14.   *Laser therapy*

INTRODUCTION

The word *laser* is an acronym for light amplification by the stimulated emission of radiation. It refers to the production of a beam of radiation which differs from ordinary light in the following ways:

1 *Monochromaticity*: lasers are of a single specific wavelength and hence of a defined frequency. In the case of visible lasers a single pure colour is produced, e.g. ruby lasers give a red light at 694.3 nm (Table 14.1). Lasers

Table 14.1 Examples of lasers

Laser type		Wavelength (nm)	Radiation
Ruby		694.3	Red light
Helium–neon		632.8	Red light
Gallium aluminium arsenide diodes	Continuous wave	650	Red light
		750	Red light
		780	Infrared
		810	Infrared
		820	Infrared
		850	Infrared
		1300	Infrared
	Pulsed injection	860	Infrared
		904	Infrared
Carbon dioxide		10 000	Infrared

are a more efficient way of producing monochromatic radiation than other methods which depend on absorbing the unwanted wavelengths. Single-wavelength laser radiation is also referred to as monochromatic in the infrared and ultraviolet regions, despite being invisible.

2 *Coherence*: laser radiation is not only of the same wavelength but also in phase, that is to say the peaks and troughs of the electric and magnetic fields all occur at the same time. This is called 'temporal coherence'. Furthermore they are all travelling in the same direction; this is called 'spatial coherence'.

3 *Collimation*: as a consequence of spatial coherence lasers remain in a parallel beam. Because the radiations do not diverge the energy is propagated over very long distances. This property makes it invaluable for measurement and aiming purposes.

The analogy is often made between lasers and an army of soldiers marching in step, in the same direction and wearing the same uniform.

When lasers interact with matter the effects are the same as any other equivalent electromagnetic radiation—reflection, refraction, absorption and hence scattering. In this way collimation and coherence are diminished or lost. The extent to which this happens will depend on the nature and density of matter present so that lasers will pass unaffected through space and be only slightly altered in air (for visible radiations) but be markedly altered on entering a more dense material such as the tissues.

The production of lasers involves the storage of energy in the atoms of the material and this can be released as an extremely short, almost instantaneous, pulse of energy. The laser can also be focused like any radiation, which means that the intensity or power density (W per cm^2) can be very high. It can therefore be used to deliver large amounts of energy to a small region over a very short time. However lasers are not notably efficient, the best only convert some 20% of the energy that powers them into laser radiation and many less than 1% (Hecht, 1989).

When laser radiation is absorbed by the tissues it will cause heating if it is of sufficient intensity, but it is also considered to have specific biological effects due to the special nature of laser radiation.

Principles of lasers

It will be recalled that electrons of an individual atom exist as a 'cloud' of negative charges circling the positively charged nucleus. According to quantum theory electrons can only occupy certain energy levels or 'shells' around the nucleus. The electrons in the outermost orbit or shell are most easily affected by outside forces. If the atom is given additional energy, say by heating, these outer electrons can be made to occupy higher energy levels and if enough energy is added to the atom an outer electron may gain enough energy to detach itself, freeing itself from the pull of the nucleus. The atom then becomes a positively charged ion and the electron is a free negative charge. (The amount of energy needed to remove an electron is called the ionization energy and is measured in electron-volts; it is different for each kind of atom.) When the outer electrons are in one of the higher energy states but not free from the atom, they will always tend to return to a lower energy state, sometimes to their lowest energy state which is the most stable and is known as the ground state (Fig. 14.1). An electron may do this by cascading down from one energy level to the next or it may jump directly to the ground state. In all cases the additional energy from the higher energy levels must be given up and this is done by giving off a photon (quantum) of radiation (Fig. 14.2). Each step from one energy level to the next is known as a transition and the wavelength (and thus the frequency) of the emitted photon depends on the energy difference between the two energy levels; the more the energy difference, the shorter the wavelength and higher the frequency. (A photon of red light, for example, has an energy of about 2 eV; Silfvast, 1973.)

While an electron is in a higher energy state the atom is said to be excited and this state will last a very short time, characteristically about 10^{-8} s, before

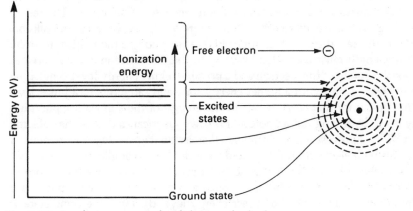

Fig. 14.1 An electron energy level diagram for hydrogen.

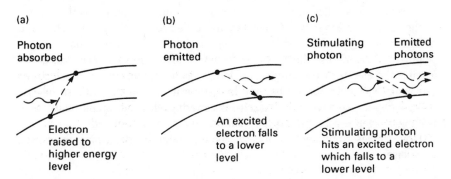

Fig. 14.2 Absorption and emission of photons. (a) Absorption; (b) spontaneous emission; (c) stimulated emission.

the electron falls to a lower energy level emitting a photon. There are some excitation levels in all atoms from which electrons cannot easily leave spontaneously but need to give up their energy on collision with other atoms. Such electrons remain in their higher energy state for much longer average times, e.g. 0.001 s $(10^{-3}$ s) and are referred to as being metastable states (Silfvast, 1973).

Energy can be introduced into matter in various ways. Heat, for example, leads to molecular collisions which alters the complex energy levels sustained by molecular interaction causing excitation. Electrons falling back to their stable states emit photons at numerous different wavelengths giving a continuous spectrum in the infrared and visible spectrum (i.e. the way infrared lamps work). An electric charge applied to a gas of a single element causes collisions of atoms with ions. This causes certain permitted transitions (allowed for that particular element) so that electrons returning to their ground state emit photons of a few particular or characteristic wavelengths only, hence a line spectrum. Now photons themselves, if absorbed, can give energy to the atom causing excitation. Sometimes the excited electron falls to the ground state emitting a photon of less energy (longer wavelength) than the exciting radiation in a process called fluoresence; see Chapter 11. (The rest of the energy is transferred to other atoms or molecules by vibration or collision; this is called radiationless transitions.) For absorption of the photon to occur its wavelength must correspond exactly to the difference in energy between the existing state of the electron and a possible higher energy level. Similarly if the electron is already in a higher energy state and can move to a lower level with a difference that corresponds to the energy of the stimulating photon it may do so by giving out a photon of its own identical to that of the colliding photon. This process is called stimulated emission (Fig. 14.2c). A large number of atoms with electrons in the excited state can lead to amplification since one photon releases a second and these two can release two more and so on—a kind of cascade or avalanche effect. Such a system can only emit photons if there are more electrons at a higher energy level than in the ground state. If this does not occur all the photons released from electrons falling from high-energy states are absorbed in the molecules, raising the energy of electrons in the low-energy (ground) state. Having more atoms in the upper energy state than the lower is called 'population inversion', simply because it is the reverse of the usual situation in which there are more electrons in the ground state and at lower energy levels. For lasers to operate it is necessary to have such a population inversion which can be achieved under some circumstances by forcing the electrons of many atoms into their metastable state. As electrons remain in this state for a relatively long time it is possible, with an intense energy input, to have more electrons entering the metastable state than leaving it. Hence a temporary population inversion is achieved.

How the laser apparatus works will be illustrated by describing the pulsed ruby laser.

The ruby laser

This consists of a small synthetic ruby rod made of aluminium oxide with a trace of chromium oxide; it is about 10 cm long and about 1 cm in diameter. A helical xenon flash tube is wound around it. This latter is an electric discharge tube which will give an intense flash of white light. Both ends of the rod are made flat and silvered to provide a reflecting surface; one end is totally reflecting and the other partially transparent so that some radiation can be emitted.

A brief light pulse, e.g. 0.5 ms, is provided by the xenon flash tube which excites the ruby molecules and raises many electrons to higher energy levels which they occupy for very short average times before falling to the metastable level where they remain for much longer average times. Thus, for a time, there are more electrons in the metastable level than the ground level and so population inversion has occurred. When the transition from metastable to ground state does occur a photon with a wavelength of 694.3 nm is emitted. This photon would have exactly the right energy to raise a ground state electron to the metastable level and be reabsorbed but as there are relatively few ground-state electrons the photon is much more likely to interact with other metastable electrons, stimulating them to return to the ground state and so emitting an identical photon. The process rapidly accelerates as more and more photons are released; i.e. stimulated emission of radiation occurs. The photons, having a wavelength of 694.3 nm, which is of course red light, are reflected up and down the short ruby rod, rapidly increasing the effect so that all the energy stored in the ruby molecules is released in a very brief time, as a pulse of red light of identical photons and so of a single wavelength of coherent radiation: this emerges from the rod at the partially transparent end (see Holwill and Silvester, 1973).

Measurement of laser energy

Energy is expressed in joules and the amount of energy falling on a surface is expressed in joules per square metre (J/m^2) or joules per square centimetre (J/cm^2), so often termed energy density.

The rate at which laser energy is produced is measured in joules per second, hence in watts (1 W = 1 J/s). Most lasers used in physiotherapy have output powers of milliwatts; see Table 14.2.

If the laser is pulsed the temporal average power must be distinguished from the temporal peak power (see discussion in Chapter 10). The temporal peak power is that of each pulse but the average or mean power depends on the pulse length and the pulse frequency. To express the average power per unit area the term 'power density' is sometimes used. This would be given in watts per square centimetre or per square metre.

The divergence of the laser beam may also be described in terms of an angle, expressed in degrees.

Table 14.2 Classification of lasers

Effect	Number	Range of power	Usage
No effect on eye or skin	1 2	Low power	Blackboard pointer Supermarket barcode reader
Safe on skin, not on eye	3A 3B	Mid power	Therapeutic—physiother-apy models; up to 50 mW mean power (physiotherapy with 3A and 3B lasers is also called low-level laser therapy; LLLT)
Unsafe on eye and skin	4	High power	Surgical—destructive

The uses of lasers

The idea of a 'magic ray' which can be used for destruction at a distance has long been part of science fiction. This has, perhaps, led to certain expectations concerning the properties and destructive power of lasers. Certainly large quantities of energy can be applied to small areas and transmitted through space but a major use has been in ranging and measurement. The fact that radiations are held in a narrow parallel beam has allowed the laser to be used for making extremely accurate measurements over considerable distances; thus it is used for the precise alignment of bridges and tunnels and perhaps most dramatically, making exact measurements of the distance between the earth and the moon.

The moon-landing on 20 July 1969 allowed a reflector to be positioned on the moon that would greatly increase (by 10–100 times) the amount of laser energy reflected back to earth. Later that year the time taken for laser pulses fired at the moon to return to earth was accurately timed. It takes about 2.5 s for the radiations to travel the 240 000 miles (380 000 km) to the moon and back again. Knowing the velocity of light (299 792 500 m/s), it was possible to calculate the distance to an accuracy of about 15 cm (Faller and Wampler, 1970).

In medicine lasers have been used for heating very small precise areas. Thus they are used to 'weld' back detached retinas as well as for surgical incisions and tumour destruction.

Low-power lasers which cause no significant heating are used in physiotherapy.

Modern laser technology is widely used for information processing and handling such as some computer printers for fibreoptic telephone links. In these, laser pulses encode the signal and boost it as it is transmitted hundreds or thousands of miles. There is now even a transatlantic fibreoptic telephone line.

In the home, compact disc audio players use small semiconductor lasers focused on a tiny area of the reflective disc.

Lasers are also used in industry to make controlled cuts in metals and other materials.

Military uses of lasers include many aiming devices for bombs and missiles as well as the dramatic use of very powerful lasers to shoot down enemy missiles. An infrared laser that generates more than 2 MW for a few seconds is currently under development in the USA for this purpose (Hecht, 1989).

Types of low- and mid-power lasers

Helium–neon lasers

Helium–neon lasers consist of a long tube containing these natural gases at low pressure surrounded by a flashgun tube, as described for the ruby laser. Excitation of these atoms leads to different energy levels between them and the transfer of energy, giving off a photon of wavelength equivalent to the energy gap. These photons are reflected to and fro along the tube giving rise to further photon emission and emerging as a narrow beam (of about 1 mm diameter) from the partially transparent end. Helium–neon lasers give radiation in the red visible region at 632.8 nm (see Fig. 14.3 for comparison of helium–neon laser output with the infrared lamp). The output is usually applied to the tissues via an optical guide—a fibreoptic cable—the end of which is held in contact with the tissues. There are, of course, some energy losses in the glass fibre of the cable and the laser beam may diverge somewhat as it emerges at the end of the optical fibre.

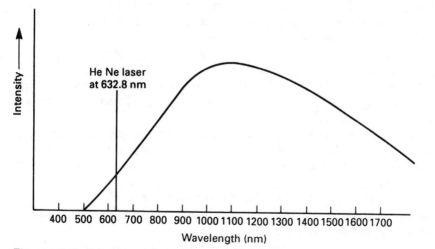

Fig. 14.3 Comparison of laser output with infrared lamp. (Infrared and visible radiations were emitted from typical luminous infrared lamp giving radiations at a range of wavelengths; peak emission around 1000 nm.)

Electrotherapy explained

Semiconductor diode lasers

These are of various kinds, involving gallium aluminium arsenide (GaAlAs). In these, electrons can flow more readily in one direction than in the other (see Chapter 3). The electrons are excited by the application of a suitable electrical potential and their occupation of 'holes' in the crystal lattice arrangement may lead to the emission of a photon which may then stimulate identical photons in the manner already described. The photons are reflected to and fro and emitted as a laser beam from one partially transparent end. Such devices, which are relatively cheap to make, extremely robust and conveniently small, are becoming more widely used.

Perhaps the greatest asset of these devices is the fact that some types can be made to emit laser beams at a range of different wavelengths. Gallium aluminium arsenide can be built to give specific wavelengths by varying the ratio of gallium to aluminium and constructing the diode in a precisely controlled manner (called molecular beam epitaxy). In this way laser diodes have been made that will emit at a whole range of wavelengths (see Table 14.1).

Semiconductor laser diodes can give either a continuous or a pulsed output. Continuous wave diode lasers are usually of relatively low power, i.e. a few milliwatts. They can be made to give up to 200 mW but are expensive to make for higher-power operation. Alternatively they can be pulsed electronically; that is, the continuous output is divided into a series of pulses each having the same low power as the continuous emission.

Pulsed injection laser diodes have high peak power outputs but relatively low average power. The average power is altered by changing the pulsing frequency. King (1989) comments that peak power, although of interest for some applications, tells us nothing about average power even if the pulse length is known, because the peak power is attained for only a fraction of the total pulse length. Some studies have compared different pulse frequencies but have used a constant pulse power and thus different average powers, invalidating any conclusions (King, 1989).

Due to their small size semiconductor lasers can be applied directly to the tissues in a hand-held applicator.

Sometimes several laser diodes of assorted wavelengths are mounted together to form an emitter which can be used to treat a larger area. These are known as 'cluster probes'.

For all these forms of low-power laser a suitable electronic circuit is provided to generate the appropriate current intensities to drive the laser diode or power the flashtube. Pulsing and timing are also done electronically on the principles considered in Chapter 3.

Carbon dioxide lasers are used to produce high-intensity laser beams (up to 20 000 W) in the infrared region around 10 000 nm. These are used surgically for tumour destruction.

EFFECTS OF LASERS ON THE TISSUES

The interaction of lasers with the tissues is essentially the same as any other radiation in that it can be reflected from the surface or penetrate the tissues in proportions that depend on the angle of incidence, the wavelength of the radiation and the nature of the tissues. When the radiation is applied at right angles to and in contact with the surface, reflection is at a minimum so penetration is maximized (see Chapter 11).

Once any radiation enters the tissues it can be absorbed or transmitted further in proportions which depend on the wavelength and nature of the tissues. The penetration depth (i.e. the depth to which some 37% of radiations penetrate) of red visible and near infrared radiation is considered to be a few millimetres. It is sometimes stated that for monochromatic radiations the penetration depths are greater: red visible is considered to have a penetration depth of 3–7 mm and near infrared of wavelength 800–900 nm about 30–40 mm (cf. Table 13.2). The suggestion is that coherent lasers penetrate further than non-coherent infrared but as coherence is lost on entering the tissues (see below) there seems to be no evidence to support this point. In an excellent authoritative review of the subject King (1989) concludes that the penetration depth of red light in soft tissue is about 1–2 mm and about 2–4 mm for infrared of 800–900 nm. It is considered that 1% or so of the energy may penetrate to 5–10 mm and hence only a tiny fraction to 30–40 mm.

Radiation entering the tissues may be reflected and refracted at various interfaces beneath the skin which will lead to scattering and loss of penetration. This occurs much more easily when the radiations are not applied at a right angle, when refraction may occur.

Different wavelengths have different penetration depths so it is possible to adjust the relative amounts of energy absorbed at different depths by selecting an appropriate wavelength. Thus radiations which penetrate furthest, i.e. those in the near infrared, such as 904 nm, are chosen to treat deeply placed structures, whereas skin lesions or superficial wound surfaces are appropriately treated by one of the red lasers which will be absorbed largely in the skin.

Since the beam of radiations is very narrow—often about 2 or 3 mm—treatment can only be applied to a small zone of tissue at a time. Although the radiations diverge somewhat in the tissues with distance and considerable scattering, the area treated must still be fairly small. Treatment therefore involves a series of separate applications at discrete points, each for fairly short periods of a few seconds to a few minutes. The cluster probe, already mentioned, treats larger areas if required, the area between the diodes is treated because of the scattering (Gourgouliatos, 1990). Scanning lasers can also be used to increase the area irradiated.

As noted already the laser may be applied as a continuous output or pulsed at different frequencies. The pulsing frequency can be varied and is considered by some to be an important parameter of treatment (see below). The pulse length can vary although it may be fixed for a particular machine; it is often of the order of 100–200 ns. Although each pulse may have a few watts power (some are of 5 or 6 W) the average power is very low at less than 1 mW because of the extremely short pulses. Continuous-output low-power laser sources usually emit around 1 mW. Therefore in all cases there is insufficient energy introduced into the tissues to cause detectable heating.

THERAPEUTIC USES OF LASERS

There are two major areas for which laser therapy is used: tissue healing and pain control. Currently the efficacy of the former appears to be better supported than that of the latter.

Tissue healing

The use of radiations of all kinds to accelerate wound healing has a long history but radiations in the red part of the visible spectrum have been particularly employed and found to be effective. In fact it is suggested (Karu, 1987) that the advent of the helium–neon laser led to the rediscovery of the therapeutic benefit of 'red light therapy', at least in respect of accelerating tissue healing. The observed benefit of laser therapy has been attributed to its coherence but this idea is not supported by the evidence (Karu, 1987). However Colver and Priestley (1989) found a failure of the helium–neon laser to affect components of wound healing *in vitro*.

One of the major determinants of accelerated wound healing is probably wavelength. The evidence relating wavelength of radiation to specific biological effects is extensive, covering tissue and cellular experiments in the laboratory, but it is inconsistent. However, Young *et al.* (1989) showed that 660, 820 and 870 nm wavelengths encouraged macrophages to release factors that stimulated fibroblast proliferation above the control levels whereas the 880 nm wavelength was inhibitory. Only the 820 nm wavelength was coherent and polarized, showing that at certain wavelengths coherence and polarization are not essential. In general, it seems that responses to visible radiations occur at both cellular and organismal levels; that laser stimulation is of a photobiological nature and that effects are due to both coherent and non-coherent radiation (Karu, 1987).

Another important factor is pulse frequency. Dyson and Young (1986) found that when using a Space Mix 5 laser (combined infrared at 904 nm 200 ns pulses and helium–neon at 632.8 nm) on surgical skin lesions of mice, there was greater wound contraction at 700 Hz infrared pulse frequency compared to 1200 Hz. By 11 days after injury there was greater cellularity and more and better organized fibroblasts in the 700 Hz group. King (1989) draws attention to the fact that no significant differences in contraction were found on many days in the time series.

Additional factors involved in the acceleration of wound healing by laser may include a marked increase in collagen formation, vasodilation and DNA synthesis (Mester *et al.*, 1985) and an increase in RNA production (Gamaleya, 1977).

Laser treatment is recommended for the treatment of indolent wounds and trophic ulcers to promote more rapid healing and it is considered that low-intensity visible radiation has an effect in accelerating or stimulating cell proliferation. In such wounds cell proliferation may be inhibited by low oxygen concentration, abnormal pH or other abnormality such as deficiency of nutrients. In these circumstances light may act as a signal to increase proliferation. Any physiotherapeutic effect may be much less evident, or non-existent if the wound is healing at the optimum rate (Karu, 1987).

Pain control

Laser therapy is used for the relief of pain in many conditions, both acute and long-term (England, 1988). Rheumatoid arthritis, osteoarthritis, bursitis and various aspects of back pain (nerve inflammation, muscle spasm, osteophytosis) are found to have benefited from laser treatment (Seitz and Kleinkort, 1986). The laser treatment of rheumatoid arthritis has also been studied by Colov *et al.* (1987) and was found to have a significant pain-relieving effect and reduction of joint swelling as well as objective improvement in hand function (Goldman *et al.*, 1980).

Neurogenic pain (trigeminal, postherpetic neuralgia and others) has been found to be relieved in some patients by laser applications (Walker, 1983). This was thought to be due to the laser affecting serotonin metabolism.

Pain is also often treated by application of the laser source to trigger or acupuncture points (Ong, 1986), both on their own and in conjunction with local treatment. Such points show a lower than normal skin resistance when tested with a small current (see Chapter 3). It is further considered that resolution of the condition is associated with a return to normal skin resistance. A randomized, double-blind study (Snyder-Mackler *et al.*, 1986) of the skin resistance over trigger points before and after three successive treatments of helium–neon laser showed a statistically significant increase in skin resistance after treatment. This suggests that the laser treatment has some therapeutic effect on the underlying musculoskeletal trigger point and may aid resolution of the pathological condition. In two groups of healthy subjects given therapy to auricular acupuncture points, an increase in pain threshold at the wrist was found only in those treated with laser (King *et al.*, 1990).

There is also a considerable body of experimental work which has found no effect from laser applications; for further reading see King (1989).

Other therapeutic effects

Low-power laser therapy has been used for other therapeutic effects both clinically and experimentally. For example, fracture consolidation has been found to be accelerated (Trelles and Mayayo, 1981) and post-traumatic nerve degeneration prevented (Nissan *et al.*, 1986; Schwartz *et al.*, 1984). An investigation of nerve conduction latency, amplitude and temperature around the nerve (Greathouse *et al.*, 1985) could find no change as a consequence of either 20- or 120-s infrared laser application. However recent studies (Baxter *et al.*, 1990) found a small but reproducible, increase in nerve conduction latency due to laser irradiation at therapeutic doses in humans. Such an effect can hardly be due to heating—which would decrease nerve latency—and could perhaps account for the analgesic effects claimed for laser therapy.

PRINCIPLES OF APPLICATION

Most low- or medium-power laser sources are applied to the skin by a hand-held applicator about the size of a large marker pen. The laser diode is close to the tip, which is a small lens. The applicator is sometimes called a wand (the association with magic is presumably unintentional!). In other types of laser the applicator may be held in a rigid but mobile stand and applied about 30 cm away from the patient. This latter type may provide several sources of laser output to cover a relatively large area. In one type, a helium–neon red light laser is allowed to emit a beam spreading to a circular area of some 10 cm diameter into which five infrared lasers are directed, giving a large treatment area (Forster and Palastanga, 1985). Some versions use laser diodes, called cluster diodes, which all emit at different wavelengths to take advantage of any different effects that may ensue from the use of different wavelengths.

The position of the patient should be chosen so that the area to be treated is accessible and supported. The surface of the skin to be treated should be inspected and cleaned with an alcohol wipe. The nature of the treatment and the need to wear goggles are explained to the patient. Protective goggles or spectacles are usually worn to obviate any risk of accidental application of the laser beam into the eye (see below).

A key usually activates the machine and ensures that unauthorized people do not switch the laser on. The laser applicator is applied to the surface before switching on. There is sometimes a switch on the applicator itself and usually an indicator light to show that the infrared laser—which is, of course, invisible—is on. It is important to maintain the laser applicator in contact with the tissues so that the beam is applied at right angles in order to achieve maximal penetration.

If contact is not desired, for example because of an infected wound, the applicator may be held just off the surface or covered with transparent non-reflective film. In all other circumstances firm contact should be maintained throughout treatment but should not provoke pain where tenderness is present. The position is maintained for the necessary time. If a larger area is to be treated the applicator is removed and repositioned on a new site, turning off the output during the transfer.

DOSAGE

The treatment dose is in terms of J/cm^2 or mJ/cm^2, i.e. the energy density. (1 J = 1 Ws or 1000 mWs). If the mean power output is given in milliwatts the required number of joules can be given by applying the laser for the appropriate time, e.g. 20 mW for 50 s is 1 J of energy. It is important to differentiate between power output at the source and power density, which is the wattage per square centimetre. If power output alone is given this must be divided by the area of the beam at its source. For example, if mean power output = 10 mW and area of beam is 0.125 cm^2, 10/0.125 = 80 mW/cm^2 (power density). Therefore, energy density = 80 mW/cm^2 × 60 s (say) = 4800 mJ/cm^2 or 4.8 J/cm^2.

There is wide variation in the recommendations for the optimal energy for different conditions. The usual ranges are from 1 to 10 J/cm^2 but doses as low as 0.5 J/cm^2 and up to 24 J/cm^2 have been suggested. Mester *et al.* (1985) suggested that there was a 'saturation energy density of 4 J/cm$^{2'}$ in open wound experiments. Higher doses are usually recommended for subcutaneous tissues. Some machines have variable power outputs; others are fixed.

Half-value depths and penetration depths, which have specific meanings, are not usually stated for lasers and their 'penetration powers' are rather ambiguous, as discussed earlier. England (1988) states that the human epidermis appears to absorb 99% of laser radiation, varying with skin pigmentation but Diamantopoulos (personal communication) gives the absorption figures as 80% in the dermis with 20% reaching the subcutaneous tissue, suggesting that the surface energy density is multiplied by 5 (i.e. 5 times the time required at the surface) to achieve a comparable dose in the subcutaneous tissues.

Where pulsed lasers are concerned, the pulse frequency has to be considered. On some machines the mean power output is always the same regardless of pulse frequency. This is achieved by adjusting the pulse width so that the low pulse rates have long pulse lengths and the high rates have shorter pulse lengths. It is generally recommended that the low pulse frequencies are used for acute conditions and the higher ones for chronic conditions but note that on machines where the mean power output is said to be constant the energy introduced into the tissues will not be altered by this pulsing difference. Where the duty cycle (percentage of time the laser is on) varies, the mean power will also vary as the same proportion (i.e. as the duty cycle) of peak power. The arguments for pulsed versus continuous beam lasers are similar to those for ultrasound except there is no heating effect from therapeutic mid-power lasers.

For wounds and large areas, the part is divided into centimetre squares (like a grid) and each area is separately stimulated, or a scanning technique may be used in which the laser is moved continuously over the wound surface; adequate dosage is achieved, it is suggested, because granulation tissue has higher absorption than intact skin (Ohshiro and Calderhead, 1988). Alternatively the healthy skin at the edge of the wound can be stimulated with a series of applications at 1–2 cm lengths.

Painful areas are usually treated at the point of maximal pain, for example, a trigger or acupuncture point (Ong, 1986). If possible pain relief should be obtained during the treatment. When treating chronic lesions it is possible to provoke an exacerbation of pain. The part probably should not be treated with laser again until this reaction has subsided. The subsequent dose should be either reduced or repeated if the exacerbation was not too severe.

Discrete lesions should obviously be treated directly over the affected part. It is sometimes advised that neurogenic lesions should be initially treated with low doses as a reaction can be pronounced. Usually contractures and scars require higher doses, e.g. at least 3 J/cm^2.

If there is no response to treatment the dose should be increased. Five to six treatments are said to be sufficient to establish some response to treatment.

DANGERS AND CONTRAINDICATIONS

The main danger involving low-level laser therapy is a risk of eye damage if the beam is applied directly into the eye. As therapeutic lasers have very little power there is normally no thermal effect when it is applied to the skin. However if it passes through the lens of the eye, the beam can become focused on a very small area, causing intense heating. Various reported studies on rabbits and monkeys (Seitz and Kleinkort, 1986) have indicated that this mechanism does cause burns of the retina but that at least 7 mW power at the cornea was needed to produce irreversible damage in monkeys. Although the risk to humans would seem to be small, shining a laser into the eye or looking directly into the laser beam should be strictly avoided.

It must also be recognized that the laser beam can be almost totally reflected from any shiny surfaces. It is recommended that reflecting surfaces should be removed from the area or covered. The laser beam should only be switched on when the applicator is in contact with the skin; some units have a switch on the applicator itself to facilitate this. Further precautions include wearing protective goggles. Treatment in a well lighted area, to ensure constriction of the pupil and thus diminish the amount of radiation that could enter the eye, is also recommended. Some authorities require a notice to be on display outside the immediate treatment area warning that a laser is in use.

Direct treatment of neoplastic tissue should be avoided on the grounds that cell stimulation may occur leading to increased rates of growth or metastases.

In the interests of prudence the use of lasers over the unclosed fontanelle of infants and over the pregnant uterus should be avoided (Seitz and Kleinkort, 1986) but there is no evidence that damage could occur in either brain or fetal tissue.

It the applicator is used in contact with infected skin areas it will need to be cleaned and sterilized with a suitable solution after use.

Treatment over the cardiac region of patients with pacemakers should be avoided (Forster and Palastanga, 1985) but the reason for this are not clear.

England (1988) added venous thrombosis, phlebitis and arterial disease to the list of areas to be avoided.

REFERENCES

Baxter G. D., Bell A. J., Allen J. M. *et al.* (1990). Laser mediated increase in median nerve conduction velocities. The 4th International Biotherapy Laser Association. Seminar on Laser Biomodulation, Guy's Hospital, London.

Colov H. C., Palmgren N., Jenson G. F. *et al.* (1987). Convincing clinical improvement of rheumatoid arthritis by soft laser therapy. *Lasers Surg. Med.*, **7**, 77.

Colver G. B., Priestley G. C. (1989). Failure of a helium–neon laser to affect components of wound healing in vitro. *Br. J. Dermatol.*, **121**, 179–86.

Dyson M., Young S. (1986). Effects of laser therapy on wound contraction and cellularity in mice. *Lasers Med. Sci.*, **1**, 125.

England S. (1988). Introduction to mid laser therapy. *Physiotherapy*, **74**, 100–2.

Faller J. E., Wampler E. J. (1970). The lunar laser reflector. *Sci. Am.*, **222**, 38–49.

Forster A., Palastanga N. (1985). *Clayton's Electrotherapy: Theory and Practice*. Eastbourne: Baillière Tindall.

Gamaleya N. F. (1977). Laser biomedical research. In *Tae-MSSR Laser Applications in Medicine and Biology*. New York: Plenum Press.

Goldman J. A., Chiapella J., Casey H. (1980). Laser therapy on rheumatoid arthritis. *Lasers Surg. Med.*, **1**, 93–101.

Gourgouliatos Z. (1990). Application of the Monte Carlo model in the investigation of the direct penetration of light produced by single and multiple wavelength diode cluster probes. The 4th International Biotherapy Laser Association. Seminar on Laser Biomodulation, Guy's Hospital, London.

Greathouse D. G., Currier D. P., Gilmore R. L. (1985). Effects of clinical infrared laser on superficial radial nerve conduction. *Phys. Ther.*, **65**, 1184–7.

Hecht J. (1989). Lasers. Making light work. *N. Scientist*, **122**, 1669.

Holwill M. E. J., Silvester N. R. (1973). *Introduction to Biological Physics*. London: John Wiley.

Karu T. I. (1987). Photobiological fundamentals of low-power laser therapy. *I.E.E.E. J. Quant. Electronics*, *QE23*, **10**, 1703–17.

King P. R. (1989). Low level laser therapy: a review. *Lasers Med. Sci.*, **4**, 141–50.

King C. E., Clelland J. A., Knowles C. J., Jackson J. R. (1990). Effects of helium–neon laser auriculotherapy on experimental pain threshold. *Phys. Ther.*, **70**, 24–30.

Mester E., Mester A. E., Mester A. (1985). The biomedical effect of laser application. *Lasers Surg. Med.*, **5**, 31–9.

Nissan M., Rockind S., Ralon N., Bartal A. (1986). He-Ne laser irradiation delivered transcutaneously: its effect on the sciatic nerve of rats. *Lasers Surg. Med.*, **6**, 435–8.

Ohshiro T., Calderhead R. G. (1988). *Low Level Laser Therapy: A Practical Introduction*. Chichester, John Wiley & Sons.

Ong K. L. T. (1986). Handling the patient in pain. *Physiotherapy*, **72**, 284–8.

Schwartz M., Doron A., Erlich M. *et al.* (1987). Effects of low energy He-Ne laser irradiation as post-traumatic degeneration of adult rabbit optic nerve. *Lasers Surg. Med.*, **7**, 497–505.

Seitz L. M., Kleinkort J. A. (1986). Low-power laser: its application in physical therapy. In *Thermal Agents in Rehabilitation* (Michlovitz S. L., ed.). Philadelphia: F. A. Davies, pp. 217–37.

Silfvast W. T. (1973). Metal-vapor lasers. *Sci. Am.*, **228**, 89–97.

Snyder-Mackler L., Bork C., Bourbon B., Trumbore D. (1986). Effects of helium–neon laser on musculoskeletal trigger points. *Phys. Ther.*, **66**, 1087–90.

Trelles M., Mayayo E. (1981). Bone fracture consolidates faster with low power laser. *Lasers Surg. Med.*, **7**, 36–45.

Young S. R., Bolton P., Dyson M., *et al.* (1989). Macrophage responsiveness to light therapy. *Lasers in Surgery and Medicine*, **9**, 497–505.

Walker J. (1983). Relief from chronic pain by low power laser irradiation. *Neurosci. Lett.*, **43**, 339–44.

15. *Ultraviolet radiation*

The radiations between the visible and X-ray sections of the electromagnetic spectrum (see Frontispiece and Chapter 11) were originally termed ultraviolet by Johann Ritter in 1801. They are so called because they are invisible radiations beyond the violet end of the spectrum. In view of the evident effects of sunlight on plants and on the skin it is hardly surprising that radiations from the sun have been considered to be therapeutically valuable throughout history.

It is worth considering here the meaning of some words. *Radiation* can be used to refer to any electromagnetic waves but is not customarily used for radio waves. The word is thought to arise from the Egyptian sun god, Aton Ra (2760 BC). Similarly Helios, the Greek god of the sun, is invoked in the term for treatment by the sun's radiations—*heliotherapy* (Diffey, 1982b). Another Greek word *actis*, a ray, is used in combination to give *actinotherapy* which implies treatment by any rays but is usually used to indicate radiations with wavelengths near the visible. *Phototherapy* implies treatment by radiations in the ultraviolet and visible regions. The word 'light' indicates visible radiations but is often extended casually to both the ultraviolet and infrared regions, as in references to 'ultraviolet light' or 'laser light' (from infrared lasers) as well as simply 'sunlight' which indicates all the radiations from the sun.

NATURE OF ULTRAVIOLET RADIATION

Ultraviolet radiations (UVR) are well recognized as the wavelengths that cause sunburn and tanning on exposure to the sun. It must be realized that a range of radiations is embraced by the title but only some of them produce these effects. Generally UVR behave in a similar way to visible radiations in the way they are reflected, refracted or absorbed, except that they are more strongly absorbed in air, in particular the short-wavelength ultraviolet. Thus much of the short UVR emitted by the sun never reach the surface of the earth (see Chapter 11). A further difference, of course, is the fact that UVR transmit much more energy than visible radiations (see Chapter 11) so that they are able to provoke chemical changes and not simply heat at sites where they are absorbed.

As already noted, UVR are usually defined in terms of their wavelengths, extending from the violet end of the visible at 390–400 nm to the soft X-ray region; the division here is variably defined. The ultraviolet spectrum is divided into three regions: A, B, and C. The wavelengths limiting these regions are internationally agreed and are those endorsed by the National Radiological Protection Board in the UK (Table 15.1). Some variations are given in other sources.

Radiations of wavelengths between 200 and 100 nm, and indeed below, are often called 'vacuum UV' because, being rapidly absorbed in air, they can only be effectively passed in a vacuum. It is also suggested that the lower limit should be set at about 180 nm. This is the usual lower limit for therapeutic radiation because shorter wavelengths are not transmitted through the quartz envelopes of the therapeutic sources used.

Table 15.1 Classification of ultraviolet radiation

Region	Wavelength	Other names
		Biotic
UVA	400–315 nm	Long UV, blacklight
UVB	315–280 nm	Medium UV, erythemal UV
		Abiotic
UVC	280–100 nm	Short UV, germicidal UV

(The frequency therefore ranges from 0.75×10^{15} at 400 nm to 3×10^{15} at 100 nm.)

PRODUCTION OF UVR

The sun is the most obvious source of UVR; solar radiations are considered later. Incandescent sources, like the sun, can produce UVR if the temperature is high enough (Wien's law: increasing temperature leads to the peak emission moving to shorter wavelengths; see Chapter 11). It will be recalled that the tungsten filament infrared source emitted some ultraviolet which was absorbed by the glass (see Chapter 13). The amount of ultraviolet generated is actually very small (about 0.17% in a 1000 W lamp), so that it is an unsatisfactory way of producing ultraviolet for therapeutic purposes. Therefore it is produced by the passage of a current through an ionized vapour— usually mercury vapour. Gases do not conduct current well at normal temperatures and pressures but can be made to do so at low pressure or high temperatures. They will, of course, conduct a current dramatically if the voltage is sufficiently high, as in lightning.

Low-pressure mercury vapour discharge tubes

The tube or envelope must be made of quartz (or special glass) to allow UVR to pass through it. Metal electrodes are sealed into the ends (Fig. 15.1). As the pressure in the tube is very low (around $400 \, \text{N/m}^2$) the mercury will be in vapour form. (Atmospheric pressure is approximately $100\,000 \, \text{N/m}^2$.) Some electrons will be detached from their parent atoms by natural radiation, thus leaving some mercury ions, and will then recombine. If a strong voltage is applied across the electrodes electrons can be accelerated and collide with other atoms, splitting off further electrons and leaving many free ions. Recombination of electrons and ions occurs and a steady current flows with electrons being added at one electrode and removed at the other. This process needs a high voltage to start it but will continue with a lower voltage and is regulated by limiting the current that is allowed to pass through the tube. As mains alternating voltage is applied the process reverses 100 times every second. Now, when many free electrons are being accelerated in the tube many collisions with neutral mercury vapour atoms will occur; some will simply be elastic collisions and will not affect the atom, some will cause ionization (knocking an electron off the atom) and some will cause excitation (moving one of the electrons off the atom to a higher energy level). When these excited electrons return to their normal energy level the energy they lose is emitted as a photon of a characteristic wavelength for that particular transition (see Chapter 14). Similarly electrons recombining with ions will give the same effect. The characteristic photon wavelengths given off by mercury atoms are in the green–blue–violet end of the visible spectrum and in the ultraviolet. Thus a line spectrum is produced; see Table 15.2 for the wavelengths of some, typical of mercury. The wavelengths and intensities emitted are modified at different lamp pressures and filtered by the quartz or special glass envelope.

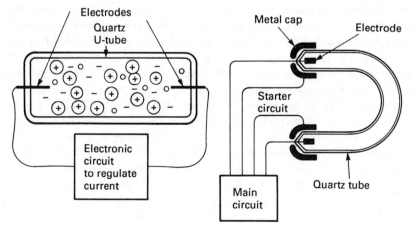

Fig. 15.1 Mercury vapour gas discharge tubes.

Table 15.2 Wavelengths of mercury atoms in the green–blue–violet end of the spectrum and in the ultraviolet

Wavelength (nm)	Radiation	Intensity
253.7	Short UVC	High
313	Medium UVB	Low
365.5	Long UVA	Low
404.7	Violet visible	Low
435.8	Blue visible	Moderate
546.1	Green visible	Moderate–low
578	Green visible	Low

Fluorescent lamps

These are low-pressure mercury discharge tubes with a phosphor coating on the inside. This layer absorbs short UVR, notably the spectral line at 254 nm, which causes excitation of the phosphor atoms and re-emission at a longer wavelength, i.e. fluorescence. The particular wavelengths and the amount of each emitted will depend on the composition of the phosphor used. (These phosphor coatings are actually mixtures of phosphates, borates and silicates.) The output of these lamps also varies with their temperature. Most give an optimal output with the outside of the tube at about 40°C. Such tubes are familiar as standard fluorescent lighting tubes. The tubes used for ultraviolet treatment in physiotherapy are identical in size and shape but have a special phosphor coating in the tube that makes it produce a continuous spectrum between 250–280 nm and 380 nm (with a peak at 313 nm) and lines in the blue and green visible (Fig. 15.2; Diffey, 1982b). This gives a considerable UVA and UVB output but no UVC.

For the treatment of patients, four 120-cm length tubes made of a special glass that transmits ultraviolet are mounted in a semicircular tunnel-type frame. Each tube is backed by a curved reflector along the whole length of the tube. The whole assembly can be supported by wires passing over pulleys secured to an overhead beam and attached at the other end to counterweights. The tunnel can thus be easily raised and lowered to manoeuvre it over the patient in the lying position. The tunnel may also be supported on a wheeled frame or two tubes may be mounted in a kind of quarter-circle frame mounted on a stand. All these arrangements are referred to as Theraktin lamps.

The same type of tube is used to produce large amounts of UVA radiation for use in the treatment of psoriasis in conjunction with a psoralen sensitizer (see below) as PUVA treatment. In these the phosphor coating is different and leads to emission from 315 to 400 nm and several lines in the blue and green visible region (Fig. 15.2). A reflecting layer is applied between the glass envelope and the phosphor layer over more than half the circumference of the tube along its length. This ensures that the radiations are largely directed forwards and when several of these tubes are packed together side by side they provide an approximately uniform emission. A number of tubes (48 in

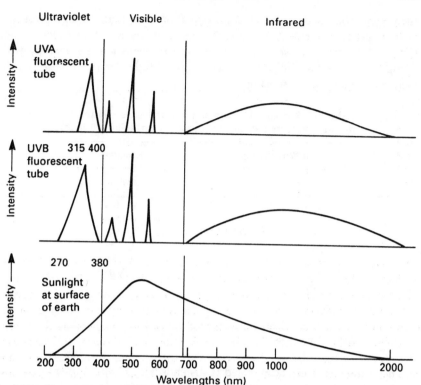

Fig. 15.2 Spectra distribution of UVA and UVB fluorescent lamps and sunlight (not in proportion).

one type) are fixed in the walls of a treatment cabinet in which the patient stands to receive all-round body irradiation.

All these fluorescent lamps emit visible radiation giving a bluish-white light when the tube is operating but it must be realized that the visible emission has no relation to the ultraviolet being emitted. All fluorescent tubes have a slight fall in output during their working lives. This is trivial for fluorescent lighting tubes but the ultraviolet lamps use less stable phosphors so that their useful life is usually limited to about 1000 h.

The low-pressure mercury vapour discharge lamps so far discussed are often called 'cold' ultraviolet lamps to distinguish them from the 'hot' lamps which work at higher temperatures and pressures. At these higher temperatures the discharge occurs largely in the space between the two electrodes and hence are called 'arcs'. These arcs also produce a continuous spectrum of radiations superimposed on the characteristic line spectrum.

Medium-pressure mercury arc lamp—Alpine sunlamp

This lamp is very widely used in physiotherapy departments in the form of a U-shaped tube working at a pressure of a few atmospheres (Fig. 15.1b). (Up to 10 atm is described as a medium-pressure tube; 10–100 atm is a high-pressure tube. Some sources describe all lamps operating over 1 atm as high-pressure.) UVB is produced at 297, 302 and 313 nm and several other spectral lines (Table 15.3) as well as some continuous spectral emission. By analogy with sunlight (see below) they are called 'high-altitude' lamps (*Höhensonne* in German), hence Alpine sunlamp.

Table 15.3 Some of the major spectral lines emitted by medium-pressure mercury vapour arc lamps (Diffey 1982b)

Wavelength (nm)	Radiation
578	Visible
546	Visible
436	Visible
405	Visible
365	UVA
334	UVA
313	UVB
302	UVB
297	UVB
265	UVC
254	UVC

From Diffey (1982).

The U-tube has electrodes sealed at the ends (Fig. 15.1b). It operates in the same manner as the low-pressure mercury vapour lamp—characteristic radiation lines are produced by specific energy transitions due to excitation in the mercury atoms. As well as this, recombination of ions with electrons causes the emission of photons of many different wavelengths, leading to the emission of a continuous spectrum of wavelength. As well as visible radiations these tubes, operating at higher temperatures, produce infrared radiation. This precludes placing them close to the skin unless they are cooled. The Alpine sunlamp is air cooled.

The U-tube of the Alpine sunlamp is set at the centre of a parabolic reflector made of a special aluminium alloy supported on a strong stand. As a U-tube it acts more like a point source of radiation. The reflector and tube can be easily raised and lowered on the vertical stand because there is a counterweight system and can be adjusted at two pivotal points as well as rotated about the vertical stand to allow it to be suitably positioned. It is usually applied at a distance of 45 or 50 cm.

All mercury vapour lamps contain a small quantity of the inert gas argon to facilitate starting up the lamp and help control electron mobility. It also helps to prolong the life of the metal electrodes.

In order to start up the medium-pressure burner a high voltage is applied to metal caps (Fig. 15.1b) fitted outside the quartz envelope by means of a separate step-up autotransformer. Pressing a button on the control panel applies a charge of 400 V or so to the metal caps, causing ionization of the argon atoms. The high charge displaces an outer orbital electron from several argon atoms leaving them as positive ions. The presence of sufficient free positive ions and electrons allows the flow of a convection current in which positive ions gain electrons from the negative electrode and electrons move to the positive at the (lower) mains voltage. The small quantity of mercury—which is a drop of liquid at normal temperature—is rapidly vaporized due to the heat generated by the passage of current. Mercury atoms of the vapour become ionized giving the spectral emission described above. This process takes about 5 min for the temperature to reach its stable operating level and hence for the emission to become stable at its standard output.

Short UVR react with oxygen in the air to produce a small quantity of ozone (O_3), which is evident from its smell, even at low concentrations. Ozone is toxic at high concentrations so ventilation should be adequate around these lamps. In some modern lamps the burner envelope is modified so that it does not emit ozone-producing ultraviolet below 270 nm.

The Kromayer lamp

The Kromayer lamp is a medium-pressure mercury vapour ultraviolet lamp designed to be used in contact with the tissues, both on the skin surface and in body cavities. This is achieved by enclosing the emitting tube in a water jacket which cools it and filters out the infrared which would otherwise cause a heat burn, but allowing the visible and ultraviolet to pass. The lamp was originally designed in 1905 by Dr E. L. Kromayer, hence its name. Forced air-cooling has also been used in a system called Aero-Kromayer. The mercury vapour U-tube works in the same way as described above but is enclosed in a waterproof metal container with a quartz window in front. Surrounding this is another metal container and quartz window: water is pumped between the two windows (Fig. 15.3).

The whole assembly, with an outer case and handle, is connected to the water pump and cooling system in the base of the machine by flexible pipes. The water is contained in a tank mounted in the body of the lamp and constantly recirculated. To avoid deposits forming on the quartz windows and in the pipes distilled water is recommended. The water passing between the two quartz windows absorbs infrared, becomes warmer, and is pumped to a radiator in the body of the machine over which air is passed by a fan.

This lamp will also require about 5 min to reach operating temperature. When the Kromayer lamp is switched off the water pump should be left running for a few minutes to lower the temperature. If the cooling water flow is stopped while the lamp is still hot it may damage the seals between the quartz window and metal case or other parts.

The UVR emitted from the Kromayer lamp are inevitably reduced by passing through two quartz windows and about 1 cm of water as well as the quartz envelope of the lamp (Fig. 15.3). However, application directly to the tissues or a few centimetres away ensures that the output is many times stronger than that of the Alpine sunlamp, applied at 50 cm. Thus doses of a few seconds with the Kromayer can achieve the same effect as those of a few minutes with the air-cooled lamp—but only to a very small area. Although the

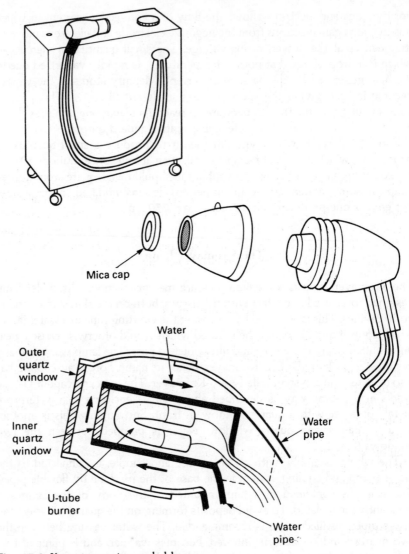

Fig. 15.3 Kromayer water-cooled lamp.

output of the tubes is the same in both lamps there is relatively more UVC from the Kromayer since short UVR are particularly attenuated in air. This is useful if the Kromayer is being used for a bacteriocidal effect.

In both these 'hot' mercury arc lamps the quartz envelope becomes gradually changed by the heat into tridymite, which is a different form of silica. Quartz is used for these lamps because it allows the transmission of all ultraviolet down to a wavelength of 170–180 nm but tridymite is opaque to ultraviolet and therefore the effective output of the lamp gradually diminishes with use. This problem is overcome by incorporating a resistance in the circuit which can be reduced in steps as the lamp ages. (Reducing a series resistance allows a higher current to the lamp, thus increasing the output to compensate for the loss of transmission through the quartz envelope.) This resistor sometimes called the intensity stabilizer can be moved over a scale marked in elapsed hours. A record of the total time during which the lamp has been in use (i.e. burning hours) should be kept and the resistance altered accordingly. After 1000 h the quartz tube has to be replaced.

The outer quartz window of the Kromayer is covered by a mica cap which is removed when the lamp is used. This completely obstructs the emission of all UVR allowing only some green visible radiations to be transmitted, and thus prevents any inadvertent application of ultraviolet.

Various filters can also be used with the lamp. A special holder can be fitted to the front window of the Kromayer to support various-shaped quartz rods, often called applicators. These will transmit UVR to the deeper part of a sinus or ulcer or into a body cavity. While there is considerable attenuation of radiations in these rods, so that the dose has to be markedly increased to compensate, most of the ultraviolet is conveyed, even in curved applicators, due to the strong refraction of ultraviolet between quartz and air which leads to total internal reflection of the ultraviolet (see Chapter 11).

Measurement of UVR

The energy transmitted by UVR can be measured to investigate the output of UVR lamps and quantify treatment. Photodiodes are most widely used as they are rugged and relatively cheap. Coupled to a suitable electronic circuit they register the photon emission and with added filters can determine the output of different wavelengths. The measurement is of the power of the radiation or intensity of radiation at a specific point (more properly called the irradiance) measured in watts per square metre or watts per square centimetre. The amount of energy applied is the irradiance (in W/cm^2, say) multiplied by the time of exposure in seconds giving a dose or 'radiant exposure' in joules per square centimetre (J/cm^2).

PHYSIOLOGICAL EFFECTS OF ULTRAVIOLET

The well known acute effects of the sun, i.e. sunburn, are really the effects of UVB radiations. Under normal physiological conditions it takes huge doses of UVA to provoke any kind of reddening and UVC is not normally found in significant quantities in the sun's radiation reaching the earth's surface. UVR is largely absorbed in the outer layer of the skin so that the direct effects are limited to those on the skin and the eyes. These effects can be considered in two groups: the immediate or acute effects occurring within hours, days or weeks and the long-term chronic effects noted only after years.

The immediate, acute effects of ultraviolet on the skin

An erythema, or reddening, appears some time after the application of the ultraviolet. This is often a matter of hours and is called the latent period. Over some hours the erythema increases and then fades during the subsequent hours or days. Oedema and irritation of the skin are evident if the application of ultraviolet is sufficiently intense, as well as desquamation (peeling) of the superficial epidermis. If the same dose of UVB is repeated after these changes have recovered it provokes a less strong reaction due to the pigmentation (tanning) and skin thickening that occurs. This protective pigmentation and thickening can last 30–40 days and occurs not only as a result of a single erythematous exposure but also after a series of exposures each insufficient to provoke visible reddening (Nonaka *et al.*, 1984), hence called suberythemal doses.

The degree to which these effects occur depends on the amount of UVB energy applied, the radiant exposure, and the reactivity or sensitivity of the skin of the subject. Thus the fair-skinned person will exhibit a more marked reaction than the dark-skinned given the same radiant exposure. These changes are summarized in Table 15.4. During the recovery period after strong applications some itching of the skin may occur.

Other effects will occur in the skin that are not immediately detectable, the best known being the formation of vitamin D from 7-dehydrocholesterol in the sebum. Vitamin D is important for the absorption and utilization of calcium (see below). There is also evidence that UVR leads to immunosuppression for a short time, affecting Langerhans cells in the skin (Räsänen *et al.*, 1989). All these effects are discussed further below.

Effects on the eyes

Strong doses of UVB and C radiation to the eyes can lead to conjunctivitis (inflammation of the tissue over the cornea and lining of the eyelids) and to photokeratitis (inflammation of the cornea). This results in irritation of the eye, a feeling of grit in the eye, watering of the eye and aversion to light (photophobia). In severe cases intense pain and spasm of the eyelid may be present. This is also known as 'snow blindness' when it arises due to solar UVB and C reflection from the snow. It can also occur due to reflection from sand and from using welding arcs without eye protection. The condition usually recovers in about 2 days without permanent damage but the eye, unlike the skin, does not develop tolerance to ultraviolet radiation. In fact the reverse seems to occur in that subsequent applications seem to provoke conjunctivitis more readily, but this may simply be that initial recovery is apparent but not complete for several days longer. Although all UVB and C radiations will produce these effects the most damaging seem to be those of 270 nm.

While UVB and C are absorbed in the cornea, UVA can pass through to be absorbed mainly in the lens of the eye. It has been suggested that strong doses of UVA may be implicated in the formation of cataracts.

Long-term chronic effects of ultraviolet on the skin

Prolonged exposure over many years to strong solar radiation can lead to premature ageing of the skin; this is especially so in the fair-skinned. The skin

Table 15.4 Description of degrees of erythema

Degree of erythema	Approximate latent period	Appearance	Approximate duration of erythema	Skin oedema	Skin discomfort	Desquamation of skin	Relation to dose causing E_1
E_1	6–12 h	Mildly pink	<24 h	None	None	None	1
E_2	6 h	Definite pink-red Blanches on pressure	2 days	None	Slight soreness, irritation	Powdery	2.5
E_3	3 h	Very red Does not blanch on pressure	3–5 days	Some	Hot and painful	In thin sheets	5
E_4	<2 h	'Angry' red	A week	Blister	Very painful	Thick sheets	10

becomes wrinkled, dry and leathery and there is decreased function of sebaceous and sweat glands with loss of elastic tissue. Such changes are most often seen in those who have spent much of their working lives in strong sunlight, such as farmers, fishermen or other outdoor workers. It is a particular problem in locations where fair-skinned populations have emigrated to sunnier climates, such as Australia, South Africa or Israel.

Exposure to high levels of UVR over many years also increases the risk of certain skin cancers, basal cell and squamous cell carcinomas. This is evidenced by the fact that these develop on body areas exposed to sunlight, and that the incidence is higher in outdoor workers and fair-skinned people working in places that have much sunshine, as well as from laboratory studies on mice. For a given genetic susceptibility to non-melanoma skin cancer it has been shown that age and annual ultraviolet exposure are the two most important risk factors; in fact the risk is proportional to age[5] times annual dose of UV[2] (Fears *et al.* 1977). Diffey (1989) states that the occupational risks associated with working with UVR are small provided that good working practices are adopted so that acute erythema develops no more than once or twice a year.

The erythema due to ultraviolet radiation

The redness of sunburn is familiar and unmistakedly different from that due to heat in that the redness is uniform, not mottled, and there is a sharp distinct edge at the junction with an unexposed area. This indicates that it is capillaries in the dermis that primarily dilate and not the arterioles. Since UVB and C are largely absorbed in the epidermis it is considered that the reaction is due to the release of chemical substances. Histamine substances are invoked especially during the early development as are certain prostaglandins which may be released from epidermal keratinocytes (De Leo *et al.*, 1984) as well as prostacyclin from epidermal cells in the blood vessels of the dermis. The histamines, kinins and other agents associated with the inflammatory response are released from mast cells in the dermis.

It has been explained in the past that these chemicals were formed by a long chain of reactions and diffused slowly from the epidermis, which would account for the latent period. However, it has recently been clearly shown that the latent period is an artefact because the early, very slight erythema cannot be seen by the eye (Diffey and Oakley, 1987). Vasodilation appears to begin very soon after the irradiation is applied.

The erythema appears to differ somewhat depending on the ultraviolet wavelength. This has led to descriptions of an 'action spectrum', that is a graph of wavelength against erythemal effectiveness. For many years it was accepted that radiations around 297 nm were most effective at producing erythema with a lesser peak in the UVC around 250 nm and a trough of minimal effectiveness at about 280 nm. This, however, has not been supported by other investigators who produced different graphs, e.g. Sayre *et al.* (1966). For discussion of this see Diffey (1982a). One major reason for the disagreement is the uncertainty of defining the erythema response. It seems probable that, in general, the effectiveness of the radiation in provoking erythema increases with decreasing wavelength, as might be expected, conforming with the energy carried. However, there is evidence that the mechanism producing erythema due to short UVC may be different from that due to longer UVB (Farr and Diffey, 1985).

The erythema due to UVA seems to be rather different in several respects. There is some immediate erythema merging into a much later developing erythema which may last several days. It is considered that UVA may directly affect blood vessels in the dermis. It takes about 1000 times the dose of UVA to give an erythema equivalent to that of UVB.

About 20 mJ/cm^2 of 300 nm UVB are required to produce minimal erythema in a fair-skinned individual.

Pigmentation

Pigmentation of the skin occurs as a result of both the formation of melanin in the deep region of the epidermis and the migration of melanin already formed into more superficial layers. This process takes a little time and is usually noticeable about 2 days after exposure. In already pigmented individuals some immediate tanning may occur within as little as 10 min of exposure, due to darkening of existing melanin by photo-oxidation, it is believed. Pigmentation is strongly stimulated by erythema-producing UVB at about 300 nm and also, to a lesser extent, by longer wavelengths in UVA and even into the visible (Diffey, 1982b). Thus sunbeds which emit UVA and visible radiations are able to induce a tan without the erythema, although an erythema will occur at sufficiently high doses or if the patient has taken a sensitizer (see PUVA later). The increased melanin content of the skin affords protection by preventing UVR reaching the lower layers of the epidermis where the dividing keratinocytes are situated. This protective effect is aided by the skin thickening that also occurs.

Increased skin growth

Stimulation by UVR provokes increased keratinocyte cell turnover so that the skin grows more rapidly for a time, leading to shedding of the most superficial cells at an earlier stage in their development than usual so that they remain in pieces, or even sheets, and can be peeled off. This peeling or desquamation varies with the intensity of applied UVR (see Table 15.4). As the skin recovers the growth continues so that the final result is skin thickening which adds to the protection due to pigmentation. Both these protective effects fade over 4–6 weeks if there is no further ultraviolet application.

Vitamin D production

UVB is able to convert sterols in the skin, such as 7-dehydrocholesterol to vitamin D (calciferol, cholecalciferol) which, after changes in the liver and kidneys, is able to facilitate the absorption of calcium from the intestine. (Insufficient vitamin D coupled with undernourishment leads to rickets in babies and osteomalacia in adults.) The UVB radiations most effective in producing vitamin D are in the 280 and 300 nm regions. Suberythemal doses of UVB are adequate to promote vitamin D synthesis but otherwise-healthy individuals living in higher latitudes may have insufficient vitamin D in winter, as may the bed-bound both in hospital and at home.

SKIN—STRUCTURE AND ACTIVITY

Before further consideration of the effects and therapeutic uses of UVR it is useful to review normal skin.

Keratinization

The epidermis is supported on, and receives nutrition from, the vascular dermis which provides a strong flexible base. The epidermis is continuously producing keratin by means of cell division in the basal cells (stratum germinativum). These basal cells gradually grow up through the prickle cell layer, lose their nucleus, die and become converted to pieces of flattened keratin. These pieces of keratin are steadily lost from the skin surface, especially when the surface is rubbed or washed (Fig. 15.4a).

After mitosis in the basal layer each daughter cell may:

1 differentiate and grow through the prickle cell layer to die and form keratin;
2 enter a resting phase, becoming inactive for a time;
3 proceed to another cycle of mitosis to form two daughter cells.

The time taken from mitosis to mitosis is known as the cell turnover time and is, on average, about 6 days. The average time taken for a cell to pass from the basal layer to be shed as a keratin flake at the surface is called the epidermal transit time and may be about 28 days (Burton, 1979) or longer—45–70 days. If the transit time remains constant but the rate of mitosis speeds up, i.e. the cell turnover time is decreased, the skin will be thickened. The rate of basal cell division seems to be controlled by a variety of factors, some of which must be local since friction on the surface or the loss of some epithelial surface provokes keratinocyte synthesis, as does UVR.

Keratin itself is formed of folded, cross-linked polypeptide chains; it also forms hair and nails. Keratinized epithelium is pliable while it is wet but becomes harder and more brittle on drying, thus trapping moisture in the surface. Putting oils or grease on the skin will make the surface soft, as described in connection with wax treatment in Chapter 8.

(a) Cross-section of the epidermis

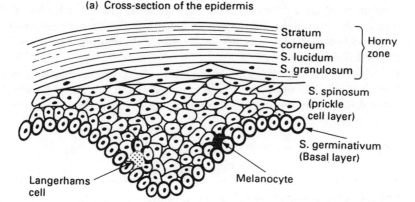

(b) A melanocyte

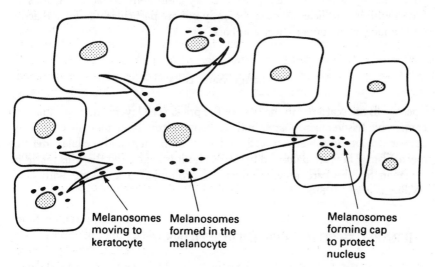

Fig. 15.4 The skin. (a) Cross-section of the epidermis; (b) a melanocyte.

Pigmentation

The pigment melanin is produced by melanocytes in the basal layer of the epidermis. It is formed from the amino acid tyrosine by special organelles, called melanosomes, in the cell. These melanosomes are able to pass along dendritic processes of the melanocytes to enter the neighbouring keratinocytes. In the keratinocytes they cluster over the nucleus forming a protective cap—a sort of umbrella—which absorbs UVR before it can reach the DNA of the nucleus (Fig. 15.4b). As the keratinocytes migrate to the surface the melanosomes and their contained melanin disintegrate and are lost with the keratin flakes from the skin surface. In darker skin there are the same number of melanocytes but they produce larger, longer-lasting and more widely dispersed melanocytes.

Melanocyte activity is stimulated by ultraviolet. The mechanism is not fully understood but involves enzymic activity and hormones, melanocyte-stimulating hormone from the pituitary, adrenocorticotrophic hormone and oestrogen.

Sebaceous glands

Sebum is produced in sebaceous glands by the complete breakdown of cells in the gland turning into fatty material which passes via the sebaceous duct to the hair follicles and thence to the skin surface. This 'greasing' of the skin helps waterproofing and is mildly fungicidal. The rate of sebum production is controlled by hormones, being increased by androgens. Sebaceous glands are found with hair follicles all over the body but are particularly large and active on the face, neck, upper chest and back.

Langerhans cells

These cells are scattered in the base of the prickle cell layer. They are similar to connective tissue macrophages and are derived from bone marrow cells. They appear to be involved in cell-mediated immunity and cellular defence mechanism. They are damaged by UVR and it is suggested that this might be a reason for the carcinogenic effects of prolonged overdosage with UVR (Williams *et al.*, 1989).

THERAPEUTIC USES AND INDICATIONS

The principal therapeutic uses of UVR are for skin diseases or to assist the healing of open wounds, particularly chronic slow-healing wounds such as venous ulcers or pressure sores. The most commonly treated skin diseases are psoriasis and acne vulgaris.

Psoriasis

Psoriasis is a widespread chronic skin disease of unknown cause affecting 2% of the population. A predisposition to it may be inherited. Chronic discoid psoriasis is the commonest form with thick pink or red plaques, sharply demarcated and covered with silvery scales. There are several other types: guttate, in which small lesions are scattered over the trunk; pustular psoriasis (the pustules are sterile); generalized pustular and erythrodermic psoriasis which are serious medical emergencies, and flexural psoriasis.

The epidermal transit time is reduced to about 5 days so that the keratinocytes do not change in the usual way. They keep their nuclei and tend to stick together forming the plaques. There is also increased mitosis and dilation of the dermal capillaries, which accounts for the redness.

This condition has been treated by UVR for many years but the tendency is for relapse. The Goeckerman regime consists of coal tar applications 2 or 3 times a day with general (total body) UVB radiation given once a day. This may be done with a Theraktin tunnel or several exposures with an Alpine sunlamp. The intensity is variously advised as a suberythemal or first-degree erythema (see below). The Ingram or Leeds regime (Ingram, 1954) is the most commonly used conventional treatment. The patient has a coal tar bath before being irradiated with a minimal erythema dose of UVB; the psoriatic lesions are covered with dithranol (a cytotoxic substance that inhibits DNA synthesis). Next day the dithranol is cleaned off with arachis oil or liquid paraffin and the process is repeated (Klaber, 1980). Although sensitizers such as coal tars have been considered an essential component of the treatment, more recent controlled studies have shown that UVB is the effective element (e.g. Le Vine *et al.*, 1979). Thus courses of whole-body UVB treatment using the Theraktin are successfully used in the treatment of psoriasis without other adjuncts. Fish oil therapy, which has been found to benefit psoriasis but is inadequate as a treatment on its own has been successfully used in conjunction with a course of UVB (Gupta *et al.*, 1989).

Photochemotherapy for psoriasis

The disease has been very successfully treated in recent years with the use of UVA accompanied by a sensitizer. If a psoralen-type drug is given to the patient some 2 h previously, he or she will become sensitive to UVA radiations which will produce an erythema at lower intensities than normal. The drug 8-methoxy-psoralen is used making the patient highly reactive to UVA once it has been absorbed, for some 6–8 h. Irradiation during this time leads to an erythema similar to, but not identical with, that of UVB in that the major erythema arises later and lasts longer and may not reach a peak for 2–4 days. Treatment may be given once or twice a week (Fusco *et al.*, 1980) or three times a week until clearance and then once a week for a further 4 weeks, once a fortnight for 3 sessions and finally three sessions every 3 weeks. The UVA dose, measured in J/cm^2, is initially determined according to skin type.

Using a combination of psoralen and UVA gives this treatment its popular name of PUVA. It has been shown to be very successful in controlling the disease. It is considered to be, in some degree, carcinogenic and there is also a question of increased risk of cataract formation.

Acne vulgaris

Acne vulgaris is a chronic inflammatory condition of the pilosebaceous unit especially affecting the face, chest and back. Mild acne arising at adolescence is so common as to be considered a normal feature. However, the more severe and long-lasting forms are disfiguring and cause serious distress. The sebaceous glands become more active at puberty being stimulated by androgens which coupled with infection by the acne bacillus (*Propionibacterium acnes*) provokes the formation of blackheads or comedones. These are clumps of keratin, sebum and bacteria which block the follicle. Subsequently an inflammatory response occurs which leads to the familiar papules and pustules.

UVR given in doses such as to cause significant peeling or desquamation— usually E_2—are used. The effects of the ultraviolet are to:

1 accelerate skin growth because peeling of the surface will remove the lesions and open the blocked ducts;
2 produce a non-specific inflammatory reaction to help control infection;
3 sterilize the skin surface temporarily;
4 cause some pigmentation which may serve to make the papules less obvious.

Improvement, which can sometimes be dramatic, is temporary but repetitions at intervals of a few months may enable the patient to remain reasonably clear during the worst year or so.

Chronic infection

Infected areas such as pressure sores and venous ulcers or any infected open wound are treated with high doses of UVR. The Kromayer lamp is usually used because it gives a relatively high proportion of UVC which is notably bacteriocidal. The doses given must be such as to kill surface bacteria and therefore an E_4 is used. While the lethal effects of UVC on bacteria, especially the 254 nm peak, have been well known for many years the effect of the usual clinically used doses given with a standard Kromayer lamp have, surprisingly, only been quantified fairly recently. Thus High and High (1983) found that the radiation from the Kromayer was universally successful in killing bacteria in vitro and the reduction in colony numbers correlated with the intensity used to the point where E_4 doses totally inhibited colony growth. Similarly Burger *et al.* (1985) cultured swabs from some pressure sores before and after an E_4 ultraviolet dose given with the Kromayer. The result was a dramatic and extensive reduction in bacterial numbers.

These studies support the clinical impression that UVR is an effective, safe and convenient way of controlling surface infection. This may be particularly valuable in circumstances where antibiotics cannot reach the area in adequate proportions, if the infection is resistant to them or if they are contraindicated.

It has been suggested that local UVR should not only be applied to the infected ulcer but also to the surrounding skin, on the grounds that the increased blood flow resulting from vasodilation will improve oxygenation of the skin. Moderate doses of UVR are therefore applied to the skin of existing and healed ulcers. A recent investigation (Dodd *et al.*, 1989) has shown that skin oxygenation is increased for some 48 h after treatment; however, subsequent return of vasoconstriction lowers the skin oxygen tension for some 2 weeks so that, in this respect, the effect is not beneficial.

Other skin afflictions for which UVR has been used

Historically, local ultraviolet treatments were first developed by Niels Finsen in Denmark during the 1890s. He used a carbon arc as a source of ultraviolet, passing through tubes filled with blue-coloured solution to absorb the infrared radiation. There were quartz windows at each end and the lesion to be treated was pressed against the distal quartz window. Treatment times were of the order of 1 h. The major condition treated at that time was tuberculosis of the skin. This treatment was very successful in its day but is no longer used because the incidence of this disease has fallen dramatically.

Accelerating the healing and repair of uninfected wounds

In these wounds, such as surgical incisions or clean traumatic skin injuries, E_1 or E_2 doses of UVR are used to increase the rate of skin growth and promote a reaction causing vasodilation in the skin. The UVR also helps to maintain sterility by destroying some surface bacteria. Both granulation tissue and the surrounding skin may be treated. There seems to be no supporting evidence for accelerated healing; in fact given optimum conditions, healing cannot be accelerated (Evans, 1980). However, if conditions are not the best possible, it seems a reasonable expectation that UVR will facilitate healing given the effect it has in stimulating mitosis in the germinal layer of the skin; clinical impressions seem to confirm this. Higher doses would seem likely to be counterproductive in that more skin damage would occur. Areas in which new epithelium is growing, at the edge of the wound, should be completely avoided for this reason.

Vitiligo

Vitiligo is a condition in which destruction of melanocytes in local areas causes white patches to appear on the skin. It is not uncommon and is considered to be an autoimmune disease (anti-melanocyte antibodies have been found). For the fair-skinned this disease may be of little consequence except for the need to protect the depigmented patches from excessive sunburn. In the darker-skinned it becomes a serious cosmetic problem which can be treated with topical psoralens and UVR to try to induce repigmentation. In climates with reliable natural sunshine, advice on gradual exposure may be sufficient but in higher latitudes artificial UVR is used to effect pigmentation. Both UVA and B stimulate melanocyte activity but there seem to be some differences in that UVA seems to provoke a darker and longer-lasting tan (at least in normal skin) although the protective effects do not seem to be so marked, perhaps because

UVB provokes more thickening. It would seem sensible to apply graded doses of either or both UVA and B. The surrounding normally pigmented area should be protected since darkening the contrasting area must be avoided. The fluorescent tube Theraktin lamp or the air-cooled Alpine sunlamp could be used, or even the water-cooled Kromayer if the patches were small, but it may be best to filter the short UVC out with, for example, a thin sheet of polythene.

Protection for hypersensitive skin

Normal tolerance to increased sunlight develops slowly as the seasons change, increasing over a 6-month period. However modern air travel allows a complete climatic change over a few hours. The very fair-skinned and those hypersensitive to UVR who need to go to work (or even holiday) out of doors in regions of strong sunshine can have the risk of sunburn much reduced by a course of general UVB (Theraktin) with gradually progressed dosage (see below). Even though only the face, neck and arms are customarily exposed it is sensible to treat the whole body.

Alopecia

Alopecia means baldness (from bald foxes; Greek *alopex* = fox). Male-pattern baldness, due to genetic factors, increasing age and adequate androgen levels is, of course, not amenable to treatment. Alopecia areata is a relatively common condition in which the hair falls out in patches. If the hair loss includes the whole scalp it is called alopecia totalis and if it includes all body hair, alopecia universalis. The cause is unknown but it may be an autoimmune disease. Formerly the condition was treated with mild or moderate doses of UVB (E_1 or E_2) on the grounds that it might stimulate new hair growth in association with the increased epithelial cell mitosis. There seems to be no evidence that UVR has any direct effect partly because hair growth usually recovers spontaneously in a few weeks or months. This treatment is rarely used these days except as a placebo.

Other affections for which UVR treatment is applied

Historically the application of mild general UVB radiation was considered to have a tonic effect which accounted for the increased metabolism, improved general health and increased resistance to infection. This supposed increased resistance to infection is sometimes called the 'esophylactic' effect but there appears to be no hard evidence to support this effect, so that the application of UVB for any general tonic effect on, for example, chronic respiratory disease is no longer given. (However, as the role of the skin in the immunological system of the body becomes better understood it would not be so surprising to find more rational explanations for some of the effects claimed by earlier clinicians.)

Treatment of vitamin D deficiency

As explained earlier, cholecalciferol (vitamin D_3) is formed in skin by the action of UVB and UVC on 7-dehydrocholesterol. This vitamin is also taken in the diet, notably in animal fat products. It has been understood for many years that exposure to either artificial UVR or, if available, natural sunlight is curative for vitamin D deficiency diseases. The dietary improvement, especially the consumption of fats, in developed countries over the past century has almost, but not quite, eliminated this disease. People moving to countries like the UK with less natural sunlight and retaining customary dietary habits sometimes show vitamin D deficiency. Further some bed-bound elderly patients, it is thought, may benefit from artificial UVB to maintain vitamin D and calcium levels to counteract senile osteoporosis (Corless *et al.*, 1978).

Treatment of pruritus due to biliary cirrhosis or uraemia

The intractable and serious itching that can occur due to raised bile acid level can be successfully treated by suberythemal whole-body UVB either alone or in combination with the drug cholestyramine (Cerio and Low, 1987; Cerio *et al.*, 1987). Pruritus due to uraemia in patients with chronic renal failure has also been successfully treated by suberythemal UVB (Gilchrist *et al.*, 1977). In this study some patients were also treated with UVA at somewhat higher doses but with little effect; UVB appears to be the effective radiation. It has been suggested (Diffey, 1982b) that this useful effect of UVB may be worth trying in other situations where pruritus is a significant problem.

Uses of UVR in diagnosis

Some skin lesions may be suspected photodermatoses, that is caused by visible or UVR due perhaps to the action of a sensitizer either ingested or on the skin. Many chemical substances, including drugs, can act in this way; psoralens have already been noted and may be found in some perfumes. Some allergic reactions seem to be triggered by the synergic action of the chemical and UVR. This may be tested by applying the suspected sensitizer and graded doses of UVR to see if the skin eruption is reproduced. Photopatch testing can be done by applying the suspected skin contact sensitizer to two patches which are then covered. After 2 days one test patch is uncovered and UVA applied, either from a special lamp or the Kromayer fitted with a suitable glass filter (a Schott WG 345, for example) to cut out the UVB and UVC. After a further 2 days both patches are uncovered. If the irradiated site only shows any reaction contact photoallergy is demonstrated (English, 1965; Diffey, 1982b).

The phenomenon of luminescence is used to help diagnose some skin conditions. When UVA radiation results in excitation of electrons to a higher energy state there is a subsequent transition back to a lower energy level. This can lead to the emission of a photon of radiation of longer wavelength and hence visible (see Chapter 14). If the emission of this visible radiation is instantaneous it is called fluorescence but if the emission continues after the original radiation ceases it is called phosphorescence. A Wood's lamp produces UVA, mainly in the region of 365 nm; a Kromayer lamp with a Wood's filter gives the same radiation. This can be used to produce fluorescence by shining the lamp on the surface to be investigated in a darkened room. The following conditions can be diagnosed:

1 Tinea capitis (ringworm of the scalp) – because infected hairs will fluoresce a light green.
2 Erythrasma (a bacterial skin infection) which produces a chemical (porphyrin) which fluoresces coral red.
3 Infection of burns by a *Pseudomonas* organism (*Pseudomonas aeruginosa*) because it produces a yellow–green fluorescent pigment.

Wood's light is also used in dentistry to visualize plaque and early dental caries and for other purposes.

Psychological benefit

Considerable psychological benefit has been claimed as an effect of UVR (Scott, 1983) on the grounds that patients expect to feel better and the consequent tanning makes them look better. (Such an effect is certainly exploited by the makers of sunbeds.) The same writer also suggests that patients suffering from rheumatoid arthritis seem to benefit particularly from general UVR, but offers no rationalization.

DOSAGE

The skin response to UVR depends on:

1 The quantity of ultraviolet energy applied to unit area of the skin.
2 The biological responsiveness (sensitivity) of the skin to which it is applied.

The first can be measured, or at least controlled to keep it constant, but the second can only be adequately assessed by trial applications of ultraviolet.

The quantity of energy

Typically about 20 mJ/cm^2 of UVB at a wavelength of 300 nm will produce minimal erythema on the moderately fair-skinned (Diffey, 1982b; Nonaka *et al.*, 1984). The amount of energy—the radiant response—depends on the output of the lamp, the distance from the skin and the angle at which the radiations fall on the skin. It also depends on the time for which the radiation is applied. This factor is used to regulate dosage, for if the intensity falling on the skin is constant then the effects are directly proportional to the time of exposure. This is in accordance with the Bunsen–Roscoe reciprocity law which states that the same photochemical effect will occur if the product of the intensity and time are constant; thus low intensity for a long time can produce the same effect as high intensity for a short time.

The output of the lamp

The output of the source includes the nature of the radiations, the principal wavelengths emitted and the intensity. Even lamps of the same make and type are likely to have slightly different outputs due to ageing and other effects. It is, therefore, necessary to use the same source throughout a course of treatment.

The distance from the skin

The distance between the source of ultraviolet and the skin is critical. It is usual to calculate the effect by presuming that the ultraviolet is emitted from a point source so that the inverse square law can be used to calculate the relationship of intensity and distance (see Chapter 11). Thus if the distance is doubled the intensity would be reduced to one-quarter, so to achieve an equivalent effect, the time of application must be four times the original. For example if the desired effect was achieved in 1 min at a distance of 30 cm, the time needed at a distance of 60 cm would be four times that − 4 min. It can therefore be said that dose = time/distance^2. If the same effect or dose is required at a different distance, new time/new distance^2 = old time/old distance^2. If the desired effect was produced in 4.5 min at a distance of 60 cm the time needed at a distance of 20 cm would be: $4.5/60^2$ = new time/20^2 = 0.5 = 30 s.

Since ultraviolet emitters are hardly a point source and are backed by a reflector it may be wondered why the inverse square law can be used. There are, of course, losses other than the spreading out of radiations due to absorption and scattering in air. These are approximately compensated by the reflector so that the inverse square law can be used as a satisfactory rule of thumb. It has been established for the Alpine sunlamp that at distances between 50 and 150 cm the intensity conforms with that predicted by the law (Goats, 1988). At distances less than 50 cm the intensity is apparently a little less than that predicted.

The angle at which the radiations fall on the skin

The effective intensity of radiation on the skin depends on the cosine of the angle of incidence of the radiation (see Chapter 11). Thus the lamp is normally applied at or near a right angle to the skin to achieve maximum and consistent effects. It follows that the intensity of radiation will 'fall off' around the curved body surfaces (see Chapter 11).

The biological response

The severity of the response to UVR depends on the nature of the skin to which it has been applied. Physiotherapists and dermatologists often classify patients by skin, eye and (natural!) hair colour as well as the patients' own account of how easily they burn in the sun. A system based on the burning and tanning history given by patients with observation of their pigmentation has been described (Wolff *et al.*, 1977) and is widely used for broad classification.

Type I: always burn, never tan.
Type II: always burn, tan slightly.
Type III: sometimes burn, always tan.
Type IV: never burn, always tan.
Type V: pigmented skin—mongoloid.
Type VI: heavily pigmented skin—negroid.

Coarse distinctions between light- and dark-skinned and their differing tolerance to UVR are fairly easily made. The amount of melanin in the skin contributes to both skin colour and protection against ultraviolet so it is hardly surprising to find that there is a strong correlation (Olson *et al.*, 1973; Shono *et al.*, 1985). However the response to UVR is so variable that it has proved extremely difficult to make accurate predictions of the response. Sayre *et al.* (1966), for example, were unable to find significant relationships between the energy needed to produce erythema and the colouring of the subject. There seems to be very little evidence concerning the reliability of these judgements of sensitivity of skin to ultraviolet. One of us (JL) ranked two small groups of 8 and 5 subjects for estimated response to UVR and subsequently ranked the ultraviolet dose for each subject needed to produce a minimal erythema. The rankings for each group were compared using the Spearman ranked correlation coefficient (Croucher and Oliver, 1979) resulting in correlations of 0.786 and 0.9 respectively ($p > 0.05$), indicating good but not perfect agreement.

Assessing the response to UVR

The features used to assess the acute response to UVR include:

1 The duration of the latent period in hours.
2 The intensity of erythema—how red it is.
3 The duration of the erythema in hours or days.
4 The severity of any irritation.

5 The presence of oedema or blistering.
6 The extent and type of desquamation.

Visual grading and somewhat subjective judgement are used to grade the skin reaction in terms of degrees of erythema. This has been described by many writers, who differ in their descriptions somewhat (Low, 1986). Typical descriptions are shown in Table 15.4 together with the recognized relationships. The E_1 response is equivalent to the minimal erythema dose (MED) which is widely used in dermatology; minimal perceptible dose (MPD) or minimal perceptible erythema (MPE) are also used to describe the same thing. This latter term, MPE, would seem to be the most accurate since it appears that the latent period is an artefact as changes occur when ultraviolet is applied but are undetected by the eye (Diffey and Oakley, 1987). Definitions, however, vary considerably. It will be noticed that the relationship between the erythema doses—E_1, E_2, E_3, E_4—has an approximately log/linear relation with the duration of erythema (Low, 1986) see Table 15.4. There is a similar relationship between these doses and the latent periods shown by measurement of the actual erythema intensity by light reflectance spectrophotometry (Farr and Diffey, 1984).

It is most important to understand that the terms 'first-degree erythema' (E_1) and 'minimal erythemal dose (MED)' refer to the *response* used to define a dose. The terms are also used to indicate the dose. This customary practice is followed here but it must be realized that these terms refer to the individual *patient*. Thus referring to 'the E_1 of the lamp' is meaningless. What is being indicated is the likely erythemal response on, say, average caucasian skin at a given distance after a specified time of irradiation.

Test doses

The only way to assess the effect on any given individual is by a test. This is either applied to find the E_1 or MED response or to find the appropriate erythema for the dose to be given. An estimate is made of the time needed to produce the erythema at the intended distance with a given lamp by assessing the likely skin response based on skin colour, eye colour etc., as considered above. Some knowledge of the effect of the lamp on average skin is also needed (see below). For the Alpine sunlamp this is about 30–90 s at 50 cm from the burner and for a typical Theraktin about 4–5 min at 50 cm.

Three (or five) holes of at least 2 cm² are cut in a piece of lint, paper or other suitable material. The test dose area (see below) is cleaned to remove surface grease and the template fixed to it securely. The rest of the patient is screened and thus protected from the UVR by suitable material; ultraviolet goggles are worn. Welsh and Diffey (1981) suggested that tightly woven fabrics offered the best protection. Wood and Reed (1990) investigated the UVR that was transmitted through various thicknesses of commonly used screening material. One type of paper allowed 10% of the UVR output to be transmitted through one thickness. A single thickness of lint allowed 13% of the UVR to be transmitted, increasing to 23% when the lint was wet.

The central hole is exposed to the estimated 'best-guess' dose and the holes on each side to a greater and lesser dose. Some suggest as much as 50% larger and smaller respectively or with the use of five holes, doses 33 and 66% above and below the best estimate. Obviously greater confidence in the estimate would encourage the use of smaller differences. It is sensible to cut the holes as different sizes and shapes (Fig. 15.5) in order to make identification of the erythema easier for the patient. The smallest should not however be less than 1 cm^2 because more ultraviolet energy has been found to be needed (Olson *et al.*, 1965). It is suggested that this effect is simply due to the thickness of the shield material (Low, 1986). It is best if the test is conducted at the same distance as that to be used for treatment.

After exposure to the UVR the patient is given a card similar to Figure 15.5 (which may be the shield itself) and instructed to report the presence or absence of erythema. It is probably best to ask only for the recognition of erythema and not trouble the patient with judgement of intensity. The 24-h reading—the key one—can often be read by the physiotherapist if the patient returns for treatment at the same time on the next day. From this information the E_1 or other dose can be deduced. By definition the E_1 or minimal erythmal dose is the 'hole' that appeared last and disappeared first, i.e. the least visible response.

The area chosen for this test is of importance. If the patient is to inspect the part at regular intervals a convenient, visible site is essential. It should be clear of skin disease and not significantly more pigmented than the area to be treated. The anterior (flexor) surface of the forearm is the most usual but the abdomen, medial aspect of the arm or thigh are also possible sites that are not

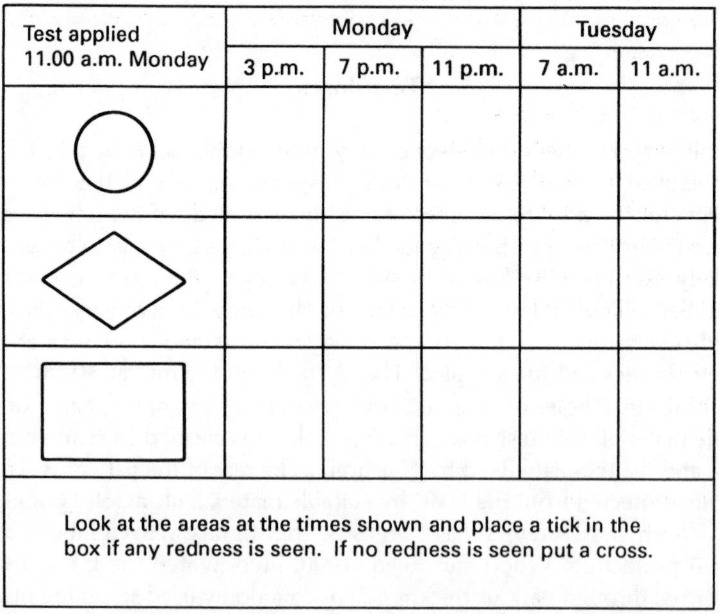

| Test applied | Monday | | | Tuesday | |
11.00 a.m. Monday	3 p.m.	7 p.m.	11 p.m.	7 a.m.	11 a.m.
○					
◇					
▭					
Look at the areas at the times shown and place a tick in the box if any redness is seen. If no redness is seen put a cross.					

Fig. 15.5 An example of a card given to a patient to record the result of a UVR test dose.

usually excessively exposed to natural sunlight. The skin of the limbs is more variable in its response than that of the trunk but the difference is small (Olson *et al.*, 1966). A thorough explanation of the test and its purpose should be given to the patient, including the warning that two or three red marks will probably be visible for a day and for those who tan readily a slight pigmented mark could be left for a week or so. Those who work in public with exposed forearms, such as waitresses, might prefer the test on some unexposed part.

Another purpose of a test dose is to determine the output of a lamp in terms of time required at a given distance for a specified erythema reaction on average skin. This is necessary for new lamps or if the output has been altered. Three staff members volunteer for the test—preferably one of average sensitivity, one slightly more sensitive (but not hypersensitive) and one slightly less so. A test dose is given to each subject in turn, as described above, and the average result determined. As already discussed, an E_1 is the minimum visible response and E_2 and E_3 responses can be judged by reference to Table 15.4.

Sensitization

Sensitization of the patient can occur with a variety of drugs, both ingested and applied topically. On some patients certain foods are said to cause this effect: strawberries have this reputation. Testing the response would take account of this effect but care needs to be exercised if a patient's drug regime has been altered during a course of ultraviolet treatments.

So many chemicals can act as sensitizers to ultraviolet in varying degrees that a comprehensive list would be prohibitively long. Commonly encountered groups are:

1 Psoralens—used as sensitizers.
2 Sulphonamides—antibiotics.
3 Tetracyclines—antibiotics.
4 Griseofulvin—antifungal agent.
5 Phenothiazine—tranquillizer.
6 Chlorthiazide—diuretic.
7 Hypnotic drugs (such as Veronal).
8 Barbiturates.
9 Gold therapy.
10 Various hormones.
11 Aspirin and derivatives.

Also substances applied to the surface:

1 Coal tar.
2 Dithranol.
3 Psoralens.
4 Eosin.

Electrotherapy explained

(See Wadsworth and Chanmugan, 1980; Griffin and Karselis, 1988 for more extensive lists.)

Progression of ultraviolet dosage

Even the smallest dose of ultraviolet which has no evident immediate effect causes a change in the skin due to pigmentation, allowing greater tolerance of ultraviolet. Thus, if the same erythemal effect is to be achieved repeatedly the dose must be increased to compensate each time. Table 15.5 provides guidance but it must be understood that the increased dose needed is dependent on the pigmentation and thickening, so that patients who pigment easily will need the full increase whereas those who do not will need less.

Table 15.5 Increased dose of UVR to compensate for increased tolerance

Original dose	Earliest time at which the dose can be repeated	Increase (%)
Suberythemal E_0	24 h	12.5
MED E_1	2 days	25
E_2	3–4 days	50
E_3	1 week	75

MED = minimal erythemal dose.

Advice on the increases used to repeat suberythemal doses varies; 10, 12.5 and 15% of the E_1 have all been suggested. This probably reflects different perceptions of what proportion the suberythemal dose is with respect to the E_1; half, five-eighths, three-quarters and just less than an E_1 have all been offered. Two-thirds is perhaps reasonable.

The earliest time given in Table 15.5 is somewhat more conservative than suggested elsewhere, e.g. Wadsworth and Chanmugan (1980). The essential point is that the erythema should have faded completely before a further dose of ultraviolet is given. There is no obvious reason for applying an E_4 dose on normal skin but if it were to be done some 2 weeks might be allowed for recovery.

As ultraviolet provokes an inflammatory reaction in the skin heavy doses involving large areas can cause systemic illness. The usual guidelines given are:

Suberythemal or E_1 may be safely applied to the whole body.
E_2 may be applied to not more than 20% of body surface area.
E_3 may be applied to not more than 4% of body surface area (about 600 cm^2).

An E_4 is not usually given on skin; if it were, maximum area would be 25 cm^2. On open wounds larger areas may be safely treated.

PRINCIPLES OF APPLICATION

General UVB application with a Theraktin

Having completed a test dose and explained the nature and effects of the treatment to the patient the ultraviolet application can be given. A suitable plinth is usually kept in position so that the Theraktin tunnel can be placed in a standard position with the tubes about 50 cm (this varies with the model) from the surface of the average patient lying on the plinth. The patient undresses completely, puts on protective ultraviolet goggles and lies down on the plinth with arms and legs straight and a little abducted. It is important not to allow the limbs to shade one another or the trunk. The head and feet protrude from the tunnel and thus receive a somewhat lower dose. The tunnel is then lowered and the correct distance from patient to tubes is measured. The position of the patient with respect to the tunnel must be repeatable from one treatment to the next. If the patient starts in prone lying with the palms facing upwards the position of the head must be made comfortable, often turned to one side. The patient is warned to keep still and not to touch the tunnel and the lamp is then switched on for the appropriate time for the required dose. After this time the lamp is switched off and the patient turns over, this time with the palms facing downwards and the head turned to the same side, to give an equivalent dose to the opposite side of the face. The lamps are again switched on for the required time and then off, and the treatment is completed.

If the patient is afflicted by modesty a suitable cloth can be used to cover the genitalia and removed by the patient as treatment begins. Wearing underwear is inefficient since it is best to expose as large an area of skin as possible. If it is considered desirable for the patient to wear a pair of briefs they must be the same pair at each treatment, otherwise a previously untreated region of skin becomes exposed late in the course so that the patient suffers perhaps an E_2 in a very inconvenient site!

Treatment may be given each day for an E_0 for the whole body, or half the body (i.e. one side only) daily with an E_1, or the whole body with an E_1 on alternate days. At each treatment the dose is increased by prolonging the time of treatment. Increasing by exactly 12.5% (one-eighth) at each treatment to repeat a suberythemal dose would be absurdly pedantic; it is sensible to increase to convenient fractions of a minute.

If an erythema occurs after treatment the dose has obviously been greater than suberythemal and should be reduced. If it is a mild erythema not progressing the dose is usually adequate. If for any reason the regular treatments are missed for a time some of the protective pigmentation and thickening is lost and a difficult judgement must be made about the appropriate dose to use. It is best to presume all protective effect is lost over 4 weeks. Table 15.6 offers suggested guidance only as people vary widely in their response.

It is evident that progression cannot be continued indefinitely since the

Electrotherapy explained

Table 15.6 Regression of general UVB treatments

If no treatments have been given for:	Dose
Up to 4 days	Usual progression
5–7 days	Repeat previous dose
8–13 days	Use the dose given at 4 treatments before this one
14–20 days	Use the dose given at 8 treatments before this one
21–27 days	Use the dose given at 12 treatments before this one
28 days or more	Use the original dose

protective changes will reach their maximum at some stage. Protection has been achieved such that the E_I (or MED) is many times the original E_I but most UVB treatment regimes are given to raise the E_I to between 3 and 5 times the original. The extent to which the dose can be progressed will depend primarily on the skin type, which is genetically determined. As any possible carcinogenic effects are dependent on age and annual ultraviolet exposure (see above) and since the only reasonable measure of exposure is the MED or E_I (Diffey, 1989) it seems sensible to limit the progression of treatment in terms of multiples of the E_I rather than an arbitrary length of course in weeks or a maximum dosage in minutes: 4-week courses and 20-min maximum applications have been recommended by some.

PUVA treatment

The use of psoralens to sensitize patients to UVA, principally for the treatment of psoriasis, was described above. Some PUVA units are like the Theraktin tunnel—the patient is treated lying; others are in vertical cabinets in which the patient stands. Patients are given 8-methoxypsoralen by mouth and exposed to the UVA some 2–3 h later. They are given grey or green glasses to wear while sensitized, i.e. from the time of taking the tablets until 8 h afterwards. They are also warned not to expose themselves to the sun for at least 8 h from ingestion (Fusco *et al.*, 1980).

If there is only a small area of psoriasis or a resistant area, a topical preparation of 8-methoxypsoralen can be applied. The concentration of the drug in the skin is much higher than that with tablets so the dose of UVA is much lower (Klaber, 1980).

A test dose is usually given to determine the patient's sensitivity and subsequently a whole-body dose of UVA is applied. This can either be sufficient to produce a mild erythema at about 3 days (the erythema due to UVA appears much later than that due to UVB) or suberythemal. Treatment may be given two or three times a week, progressively increasing the dose at weekly intervals for several weeks. The UVA dosage is measured in J/cm^2 and increases of $0.5–1 J/cm^2$ are a usual progression. The principle of basing the dosage on the response of the patient and progressing the dose is the same as for UVB, the difference being that the response to UVA is slower than to UVB.

After 2 or 3 weeks of PUVA treatment marked pigmentation can develop. This is more evident than with UVB but it is not as effective in protecting the skin from UVB radiation damage as the pigmentation provoked by UVB itself. This is possibly due to some difference in skin thickening which may be more important for UVB protection. It is important for physiotherapists to recognize this since patients who are deeply tanned by PUVA or from commercial sunbeds may not be as well protected as their colour might suggest.

There are some undesirable effects resulting from prolonged UVA treatment, notably skin changes similar to ageing of the skin after high doses, which recover after treatment is completed. There is also the possibility of promoting skin cancer and cataracts, both also associated with high doses.

The comparative benefits of UVB and PUVA have been investigated in a number of studies, e.g. Kenicer *et al.* (1981). It seems that UVB and low-dose PUVA are successful and very similar in their effect on psoriasis and that high-dose PUVA is best used on selected patients who have not improved with UVB or low-dose PUVA. Van Weelden *et al.* (1980) suggest that UVB is not only as good as UVA but safer and more economical.

Some regimes for both UVB and PUVA continue as maintenance, that is a moderate dose applied at weekly, fortnightly or monthly intervals in an attempt to prevent the recurrence of psoriasis. The value of this method is difficult to quantify and some feel that treatment should not be prolonged unless there is good evidence that cessation leads to further development of psoriasis.

Local UVB application with an air-cooled Alpine sunlamp

The majority of treatments with the Alpine sunlamp will be local—treating a defined area rather than general treatment of the whole body—although the lamp can be used for whole-body treatment using a sectional technique.

The lamp must be switched on some 5 min before it is to be used to allow the UV output to become stabilized. During this time it must be positioned so as to avoid irradiating patient or therapist. The part to be treated is exposed and cleaned to remove surface grease, either by washing or by wiping with surgical spirit. The nature of the treatment and especially the skin reaction should be fully explained to the patient as well as the necessity of keeping as still as possible during setting up and application of treatment. The patient, and in particular the part to be treated, is conveniently and comfortably positioned and supported. The dosage will have been determined by doing a test, as already described.

All areas of the patient that could be exposed to radiation when the lamp is positioned and that are not to be treated are protected with clothing or suitable screening material (see above). The part to be treated is then covered with a separate sheet of sufficient thickness and the lamp is positioned so that radiation will strike the area at right angles and irradiate the whole area intended for treatment. The distance between the burner of the lamp and the skin is carefully measured; the usual distance is 50 cm. This is more safely measured, from the physiotherapist's point of view, either from the rim of the reflector to the central point of the area to be treated or using a measuring stick. In these cases the distances measured will be 45 and 40 cm respectively (Fig. 15.6). It is critically important to record this correctly and without ambiguity as an accidental reduction in distance between test dose and treatment or between subsequent treatments could lead to a much greater dose than intended (see the inverse square law; Chapter 11).

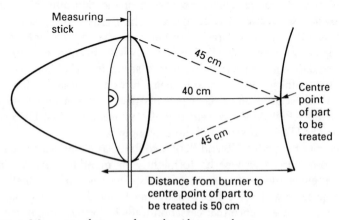

Fig. 15.6 Measuring distances from the Alpine sunlamp.

Accurate and precise timing of irradiation is also essential. After irradiation is completed the part is either immediately rescreened or the lamp switched off if not required further.

If the part is to be treated several times the dose will need to be increased (Table 15.5). It is important that the same area is treated on each occasion since the application of the higher dose to previously unexposed skin will lead to an excessive reaction. This problem is solved in many situations due to the curved shape of the body. Radiations applied to the whole surface of a limb or the rounded back will gradually reduce in intensity around the curve (see cosine law and Fig. 11.3, Chapter 11). Thus there is no sharp demarcation with untreated skin and small changes of position of the lamp will have little effect. In flat areas, such as the upper back, it is possible to produce the same gradual shading effect by moving the screening slightly during treatment; thus after, say, a quarter of the treatment time the cover is rolled down 2 or 3 cm; after half the time a further 3 cm; after three-quarters of the time it is completely removed. The result is a gradual change over the area of skin at the edge of the treatment area which is both safer for subsequent treatments and cosmetically more acceptable. The alternative is to screen the skin to the same exact line each time, which of necessity has to be a fixed point. This becomes easier if the line is subsequently marked by pigmentation.

It is important not to irradiate more than maximum skin surface, as described above.

Particular considerations for local UVR to the face

When an erythematous dose is to be applied to the face, using goggles would lead to an owl-like appearance of white encircled eyes in an otherwise red face. It is therefore usual to ask the patient to close the eyes and protect the eyelids with small pieces of cotton wool secured by a smear of petroleum jelly.

Due to the shape of the face and the distribution of the skin disease, e.g. acne, treatment may have to be applied from two or three different angles (Fig. 15.7). When treatment is applied from the front the tip of the nose is significantly nearer to the lamp than the rest of the face, so to avoid overtreatment a light smear of petroleum jelly may be applied. If the face is treated from the side, the same applies to the ears.

Determining the line on the neck which should be screened presents a problem. This can be solved by gradual shading as described above or having a fixed neckline by wearing the same top each treatment or by screening the neck up to the chinline where no sharp demarcation line is noticeable because the undersurface of the chin is not normally exposed.

Strong ultraviolet reactions in the skin around the lips may lead to discomfort so that the dose to this area is sometimes reduced by smearing on a little petroleum jelly.

In order to avoid the danger of irradiation of previously covered skin it is safer to tie the hair back so that the UVR reaches to the hairline.

Local treatment using a water-cooled Kromayer lamp

This is sometimes called 'focal' treatment. Such treatments are almost entirely applied to open wounds or the skin close to the wound. The purpose of such treatment, explained earlier, is to kill surface bacteria, promote an inflammatory reaction in the tissues to aid control of infection and to promote skin growth. It is evident that the dose needed to promote skin growth is much less than that suitable for bacterial destruction. Thus heavy doses (E_4 or $2 \times E_4$) are applied to the infected surfaces of, say, an ulcer or bedsore while an E_1 or E_2 is applied to the surrounding skin. Where new epithelium is just beginning to grow it is best to avoid treating altogether, or apply only a suberythemal dose, preferably through a blue uviol filter which filters out the red end of the visible spectrum and all UVR below 290 nm. An E_3 dose is appropriate for a clean but indolent non-skin area which is not healing.

That the ultraviolet output from the Kromayer is strongly bacteriocidal is evident (e.g. High and High, 1983) but of course, UVR cannot penetrate far into the tissues so that the main effect will be on the surface of the open wound, some of which may be necrotic. This, however, is just the region that

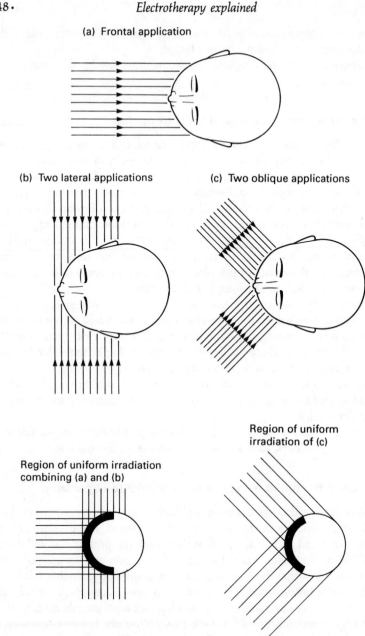

(a) Frontal application

(b) Two lateral applications

(c) Two oblique applications

Region of uniform irradiation combining (a) and (b)

Region of uniform irradiation of (c)

Fig. 15.7 Ultraviolet treatment of the face.

may not be reached by systemic antibiotics. In describing a heavy dose given to the infected surface as an E_4 or double E_4 (some refer to this as an E_5) the skin response is used as a description, although in these cases there is no skin.

The surface to be treated and the Kromayer face are cleaned with a moist swab, as far as possible, and the face is applied on, or close to, the open area. The surrounding skin must be protected when E_4 doses are being used. This can be done with an exactly cut hole in a double thickness of lint or paper or, more easily, by moulding flattened strips of wet cotton wool or gauze around the skin edge and covering the area beyond with dressing towels. Wood and Reed (in press) found that it needed 10 thicknesses of wet gauze to prevent transmission of UVR. The thickness of the cotton wool or gauze, wetted with whatever antiseptic solution is being used for cleaning the area, provides spacing, allowing the face of the Kromayer to be supported just clear of the surface (Low, 1961). As noted above, in this situation the dose is independent of the patient's skin response so that the E_4 dose on 'average' skin is used, which for a new Kromayer is likely to be about 10 s in contact. If the face is being held a short distance off the surface the dose must be increased (see below). If the open area is larger than the Kromayer face it can be treated either by a number of applications at different sites or by holding the lamp at a greater distance, allowing the radiations to diverge and hence cover the whole area.

To treat a larger area than the Kromayer face, e.g. around the open area, with an E_1 or E_2 it is usually most convenient to apply the lamp at a distance: 10 cm is often used. To hold the lamp at the correct distance a ruler or wooden spatula is temporarily taped to the side of the lamp so that when the end is touching the skin the lamp is at the correct distance (Wadsworth and Chanmugan, 1980). To calculate the dosage at different distances the inverse square law can be used as a guide. However, the times required to produce the different erythema doses in contact and at set distances should be available with each lamp from previously performed test doses (see above).

Since the dose applied to the infected area is so large compared to that given to the skin it is inconsequential that the skin dose is additionally applied to the open wound.

Reasonable precautions should be taken to avoid the spread of infection from the open wound and the quartz window may be cleaned with surgical spirit after contact with a patient. There is no need for further sterilization as the quantity of UVC emitted is lethal to bacteria on the surface.

Applicators

The Kromayer can also be fitted with quartz rod applicators in order to convey UVR into narrow sinuses or under overhanging wound edges. The applicator is fitted into a holder with a finger-operated shutter that is mounted against the quartz face of the Kromayer. Applicators are of various shapes and sizes. Ultraviolet is conveyed in the quartz without escaping due to total internal reflection (see Chapter 11). This is very effective because of the high refractive index between air and quartz (it is 1.46 which leads to a critical angle of 44°). If, however, the quartz rod is in water, which is effectively the case when it is in a sinus held against watery tissues, the refractive index is much lower (about 1.1, giving a critical angle of 65.5°; Nightingale, 1959). This means that much more UVR will leak from the sides of the applicator when it is in the tissues. A considerable proportion of the ultraviolet is absorbed in the applicator meaning that the dose must be much increased when one is used. A guide to this increase is given by multiplying the contact dose by a factor which is found from the applicator length in centimetres divided by 2.5 (Wadsworth and Chanmugan, 1980). In older units this meant one contact dose for every inch of applicator. Thus for a 7.5 cm applicator being used to deliver a contact dose of 20 s the appropriate time would be 60 s ($7.5/2.5 = 3$; $3 \times 20 = 60$). However, applicators vary a good deal and the above guide may well give an erroneous result so it is often best to test the applicator to be used with an estimated E_1 on normal skin.

When the lamp is used at a distance from the skin there is not only a change of intensity, as explained, but also a change in the relative proportions of UVB and UVC due to the greater absorption of UVC in air. This is also true of the Alpine sunlamp but is of special consequence if the bacteriocidal effect, which is largely due to UVC, is important for therapy.

Control and care of the Kromayer lamp

For safety reasons the mica cap should be kept in place at all times, except when treatment is taking place. The pump unit is switched on first and water circulation is checked by watching movement of the water in the treatment head. If an air bubble is seen in the water the window is tilted downwards to release the air. The burner can now be switched on, allowing 5 min for the output to stabilize. If the lamp is being applied at some distance from the skin the therapist and, if necessary, the patient should wear protective goggles. At the end of treatment the lamp should be switched off but the water pump left running for a few minutes to cool the lamp. Distilled water is used in the tank so that it does not leave deposits as it evaporates. The Kromayer lamp should be regularly cleaned in accordance with the manufacturers' instructions.

Records of UVR treatment

It is important to keep adequate records of all treatments but for ultraviolet treatments the information must be precise and complete both for safety and in order to give adequate treatment. For all ultraviolet treatments the following should always be recorded:

1 *Date*—it is essential to know the exact date of a given treatment for calculating progression etc.
2 *Lamp* used—the particular lamp should be clearly identified.
3 *Distance* at which treatment is applied; this must be unequivocal.
4 Exact *area treated*—and precisely where and how untreated regions were screened. The position of the patient should be noted in the case of the Theraktin.
5 *Time* for which the treatment was applied.
6 *Reaction* obtained; this should be recorded at subsequent attendance.

Other information may also be needed, such as any change in the condition (the size of the ulcer, perhaps, or the condition of the psoriatic patches etc.).

DANGERS

Since the results of ultraviolet treatment are not immediately evident, as there is no sensation and visible erythema appears only later, mistakes can easily occur.

Eyes

It is important to protect the eyes of both patient and therapist from scattered and reflected radiations. The patient should wear goggles even when not facing the source of radiation. The physiotherapist should also be aware of the cumulative effects of UVR throughout the day, e.g. six treatments of 10 s = 1 min exposure. Ordinary glasses, although impervious to UV, do not protect the eyes from lateral radiation so proper protective goggles should be worn at all times.

Overdose

1 *Too long an exposure*. It is essential to use an accurate timing device and for periods over about 1 min to have a timer with an audible warning.
2 *Too close to the lamp*. This will either occur because of inaccurate measurement or because the patient moves. Patients have been known to move closer to the lamp in the hope of receiving more effective treatment. A failure of the therapist to recognize the implications of the inverse square law is possibly the most frequent cause of excessive exposure when positioning the lamp, e.g. if an E_1 at 50 cm is 2 min, at 10 cm, just beyond the rim of the reflector, an E_1 is obtained in under 5 s.
3 *Previously protected skin* being irradiated at subsequent treatments. This can be caused by alterations in screening, different clothes, a haircut or even removal of a watch strap.
4 *Sensitizers*, e.g. change of drugs.
5 *Change of lamp*.

If an overdose is suspected it is traditionally recommended (Forster and Palastanga, 1985) that infrared should be applied to the area to produce a heat-induced erythema and hopefully disperse substances that will produce the photochemical erythema.

Ozone

Because ozone is formed it is important to ensure adequate ventilation in the area.

Electrotherapy explained

CONTRAINDICATIONS

1 Acute skin conditions—acute eczema, dermatitis and an existing ultraviolet erythema.
2 Skin damage due to ionizing radiations—deep X-ray therapy.
3 Systemic lupus erythematosus can be triggered or exacerbated.
4 Photoallergy—allergic reaction to UVR.
5 Acute febrile illness—whole-body treatment should be avoided.
6 Recent skin grafts.

HELIOTHERAPY

Heliotherapy is treatment by natural sunlight and has been used since Greek and Roman times. Early in this century heliotherapy was widely used for the treatment of tuberculosis, both pulmonary and other. This can only be effectively applied if there is a reasonable expectation of sufficient sunshine, so that many sanatoria developed in mountainous regions, notably the Swiss Alps, where the proportion of ultraviolet compared to infrared radiation is greater due to the altitude. The technique used was to expose the whole body to gradually increasing doses by graded increases of both time and area (Rollier, 1927). It was emphasized that treatment should always remain less than a sunburn dose, i.e. it should be a suberythemal dose.

The advent of artificial sources of ultraviolet (e.g. the carbon arc lamp) led to sanatoria in other than these cool, sunny climates treating tuberculosis with rest and ultraviolet. Subsequent improvements in hygiene and medication as well as other reasons have reduced the need for isolation or ultraviolet treatment of this disease.

A more recent form of heliotherapy involves the treatment of psoriasis at the Dead Sea in Israel. It is considered that the lower UVB spectrum of the sun in this region, which is well below sea level, may allow patients to receive more ultraviolet without burning; that is, the spectrum contains relatively more UVA. Some local minerals are also considered to contribute. There are claims that this is a highly effective treatment for psoriasis.

It is well known that sunburn—due to solar UVB—is only likely to occur in the summer in temperate zones. The UVB component of solar radiation is particularly dependent on the angle of the sun to the surface of the earth, thus although visible and UVA radiations increase in summer, the UVB increases proportionally much more. In fact the UVB is about 100 times more intense in summer than in winter (Diffey, 1982b). This large change occurs very slowly and it is reasonable to presume that human skin is biologically adapted to adjust to slow change.

SUNBEDS

The use of UVA-emitting sunbeds for cosmetic tanning has increased enormously in the past few years. Such sunbeds are of various types but are usually panels containing a number of fluorescent tubes giving UVA and visible radiations. An individual may lie under, and sometimes on, such a panel of tubes and it is claimed that pigmentation without erythema will occur: 'tanning without burning'. Those who already have some pigmentation tend to pigment further but for others the effect may not be marked (Rivers *et al.*, 1989). It is also important to be aware that the pigmentation induced is not a very efficient protection against later applications of UVB from the sun. There have also been found to be a high level of acute temporary, adverse effects — like irritation — as well as some possibly serious disturbances of the cell-mediated immunity system of the skin (Hawk, 1983; Rivers *et al.*, 1989).

IONOZONE THERAPY

This involves the production of ionized water vapour. The steam is produced by heating water in a tank in the body of the machine. It is passed over an ultraviolet lamp and emitted as ionized water with some ozone and oxygen. This gentle jet is applied to open wounds such as ulcers and pressure sores, and to the upper respiratory tract.

The effects are said to include a sedatory effect on nerve endings which leads to pain relief; increased blood flow affecting metabolic processes of the skin, and a bacteriocidal effect (Dolphin and Walker, 1979).

Application

Once the distilled water has been heated sufficiently to produce vapour from the nozzle of the machine the ultraviolet is turned on (it is not emitted). The nozzle is directed at the wound from a distance of 35–50 cm. The surrounding skin is protected with plastic sheeting to prevent it becoming wet. Treatment is given for 10–30 min once a day or less if the wound is clean. The moisture which accumulates in the wound should be removed before a dressing is applied.

The application should not be too close to the patient in case the surrounding skin is heat-damaged.

No controlled trials seem to have been published but a survey of 200 patients treated by this modality found that 168 had their lesions completely healed (Dolphin and Walker, 1979).

REFERENCES

Burger A., Jordaad M. J., Schombee G. E. (1985). The bacteriocidal effect of ultra-violet light on infected pressure sores. *South Afr. J. Physiother.*, **41**, 55–7.
Burton J. L. (1979). *Essentials of Dermatology*. Churchill Livingstone.
Cerio R., Low J. L. (1987). Successful treatment by general ultraviolet radiation of pruritus due to biliary cirrhosis. *Physiotherapy*, **73**, 89.
Cerio, R., Murphy, G. M., Sladen G. E., MacDonald D. M. (1987). A combination of phototherapy and cholestyramine for the relief of pruritus in primary biliary cirrhosis. *Br. J. Dermatol.*, **116**, 267–8.

Corless D., Gupta S., Switala S. (1978). Response of plasma 25-hydroxyvitamin D to ultraviolet irradiation in long-stay geriatric patients. *Lancet*, **ii**, 649–51.

Croucher J. S., Oliver E. (1979). *Statistics: an Introduction*. Australia: McGraw-Hill.

De Leo V. A., Horlick H., Hanson H. *et al.* (1984). Ultraviolet radiation induces changes in membrane metabolism of human keratinocytes in culture. *J. Invest. Dermatol.*, **83**, 323–6.

Diffey B. L. (1982a). The consistency of studies of ultraviolet erythema in normal human skin. *Phys. Med. Biol.*, **27**, 715–20.

Diffey B. L. (1982b). *Ultraviolet Radiation in Medicine*. Medical physics handbooks 11. Bristol: Adam Hilger.

Diffey B. L. (1989). Ultraviolet radiation and skin cancer. *Physiotherapy*, **75**, 615–16.

Diffey B. L., Oakley A. M. (1987). The onset of ultraviolet erythema. *Br. J. Dermatol.*, **116**, 183–7.

Diffey B., Oliver R. (1981). An ultraviolet radiation monitor for routine use in physiotherapy. *Physiotherapy*, **67**, 64–6.

Dodd H. J., Sarkany I., Gaylarde P. M. (1989). Short term benefit and long term failure of ultraviolet light in the treatment of venous leg ulcers. *Br. J. Dermatol.*, **120**, 809–18.

Dolphin S., Walker M. (1979). Healing accelerated by ionozone therapy. *Physiotherapy*, **65**, 81–2.

English J. (1965). Recent advances in ultra-violet irradiation: photosensitivity tests. *Physiotherapy*, **51**, 156–8.

Evans P. (1980). The healing process at cellular level: a review. *Physiotherapy*, **66**, 256–9.

Farr P. M., Diffey B. L. (1984). Quantitative studies on cutaneous erythema induced by ultraviolet radiation. *Br. J. Dermatol.*, **111**, 673–82.

Farr P. M., Diffey B. L. (1985). The erythemal response of human skin to ultraviolet radiation. *Br. J. Dermatol.*, **113**, 65–76.

Fears T. R., Scotto J., Schneiderman M. A. (1977). Mathematical models of age and ultraviolet effects on the incidence of skin cancer among whites in the United States. *Am. J. Dermatol.*, **114**, 479–84.

Forster A., Palastanga N. (1985). *Clayton's Electrotherapy: Theory and Practice*. Eastbourne: Baillière Tindall.

Fusco R. J., Jordan P. A., Kelley A., Samuel M. (1980). PUVA therapy for psoriasis. *Physiotherapy*, **66**, 39–40.

Gilchrist B. A., Rowe J. W., Brown R. S. *et al.* (1977). Relief of uremic pruritus with ultraviolet phototherapy. *N.Z. J. Med.*, **297**, 136–8.

Goats G. C. (1988). Appropriate use of the inverse square law. *Physiotherapy*, **74**, 8.

Griffin J. E., Karselis T. C. (1988). *Physical Agents and/or Physical Therapists*, 3rd edn. Springfield: Charles C. Thomas.

Gupta A. K., Ellis C. N., Tellner D. C. *et al.* (1989). Double-blind placebo controlled study to evaluate the efficacy of fish oil and low dose UVB in the treatment of psoriasis. *Br. J. Dermatol.*, **120**, 801–7.

Hawk J. L. M. (1983). Sunbeds. *Br. Med. J.*, **286**, 329.

High A. S., High J. P. (1983). Treatment of infected skin wounds using ultraviolet radiation—an in vitro study, 2. *Physiotherapy*, **69**, 359–60.

Ingram J. T. (1954). The significance and management of psoriasis. *Br. Med. J.*, 823–8.

Kenicer K. J. A., Lakshmipathi T., Addoh A. *et al.* (1981). An assessment of the effect of photochemotherapy (PUVA) and UV-B phototherapy in the treatment of psoriasis. *Br. J. Dermatol.*, **105**, 629–39.

Klaber M. R. (1980). Ultra-violet light for psoriasis. *Physiotherapy*, **66**, 36–8.

Le Vine M. J., White H. A. D., Parrish J. A. (1979). Components of the Goeckerman regimen. *J. Invest. Dermatol.*, **73**, 170.

Low J. L. (1961). Localization of UV dose in the treatment of varicose ulcers. *N.Z. J. Physiother.*, **3**, 20.

Low J. L. (1986). Quantifying the erythema due to UVR. *Physiotherapy*, **72**, 60–4.

National Radiological Protection Board. *Protection Against Ultraviolet Radiation in the Work Place*. Didcot: Her Majesty's Stationery Office.

Nightingale A. (1959). *Physics and Electronics in Physical Medicine*. London: Bell and Sons Ltd.

Nonaka S., Kaidley K. H., Kligman A. M. (1984). Photoprotective adaptation—some quantitative aspects. *Arch. Dermatol.*, **120**, 609–13.

Olson R. L., Sayre R. M., Everett M. A. (1965). The effect of field size on ultraviolet MED. *J. Invest. Dermatol.*, **68**, 516–18.

Olson R. L., Sayre R. M., Everett M. A. (1966). Effect of anatomic location and time on ultraviolet erythema. *Arch. Dermatol.*, **93**, 211–15.

Olson R. L., Gaylor J., Everett M. A. (1973). Skin colour, melanin and erythema. *Arch. Dermatol.*, **108**, 541–4.

Räsänen L., Reunala T., Lehto M. *et al.* (1989). Immediate decrease in antigen-presenting function and delayed enhancement of interleukin-I production in human epidermal cells after in vivo UVB radiation. *Br. J. Dermatol.*, **120**, 589–96.

Rivers J. K., Norris P. G., Murphy G. M. *et al.* (1989). UVA sunbeds: tanning, photoprotection, acute adverse effects and immunological changes. *Br. J. Dermatol.*, **120**, 767–77.

Rollier A. (1927). *Heliotherapy* 2nd edn. London: Oxford University Press.

Sayre R. M., Olson R. L., Everett M. A. (1966). Qualitative studies on erythema. *J. Invest. Dermatol.*, **46**, 240–4.

Scott B. O. (1983). Clinical uses of ultraviolet radiation. In *Therapeutic Electricity and Ultraviolet Radiation* 3rd edn (Stillwell G. K., ed.). Baltimore: Williams & Wilkins, pp. 228–61.

Shono S., Imura M., Ota M. *et al.* (1985). The relationship of skin colour, UVB induced erythema and melangenesis. *J. Invest. Dermatol.*, **84**, 265–7.

Van Weelden H., Young E., Van der Leun J. C. (1980). Therapy of psoriasis: comparison of photochemotherapy and several variants of phototherapy. *Br. J. Dermatol.*, **103**, 9.

Wadsworth H., Chanmugan A. P. P. (1980). *Electrophysical Agents in Physiotherapy*. Marrickville, NSW, Australia: Science Press.

Welsh C., Diffey B. (1981). The protection against solar actinic radiation afforded by common clothing fabrics. *Clin. Exp. Dermatol.*, **6**, 577–82.

Williams P. L., Warwick R., Dyson M., Bannister L. (eds) (1989). *Grays Anatomy*, 37th edn. Edinburgh: Longman.

Wolff K., Gschnait F., Honigsmann H. *et al.* (1977). Phototesting and dosimetry for photochemotherapy. *Br. J. Dermatol.*, **96**, 1–10.

Wood K., Reed A. (in press). A study of the intensity of ultraviolet radiations transmitted through a variety of screening materials. *Physiotherapy*.

Appendix A

NATURE OF AN ELECTRIC CURRENT

An electric current is a flow of electric charges. Electrons, protons and ions are the charges involved, although other subatomic particles may carry charges. Conductors are materials in which the outer shell electrons are free to move between constituent atoms. Normally this movement is random but if a voltage (an electric pressure) is applied to the material electrons will move away from the negative towards the positive charge. Although the motion of electrons is very rapid the movement of electrons from atom to atom (the electron drift) is quite slow. This is a conduction current and it is how charges move in metals and carbon and hence in electrical apparatus. Current is a rate of flow, that is a quantity of electrons per unit time. A rather large number of electrons (6.25×10^{18}) is the unit of quantity called a coulomb and when this quantity passes a point in 1 s the rate of flow, or current intensity, is called 1 ampere.

It is important to recognize that random electron movement occurs constantly at normal temperatures and that the electric current is super-imposed on this. It is analogous to the arrivals channel of a large international airport; aircraft deliver passengers who pass through passport control, customs etc. and eventually leave by car, bus or train. Looked at over a time-period of, say, a day the number of passengers leaving the airport is the same as the number arriving—the rate of flow may be expressed as so many thousand passengers per day—yet individual passengers have followed different pathways and spent different lengths of time at the airport. Some have been delayed by customs, some have had to wait for friends to meet them, some have gone to the restaurant for a meal and so forth, while others have passed through as quickly as they could. On a normal working day the airport is full of people as a conductor is full of electrons.

In a conductor it is only the electrons that move because the atoms are firmly held in crystalline structures which are typical of metal (and metalloid) solids; it is therefore called a conduction current. In fluids, liquids and gases, the atoms and molecules are free to move and therefore can take part in the flow of charges if they become charged. When an atom gains or loses an electron—hence it becomes negatively or positively charged—it is called an ion. Electrolytes are solutions containing ions. Body fluids are electrolytes and current can pass by the movement of these ions. Positive ions move towards the negative pole, the source of additional electrons, while negative ions move to the positive pole where electrons are being removed. Thus there is a two-way motion of ions which constitutes the current, called a convection current.

The rate of flow of charges (the current intensity) is measured in amperes. In any given conductor it will simply depend on the electric pressure or electric force, known as the voltage. It is ultimately due to the attraction of electrons for protons, that is the electric force of the atom. This is measured in volts and is known, descriptively, as an electromotive force. The difficulty electrons have in moving within a solid conductor, or ions have in moving in an electrolyte, will also determine the rate of flow and this is described as the resistance, measured in ohms. Thus a conductor with a greater resistance will allow a smaller flow of electrons. These concepts are expressed in Ohm's law which states that the current intensity (I) in amperes is directly proportional to the electromotive force (E) in volts and inversely proportional to the resistance (R) in ohms. $I = E/R$ thus $A = V/\Omega$. This is analogous to the flow of water from a tap which depends on the pressure driving it (height of the tank) and the resistance offered by the tap (how far it is turned on).

Appendix B

ELECTROLYSIS

Electrolytes are solutions containing ions. When crystalline substances dissolve in water some separation into ions occurs so that there are always a number of negatively and positively charged particles due both to the dissolved solid and dissociation of the water molecule to form OH^- and H^+ ions. If an electric field is applied by means of a pair of metal electrodes the ions will move through the solution, as shown in Figure A1. Thus positive ions move towards the negative electrode or cathode and are sometimes, rather confusingly, called cations. Negative ions move to the positive electrode or anode, hence these may be called anions. When the ions reach the metal plate or electrode they lose their charge. Positive ions gain an electron from the negatively charged metal plate and the negative ions give up their extra electron to the positive plate. The current in the solution is transmitted as ions (charges) moving in both directions. This is called a convection current. As the ions are neutralized electrically to form atoms they will act chemically. Ions 'used up' in this way are replaced in the solution by further dissociation to maintain the supply of charges. The chemical interactions that can occur at the electrodes are often complex and can involve the metal of these electrodes, so that metal may sometimes be removed from one plate and deposited on the other.

Sodium chloride solutions are utilized in transmitting current to and from the tissues for treatment purposes and will be considered, but similar effects occur where other salts, acids or bases are involved. Acid solutions are formed at the anode with the liberation of oxygen gas and alkaline solutions at the cathode where hydrogen is given off. This occurs because OH^- ions are neutralized at the anode to give OH radicals which combine to form water and release oxygen.

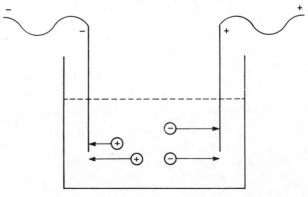

Fig. A1

Thus: $OH^- \rightarrow OH +$ an electron

$$4OH \rightarrow 2H_2O + O_2$$

Similarly Cl^- ions when neutralized react with water to form HCl and release oxygen. Consequently the excess H makes the region acidic. At the cathode H^+ ions are neutralized to form hydrogen gas and Na forms sodium hydroxide (NaOH) with the water when neutralized. Thus:

$$2Na + 2H_2O \rightarrow 2NaOH + H_2$$

The solution therefore becomes alkaline in this region and hydrogen gas is released.

These effects of altered pH and release of oxygen and hydrogen will occur whatever the salt, acid or base in solution with inert electrodes. The amount of gas produced is small in therapeutic situations and tends to remain dissolved in the water. However, if the current density is made high—say by passing a large current between two wires placed in a bowl of water—gas bubbles can be seen. These are especially evident at the cathode because of the larger quantity of hydrogen produced; in fact this can be used to determine the polarity as can the acidity/alkalinity test with litmus paper.

TRANSFORMERS

A transformer consists of two coils of insulated wire wound over one another on a common axis or on a common iron core. If a varying current is passed in one coil it will set up a varying magnetic field which affects both coils. This changing magnetic field will induce an electromotive force in the second coil and, if the circuit is completed, a current will flow. The effect between the two coils is called mutual induction; it will of course only occur as a result of a varying current. This type of arrangement is widely used to alter the voltage of the mains for many applications, hence it is known as a voltage transformer. Since there is no physical connection between the two circuits they also serve to isolate the mains from the circuit in the apparatus; as the mains supply is earthed this allows the circuit to be 'earth-free' (see Chapter 3).

A commonly employed structure is shown in Figure A2 together with the circuit symbol for a transformer (see Fig. A3). The magnetic field across each turn influences all other turns and there is an equal voltage across each turn so that the voltage across the coils is proportional to the number of turns in each coil. If the mains RMS voltage of 240 V is applied across one coil—the

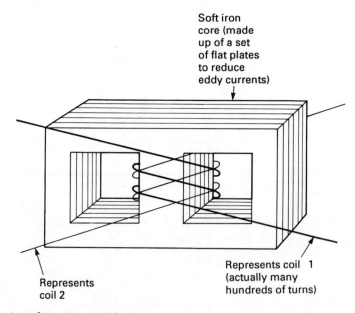

Soft iron core (made up of a set of flat plates to reduce eddy currents)

Represents coil 1 (actually many hundreds of turns)

Represents coil 2

Fig. A2 Low-frequency transformer.

primary—and the other—secondary—coil is made up of twice as many turns, the voltage across it will be doubled. Similarly if the secondary has only a quarter of the number of turns of the primary the voltage will be reduced to one-quarter of that across the primary.

The transformer is able to change the voltage but the total power output must equal the power input. Thus the maximum current from the secondary coil is limited by the power (in watts) of the primary coil. Thus: V × A (W) of primary = V × A (W) of secondary (+ small energy loss in transformer). The actual current in a circuit to which the secondary current is applied will depend on the resistance of the circuit; this is known as Ohm's law.

The energy transfer from one coil to another will only occur when the current, and hence the magnetic field, changes and depends on the rate of change. The regular sinusoidal variation of the mains current will lead to a similar sinusoidal secondary voltage, but out of phase.

(It will be out of phase because current following a sinusoidal variation will have the highest rate of change as it is reversing direction and therefore leads to the highest induced voltage in the secondary at this point. The lowest rate of change—zero—will occur when the primary current is at maximum intensity in one direction, having stopped rising and not yet started to fall. The induced voltage will thus also be zero. The variation between these two points will follow a sine curve.)

The soft iron core is used with low-frequency transformers to provide a strong magnetic field close to the coils. The magnitude of the induced effects also depends on the length and number of turns of the coils, but most critically on the rate of change. At higher frequencies so much self-induction occurs as to block the current partly or entirely. Therefore to act as a high-frequency transformer the coils are made of fewer turns. At very high frequencies such as the 27.12 MHz of the shortwave described in Chapter 10 only four or five large-diameter turns are needed, to transmit energy between the oscillator coil and that in the patients' circuit. The same principle is used, of course, to transmit energy from the coil in the drum-type applicator of a shortwave apparatus to the tissues of the patient; the tissues are behaving as the secondary coil.

Low-frequency transformers are extensively used to alter the mains voltage, both increasing it (a 'step-up' transformer) and decreasing it (a 'step-down' transformer) for the many pieces of equipment that operate on higher or lower voltages. Voltage changes are also essential for the efficient transmission of electric power (see Appendix D).

MAINS SUPPLY

The mains current is generated at power stations by dynamos converting mechanical energy into electrical energy. The mechanical energy is derived either directly, from falling water in hydroelectric stations, or indirectly from the heat of burning coal, oil gas or nuclear fission, which provides steam for turbines. The electrical energy is transmitted around the country at a very high voltage—several hundred thousand volts for the main power lines—connecting power stations in different regions and users. The high transmission voltages are reduced at transformer substations to the familiar 240 V of the household mains supply. This system allows the transmission of electrical energy to all parts of the country efficiently and economically.

The distribution is made by a single cable, the 'return' being effected by earthing both ends, i.e. at the power station, the various substations and the home or hospital supplied (see Fig. A3). The word 'return' is in quotation marks because the earth is a vast reservoir of electrons and to suggest that electrons flow back to the power station is simplistic, rather like suggesting that to remove a bucket of water from the sea at one point, run along the beach with it and empty it back will cause a current in the sea between the two points! The use of a single cable is obvious economic sense; numbers of cables can be seen suspended on pylons in rural areas but in towns they are often underground.

Transmission of high voltages is essential to obviate energy losses. The heating of a conductor, and hence the energy loss, depends principally on the current intensity. (Joule's law: $H \propto I^2 R t$; heating, H, is proportional to the current squared, I^2, multiplied by the resistance of the conductor, R, and time, t, for which the current flows.) Since any practical conductor would have significant resistance over the many miles of transmission the passage of large currents would lead to enormous losses as the wire dissipated its heat to the surroundings. What matters, fortunately, is the transfer of power which is determined by the product of voltage and current, i.e. $W = V \times A$. Thus if power is transmitted at high voltage with low currents very little energy is wasted as heat.

At the substation the voltage is reduced (see Appendix C) to the 240 V supplied to all electricity users. One terminal is earthed and is thus at zero potential to earth; the other is alternately at higher or lower potential and is called the 'live' (or sometimes the 'active' wire). These two wires pass to buildings where the neutral is again earthed. The voltage, and hence current, supplied is of an evenly alternating sinusoidal form with a frequency of 50 cycles per second, i.e. 50 Hz, and a root mean square electromotive force of

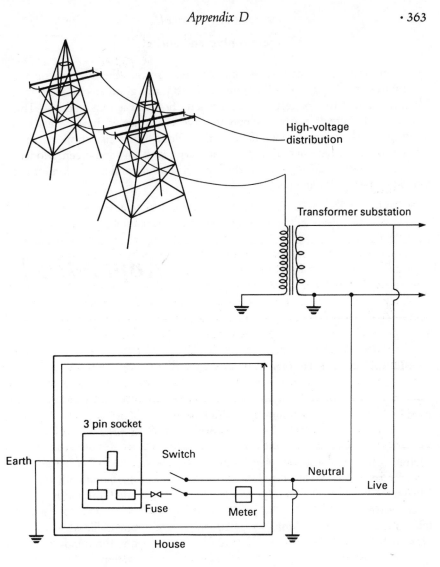

High-voltage distribution

Transformer substation

3 pin socket

Switch

Earth

Fuse

Meter

Neutral

Live

House

Mains supply

Fig. A3

240 V. Since it is a sinusoidal variation the maximum or peak voltage is only applied for a brief instance so it is more usual to give the RMS voltage, which is 0.707 of the peak voltage.

The alternating current is thus supplied to the building by two wires which pass the current through a meter, main switches, and fuses before being distributed in various circuits (Fig. A3). Circuits for the lighting carry small currents and are often protected by 5 A fuses whereas circuits designed to be used for equipment taking higher currents are protected by 13 (or 15) A fuses and connected by three-pin plug systems; most electrotherapeutic apparatus is connected by these latter.

Three-pin plug and socket

These are designed to connect in only one way so that the live, neutral and earth wires are always correctly connected and make good electrical contact. The earth pin is the longest so that it inserts first and is removed last. This ensures that there is no time when the live is connected but the earth is interrupted. The wiring is identified by the colour of the insulation, thus the live is brown, the neutral blue and the earth wire is yellow and green. Modern plugs also contain cartridge fuses which provide safety and protection for the individual piece of equipment.

Appendix E

TABLE OF SMALL UNITS

Name	Symbol	Relation to metre	Fraction of a metre
Metre	m	1	
Centimetre	cm	10^{-2}	one-hundredth
Millimetre	mm	10^{-3}	one-thousandth
Micrometre, micron	μm	10^{-6}	one-millionth
Nanometre	nm	10^{-9}	one thousand-millionth
Ångstrom unit (not an SI unit)	Å	10^{-10}	one ten thousand-millionth
Picometre	pm	10^{-12}	one million-millionth

Appendix F

BASIC GUIDELINES FOR THE APPLICATION OF ELECTROTHERAPY

Before applying any modality of electrotherapy to a patient the following questions should be considered:

1 What effect is intended and can this treatment achieve this effect? In many instances it cannot be known if treatment is effective until it is tried. Sometimes effectiveness can be seen at once, e.g. relief of pain due to transcutaneous electric nerve stimulation or ice; in other cases it cannot be recognized for days or weeks.
2 Is it safe, i.e. will the desired effect be achieved without undesirable effects? There is no effective treatment that does not carry some risks but for most electrotherapy treatment the risks are negligible provided reasonable and proper precautions are taken. Each modality has its own potential dangers and contraindications and no treatment should be considered without a thorough knowledge of these.
3 Is it the best method of treatment to achieve this effect? Is it the most economical in terms of patient and/or therapist time, or other costs?

Usually electrotherapy is part of an overall treatment plan which is selected and modified on the basis of repeated examination and assessment. However, there are some basic guidelines which can provide the framework for sound practice:

1 *Assembly of apparatus*: all the apparatus and equipment needed should be assembled and suitably positioned.
2 *Preparation of patient*
    a *Explanation.* An explanation of the treatment is an essential precursor of application. This not only reassures the patient but ensures informed consent.
    b *Examination and testing.* This refers to specific examination of the part to be treated for possible dangers and contraindications plus any relevant tests, e.g. for normal thermal sensitivity. The results should be recorded.
    c *Preparation of the part to be treated.* This involves any preparatory procedure, e.g. washing the area and positioning the patient, and in particular the part to be treated comfortably and appropriately, so that he or she is relaxed and unnecessary movement is avoided.

3 *Preparation and testing of apparatus*: this includes setting up the apparatus and any necessary testing of it prior to application. When this has been done satisfactorily treatment can begin.

4 *Instructions and warnings*: before the treatment commences it is mandatory to instruct the patient in what he or she must and must not do, e.g. keep still and not touch the apparatus, and to give essential warnings, e.g. 'If this becomes more than a comfortable warmth it can burn'. The warning given should be noted on the patient's record card.

5 *Treatment*: the patient must be observed throughout to ensure that treatment is progressing satisfactorily and without adverse effects. Accurate timing is essential.

6 *Termination of treatment*: at the termination of treatment the part treated should be examined to ensure that the desired effects have occurred if visible, e.g. superficial vasodilation, and that there are no unwanted effects. If electrotherapy is a precursor to another form of treatment, the patient is prepared for that. If it forms the whole treatment, e.g. UVR, an explanation of what to expect is given as well as instructions of when to come again and what must be done between treatments.

7 *Recording*: an accurate recording of treatment must be made for assessment, planning at the next appointment and for legal requirements.

Index

semiconductor diode 306
therapeutic uses 308–10
  fracture consolidation 309
  nerve degeneration prevention 309
  pain control 309
  tissue healing 308–9
types 304 (table)
uses 304–5
Law of conservation of energy 166
Lignocaine 19
Liminal current gradient 56, 57 (figs)
Liquids 164
Local anaesthesia 19
Low back pain 148
Low frequency currents, muscle stimulation
  by 73–5
Low-power pulsed high-frequency
  energy 254–5
Luminous light sources (radiant heat) 295

Magnetic fields
  low-frequency 256
  static 256
Magnetism 255
Mains current shock, treatment 92–3
Mains supply 362–4
Medium pressure mercury arc lamp (Alpine
  sunlamp) 319–21, 345–7
Mercury atoms wavelengths 317, 318
  (table)
Metabolism, source of heat 180
Metatarsalgia 52
Metre 365 (table)
Micrometre 365 (table)
Micron 365 (table)
Microwaves 274–85
  application principles 281–2
  contraindications 284–5
  dangers 282–3
    cardiac pacemaker 283
    eyes 283
    metal 282
    testes 283
  physiological effects 276–9
    pattern of heat in tissues 277–9
  production 275–6
  safety 283–4
  therapeutic use 280–1
Migraine 127, 129
Millimetre 365 (table)
Morphine 60–1
Motor nerve:
  action potentials in 56
  transplant 52
Motor points 44 (fig), 72 (fig), 73
Motor unit 8, 103 (fig), 104 (fig)
Mud packs (peloids) 194
Multiple sclerosis 123
Muscle:
  atrophy 51
    eutrophic electrotherapy effect 54
    retardation by electrical
      stimulation 58

blood flow in, electrical stimulation
  effect 53–4
Control facilitation 52
Denervated 55–9
Electric charges generated by 7–8
Electrical stimulation 50–9
  spasticity control 55
  splinting replaced 54–5
Fast twitch change to slow twitch 54
Innervated, stimulation of 50
Metabolism, electrical stimulation
  effect 53–4
Microwave heating 280–1
Proteins 54
Pumping action 58, 75
Spasm 209, 280, 293
  denervated muscle 55–9
  high-voltage pulsed galvanic
    stimulation 81
  innervated muscle 50
  joint motion maintenance/increase 53
  low frequency currents 73–5
  muscle strengthening effect 50–1
Strengthening 50–2, 210
Strength of contraction 29
Structure changes 54
Tear 211
Tetanic contraction 29
Transplant 52, 124
Trauma 124
Voluntary contraction force 51
Weakened/weakening 51
'Worm-like' contraction 56

Nanometre 365 (table)
Neonatal jaundice 294–5
Nernst equation 2
Nerve(s):
  afferent, stimulation of 59
  all-or-none response 45
  establishing continuity 106–7
  liminal current gradient 56, 57 (figs)
  peripheral *see* peripheral nerves
  resting membrane potential 2
  stimulation *see* nerve stimulation
Nerve conduction test 106
Nerve conduction velocity studies 115–17
Nerve fibre, myelinated 7 (fig)
Nerve impulse 3–5
  absolute refractory period 47, 48 (fig)
  all-or-none event 7
  relative refractory period 47, 48 (fig)
  saltatory conduction 5
  speed of propagation 5–7
Nerve stimulation 27–96
  by electrical pulses 44–6
  peripheral nerves 42–4
Neurogenic pain 20, 252, 293
Neuropraxia 100–1
Neurotmesis 101, 102 (fig)
Nodes of Ranvier 5
Non-luminous radiation 295
Noradraneline 63